CARING FOR THE COUNTRY

Caring for the Country

Family Doctors in Small Rural Towns

Howard K. Rabinowitz, MD
Professor of Family Medicine
Director, Physician Shortage Area Program
Jefferson Medical College
Thomas Jefferson University

Springer
New York
Berlin
Heidelberg
Hong Kong
London
Milan
Paris
Tokyo

Howard K. Rabinowitz
Department of Family Medicine
Jefferson Medical College
Thomas Jefferson University
Philadelphia, PA 19107
USA
Howard.Rabinowitz@jefferson.edu

Back Cover illustration: Illustration appearing on the back cover is courtesy of Thomas Jefferson University.

ISBN 0-387-20978-6   Printed on acid-free paper.

Printed in the United States of America.   (EB)

9 8 7 6 5 4 3 2 1   SPIN 10969038

Springer-Verlag is a part of *Springer Science+Business Media*

springeronline.com

To Carol,
the best thing that ever happened to me.

FOREWORD

It is an honor to write the foreword to *Caring for the Country: Family Doctors in Small Rural Towns*, by Howard K. Rabinowitz, MD. The stories in this book have special meaning for me: I grew up in Monongahela, a small town in southwestern Pennsylvania. My friends' parents worked in the coal mines and the steel mills. Family doctors—they were called general practitioners then—provided all my family's medical care; they treated my ear infections, removed my tonsils, and managed my sports injuries. My dad was a schoolbook salesman who called on the public schools in Nanty Glo, Bedford, and Lock Haven, PA. For more than a decade, I practiced rural medicine in upstate New York. Today I live in Oregon, a state with a large rural population and a looming crisis in the availability of rural health care services.

Health care in rural America is rich with stories—both of the physicians and the people in the communities they serve. One of every five Americans lives in a rural setting, and yet these rural inhabitants are often forgotten in discussions of the underserved in health care in the United States. Even more overlooked are the true heroes—the nine percent of the nation's physicians who have made a commitment to rural communities.[1] These doctors live the dream of service to others that was why—I thought—we chose careers in medicine.

Yet today, students and residents who share with their subspecialty professors that they plan rural family practice risk everything from solicitous but less-than-heartfelt encouragement ("Good for you. Rural people need doctors.") to high-pressure exhortations not to "waste your career."

Something seems to have happened to young American doctors over the past few decades. Altruism and service seem to be unfashionable, and *lifestyle* is a major concern. Medicine has, for many young doctors, come to mean a personal opportunity to advance one's career, rather than a commitment to care for patients.

This book tells of a program that identifies young physicians with the interest and courage to serve patients in small rural towns, and it chronicles what happened to ten of those physicians. It describes personal relationships that go beyond the examination room and tells how the doctor becomes metaphorically "part of the patient's family." Some might say that these physicians are a throwback to a time that has past. Maybe, but I think that these rural family physicians represent the best of American medicine, and we should have a lot more of them.

So, read this important book, and be inspired by the stories of the doctors. And be glad that there are programs such as the one at Jefferson Medical College that help educate the family physicians Americans need.

Robert B. Taylor, MD
Portland, Oregon

NOTE

1. Van Dis J. Where we live: health care in rural vs. urban America. *JAMA.* 2002; 287:108.

ACKNOWLEDGMENTS

I want to acknowledge the critical role of Jefferson Medical College of Thomas Jefferson University in developing and supporting the Physician Shortage Area Program (PSAP) for the past three decades. I especially want to thank Paul Brucker, President of Thomas Jefferson University and former chair of the Department of Family Medicine, for his ongoing support, mentorship, and friendship. I also want to express my appreciation to Tom Nasca, Joseph Gonnella, and Will Kellow, deans of Jefferson Medical College; Richard Wender and John Randall, chairs of the Department of Family Medicine; Clara Callahan, Bud Bacharach, and Sam Conley, Deans of Admissions; Grace Hershman, Director for Admissions; Raelynn Cooter, Registrar; and Jefferson's Alumni Association, and Office of Financial Aid—all for their invaluable and ongoing support. I want to recognize the critically important roles of Fred Markham, Associate Director of the PSAP, and Jim Diamond, Director of the Greenfield Research Center, both in the Department of Family Medicine, and to thank them for years of support in running and evaluating the PSAP. And special thanks also go to Carolyn Little, Educational Coordinator for the Department of Family Medicine, who has helped coordinate the PSAP for more than a decade and has played an important role in assuring the success of the program. I am deeply indebted to Joseph Gonnella, Jon Veloski, Mohammadreza Hojat, and Carol Rabinowitz from Jefferson's Center for Research in Medical Education and Health Care, for the use of the Jefferson Longitudinal Study, without which the PSAP outcomes studies could not have been done— and for their longstanding support of me, and of the PSAP. I sincerely thank

Christina Hazelwood and Nina Paynter, who served as research assistants and played an invaluable role in the PSAP outcomes studies. I am also indebted to my colleagues—the faculty in the Department of Family Medicine—for their ongoing support, and along with the family medicine residents at Jefferson, for caring for my patients while I was on sabbatical writing this book. Will Kellow and Sam Conley deserve special recognition for developing and initiating this unique program, as do Paul Brucker and Joseph Gonnella, both of whom I interviewed for this book.

I also want to acknowledge the important role of the Robert Wood Johnson Foundation in providing funding for this book, and to its former president, Steve Schroeder, for his support and encouragement; and to the Department of Family Medicine and Jefferson Medical College for supporting my sabbatical. I am also deeply indebted to Mike Magee and the Pfizer Medical Humanities Initiative for supporting this project. I want to thank Don Pathman and the Cecil G. Sheps Center for Health Services Research at the University of North Carolina for providing a "rural" environment for me during part of the time I worked on this book.

I greatly appreciate a number of individuals who reviewed all or part of drafts of this manuscript and provided helpful feedback, including: Jim Diamond, Fred Markham, Carol Rabinowitz, Larry Rabinowitz, Paul Brucker, Wendy Cadge, Sylvia Fields, Neil Skolnik, and a number of the current PSAP students. And I thank John Geyman, Norman Kahn, Jim Martin, Fitz Mullan, and John McPhee for their helpful advice during this project. I also want to sincerely thank Bob Taylor for his counsel, and for writing the forward to this book. A special debt of gratitude goes to Jack Colwill, whose own research, frequent advice, and constant support and encouragement has been so important throughout my career. My warmest thanks go to US Senator John D. (Jay) Rockefeller IV (WV), and his 1993–94 staff—Tamera Luzzatto, Ellen Doneski, and Mary Ella Payne—for broadening my perspective on health care policy. And I want to thank Rob Albano, and the other editors and staff at Springer-Verlag, for their help and guidance.

Personally, no words can accurately express my gratitude and feelings to the most important people in my life—my wife, Carol, and my children, Elyse and Daniel—for their love and support.

I would also like to acknowledge the important work of all the family doctors—and all the rural doctors—who are caring for the country. And finally, my greatest admiration and thanks go to those PSAP graduates who are practicing family medicine in small rural towns, including the ten PSAP graduates who I visited, and whose lives I had the opportunity to profile. They are the real heroes of this book.

CONTENTS

INTRODUCTION

> The question is, then, not merely to define the ideal training of the physician; it is just as much [to] . . . distribute [them] as widely as possible.
> —The Flexner Report, 1910

> Geographic maldistribution in rural areas is worsening.
> —The Institute of Medicine Report on Primary Care, 1996

Everyone deserves access to health care. But for the 1 in 5 Americans who live in rural areas, finding a doctor can oftentimes be difficult. Largely invisible to the majority of the population that lives in our cities and suburbs, the shortage of physicians in rural areas and small towns has remained one of the most persistent and serious problems of the US health care system for most of the past century. In some ways, today's rural physician shortage seems particularly strange—living in a global economy where you can get almost anything you want instantaneously, but unable to obtain health care because of this lack of doctors.

I first became aware of these issues more than 30 years ago when, after my internship, I spent 2 years practicing family medicine in a small rural town. The town was Sacaton, on the Pima Indian reservation in southern Arizona, and it was certainly small—the entire telephone book was on 1 side of 1 page. It was also rural. Looking out across the desert, you could see the tops of the mountains around Phoenix, almost 50 miles away, but with few people living in that vast open space. The hospital nearest to ours was 35 miles away. That contrasts dramatically with where I work today—Philadelphia, Pennsylvania—where more than five million people live in a similar area, and five other medical schools and 50 other hospitals are within ten miles of my office. So, upon joining the faculty of the Department of Family Medicine at Jefferson Medical College of Thomas Jefferson University in 1976, as the only physician with any rural practice experience, I was asked to become involved in a unique new program that had recently begun—the Physician Shortage Area Program

(PSAP)—a program to recruit and educate physicians to practice family medicine in rural areas and small towns.

· · · · ·

For more than 75 years, rural Americans have had limited access to health care. Unlike most urban areas—where there is often a large supply of physicians and where access to care is more often related to economic, social, or cultural factors—access to health care in rural areas is, in large part, related to the supply of doctors. At the same time that rural areas suffer from this serious shortage of physicians, they actually have a greater need for medical care. This phenomenon was dubbed the "Inverse Care Law" in 1971 by Welsh family physician Julian Tudor Hart, who stated, "The availability of good medical care tends to vary inversely with the need for it." People who live in rural areas of the United States are sicker, older, poorer, and more often medically uninsured than those living in metropolitan areas. Those living in rural areas are also more likely to describe their health as "fair" or "poor," and to have higher infant mortality rates, youth death rates, and adult death rates. They face longer distances to obtain health care services, smoke more, exercise less, and receive less preventive care, dental care, and mental health care. With rural populations clearly facing myriad health problems, a recent survey of people working in the field at the state and local level identified "access to quality health services" as the most important priority, by far.

Despite decades of attempting to address the rural physician shortage, including a dramatic increase in the total number of doctors trained, rural areas continue to be medically underserved. Currently, while 20 percent of the US population live in rural America, only 9 percent of physicians practice there. Primary care physicians are especially critical in rural areas, as they provide basic medical care, and also serve to coordinate access to appropriate subspecialty care, which often cannot be provided in areas with a small population. And among primary care doctors, family physicians have always been the dominant source of medical care in rural areas, and remain the key component of the rural physician workforce.

While not all rural areas are medically underserved, of the 60 million people living in rural America, more than 22 million people—almost two-thirds the total population of Canada—live in areas that the federal government has officially designated as suffering from a shortage of primary care physicians. This makes rural Americans one of the largest physician underserved populations in the country, and the majority of physician shortage areas are located there. In addition, of those rural counties that are not currently underserved, two-thirds would be if it were not for the family physicians that are already practicing there today. This is critically important as it requires that a continuing supply of rural family physicians be trained in order to replace and maintain the current supply. It also highlights how the future rural health care workforce is inextricably tied to the future of family medicine. But with fewer than 3 percent of recent medical school graduates expressing plans to practice in rural areas and small towns, as well as the recent decline in the number of physicians entering family practice, it is unlikely that people living in these areas will have an adequate supply of doctors in the foreseeable future.

This shortage of rural physicians is a serious problem in almost every state in the nation, and is particularly severe in Pennsylvania. For while Pennsylvania is primarily known for its two major metropolitan areas of Philadelphia and Pittsburgh, it actually has the third largest rural population of any state in the country (after Texas and North Carolina). In fact, according to the Census Bureau, there are more rural people living in Pennsylvania than in the eight states of North Dakota, South Dakota, Montana, Wyoming, Idaho, Colorado, Utah, and Nevada combined! In addition, almost one-half of all the physicians in Pennsylvania practice in only 3 of the 67 counties (around Philadelphia and Pittsburgh), even though almost three-fourths of the population lives in the other 64 counties.

It is within this context that policy makers, educators, and rural communities continue to face the serious challenge of finding the most effective and least costly ways to increase the supply and retention of rural primary care physicians. At its core, solving this problem will require that more physicians choose to practice family medicine in small towns and rural areas.

• • • • •

For the majority of us, the most important things in our life—in addition to our health—are our families, our friends, and our work. Outside of the family we were born into, we make personal decisions about who we want to love, live with, and be with, and the type of work we do. A critically important factor interwoven with all of these areas is where we live. It affects who we are and what we do. In fact, when we meet someone for the first time, the two questions that are often asked are: "Where are you from?" and "What do you do?" The answers—reflecting place and work—help identify us.

These same issues are also very important for physicians, as each decides what specialty they want to enter, and where they want to practice. In many instances, these decisions of specialty choice and practice location are separate and unrelated. But rural family practice is unique—it is both a profession and a place, closely interconnected with each other. It is family practice—the broadest of all the medical specialties—providing health care to everyone in the family, of all ages, and taking care of the vast majority of their medical problems. Family doctors, like other primary care physicians, differ from non-primary care specialists in that they make a commitment to care for a group of people (usually about 2,000), to help keep them healthy, and to care for them irrespective of whatever illnesses or problems they may have. Nonprimary care specialists, on the other hand, generally take care of people only after they have certain symptoms or diseases. Because of this, family doctors develop long-term relationships with their patients, know their patients and their families, and share in their life events. That is what draws many physicians to practice family medicine—caring for people, not just the disease. It is the reward of "being your doctor." And, while family practice has had its highs and lows in popularity as a career choice over the past few decades, it will always maintain a critical role in caring for patients. As Dr. David Rogers, founding president of the Robert Wood Johnson Foundation wrote, "Having access to a more effective primary-care system constitutes a profound human need." Data have also shown that the supply of family doctors, and a medical infrastructure based on family physicians—in this country, and in many other countries in the world—is related to better health and lower mortality.

Rural family practice also means rural living and a rural lifestyle. But rural family practice is more than just practicing family medicine in a rural location—in the same way that vegetable soup is more than just peas and carrots and water. Combining them together results in a new and entirely different product. Family practice is intimately related to rural areas and interwoven into the fabric of small towns. Family doctors are really the only primary care physicians that can practice in very small population areas, since there aren't enough patients to support having an internist, a pediatrician, and an obstetrician to provide primary care for the community. And most small towns don't have nearly enough people to support neurosurgeons and gastroenterologists. While all family doctors are trained in the broad areas of family medicine (e.g., including obstetrics), only those in rural areas are likely to use this training, so that their scope of family practice is much broader. In addition, their patients are their friends and neighbors, and so they live with their patients and know their lives more intimately.

$$\bullet \quad \bullet \quad \bullet \quad \bullet \quad \bullet$$

For more than half a century, foundations, government, and medical schools have tried to find ways to get doctors to practice in rural areas—and to stay there. Although critically important, this has not been easy. Most programs have either used financial incentives, provided educational experiences to medical students or residents, or have attempted to support doctors in opening or remaining in practice. One of the earliest of these programs, developed by the Sears Roebuck Foundation in the 1950s, was a program of community-based assistance—providing small towns with technical assistance, architectural plans, and advisory staffs to help them build medical clinics and recruit physicians. From 1956 until it ended in 1970, this program helped to build 165 clinics. In 1970, the National Health Service Corps (NHSC) was created, and since then has been providing scholarships and loan forgiveness to medical students and physicians in exchange for primary care practice in one of the nation's underserved communities—most of which are located in rural areas. In addition, state and other organizational programs provide physicians and other health care providers with loan forgiveness, scholarships, and assistance in exchange for medical service. Since 1976, the federal government has also provided financial support to medical schools and academic departments of family medicine and divisions of primary care through Title VII of the Public Health Service Act, to help increase the number of physicians in primary care and those practicing in underserved areas.

In 1971, the federal government began supporting Area Health Education Centers (AHECs), decentralizing certain clinical aspects of medical training and moving them into primarily rural areas at some distance from the medical schools. Today, this multidisciplinary program continues to provide ongoing educational programs in most states. Many medical schools also provide rural preceptorship training in private medical practices throughout the country, with some of these programs in existence for decades. Finally, a few medical schools have developed programs to preferentially admit and educate rural students. The University of Illinois began such a program in 1948 in order to increase the number of rural general practitioners in the state, and an evaluation of the program in 1973 showed it to be quite successful.

· · · · ·

To help address the rural physician shortage, Jefferson Medical College of Thomas Jefferson University in Philadelphia, Pennsylvania, initiated the Physician Shortage Area Program (PSAP) in 1974. Jefferson, the largest private medical school in the country at the time, had a long history of graduating practicing physicians for the area, the state, and the country. The PSAP was begun, according to current University President Paul C. Brucker, MD—who came to Jefferson in 1973 as the founding chairman of the Department of Family Medicine—because the school "appreciated the need in Pennsylvania for physicians in rural areas." And, because Jefferson's dean at the time, Dr. Will Kellow—who had previously been on the University of Illinois faculty and would have been aware of their rural program—"had a sincere desire, and thought that the school had a societal responsibility, to train the number and kinds of physicians that the state and country needed. I think the school was pretty altruistic about this." In fact, the university has been the only source of financial support for the PSAP throughout its history, even though the state has been the major beneficiary of the program. Dr. Joseph S. Gonnella, who came to Jefferson as associate dean for academic affairs with Dean Kellow, and who himself later served as dean of Jefferson Medical College from 1984–2000, echoed that "We were one of the schools at the time that was trying to do something that was good for the state. We were very proud of the PSAP."

The PSAP recruits and selectively admits medical school applicants who have grown up, or lived a significant part of their lives, in a small town or rural area, and who also are committed to practice the specialty of family medicine in a similar area, either their home town, or another small town or rural area. Only applicants who have both a rural background and a strong commitment to a career in rural family practice are given consideration for the program. Since 1980, Jefferson has worked cooperatively with six Pennsylvania colleges—Allegheny College, Bucknell University, Franklin and Marshall College, Indiana University of Pennsylvania, the Pennsylvania State University, and the University of Scranton—to help recruit and select students for the PSAP. All applicants to Jefferson are given information about the program, and those interested in applying fill out a supplemental application, submit three additional supporting letters of recommendation from people in their community, and are interviewed either by myself, the director of the PSAP, or by Dr. Fred Markham, who has served as associate director of the PSAP since 1990. Dr. Markham, who grew up in a small town himself, practiced family medicine and taught Jefferson medical students in his office for 12 years in the rural town of Berlin, New Hampshire before joining the full-time faculty. "Berlin [with the accent on the first syllable] is where New Hampshire gets narrow," he likes to say.

Throughout its history, the number of PSAP students in each class has ranged from 5 to 24, with an average of 14 per year, representing 6 percent of all Jefferson graduates. During medical school, each PSAP student is assigned a family physician as their faculty advisor, and spends time seeing patients with their advisor during their freshman year. The group also meets together on a regular basis to discuss common issues. In addition, they are given priority to participate in a summer research project between their first and second years of medical school, working with family medicine faculty. During their third year of medical school, PSAP students take their required six-week family medicine clinical clerkship at a rural or small town location in Pennsylvania. These clerkships take place at a community hospital at one of Jefferson's affiliated family practice residency programs—currently at either Latrobe Area Hospital (Latrobe, Pennsylvania) or the Guthrie Clinic (Sayre, Pennsylvania); in prior years, students had also taken this rotation at Geisinger Medical Center (Danville, Pennsylvania) or at Franklin Hospital (Franklin, Pennsylvania). During their senior year, PSAP students take their required six-week outpatient subinternship in the discipline of family medicine, usually at a private practice "preceptorship" in a rural family physician's office. Here, students live in the rural community and work one-on-one with a practicing family doctor, learning family medicine and also what it's like to be a family doctor in a small town. PSAP students do receive a small amount of financial aid, however this is almost entirely in the form of repayable loans, and represents only a very small percentage of the high tuition and expenses for medical school.

Upon completion of medical school, PSAP graduates are expected to complete a three-year residency in family practice at a training program of their choice. Like all medical school graduates they go through a formal "match" program—applying to a number of residency programs during their senior year, and ranking them in order of preference. Each residency program also ranks which applicants they would most like to have in their program, and the final results are tabulated by computer and announced at "Match Day" every spring. After completing their residency, PSAP graduates are expected to practice family medicine for their professional career, either in their hometown or in another small town or rural area. While PSAP graduates are encouraged to practice in Pennsylvania—and two-thirds do—they can and do practice in any state, currently practicing in more than half the states in the nation. And although PSAP students are required to remain in the program throughout medical school, no formal mechanism exists to ensure compliance for either residency or practice.

• • • • •

During the past 27 years, I have had the opportunity to serve as director of the PSAP, and have known each of the more than 300 students in the program. I have been actively involved in the admissions and curricular components of the PSAP. I have also studied the outcomes of the program, which have been published in the *New England Journal of Medicine* and in the *Journal of the American Medical Association* (*JAMA*), and reported in various newspapers and on *CNN Headline News*. Because of its success, the PSAP has become nationally and internationally known.

Our outcomes research has shown that PSAP graduates are practicing rural family medicine at a rate more than eight times greater than their classmates. And almost all (84%) are practicing in either a rural or small metropolitan area, or in one of the primary care specialties. From the state perspective, although the PSAP is a very small program, it has produced 21 percent of all the family doctors in rural Pennsylvania who graduated from the state's seven medical schools, even though PSAP students represent only 1 percent of the graduates from those schools.

The issue of retention is particularly critical in rural areas, because it is so difficult to get doctors to practice there in the first place. Although the words "recruitment and retention" are often grouped together in a single phrase, they represent very different phenomena. As opposed to recruitment, retention has a multiplicative effect on the physician workforce. That is, to assure that a small rural town continuously has a physician throughout a 20-year period, you would need to train 20 doctors over that time, if each stayed for only one year—compared with needing to only train one doctor if that person stayed for 20 years! That means producing 20 times as many doctors—let alone the problems involved with people having to change their doctor every year, *if* they were able to get a new doctor every time the old one left. Longer retention not only results in better patient care because of continuity, knowing your patients, etc., but data also show that there is a substantial financial cost that goes into recruiting a new family physician—estimated to be more than $200,000, or even higher in rural areas. Even then, each new physician needs to perform another complete history and physical exam to get to know each patient and has to get to know the community. All of this has a huge personal and financial cost.

The PSAP is, in many ways, the opposite of *Northern Exposure*—the Hollywoodized TV version of rural family practice, where a New York City doctor goes to practice in a rural area in order to pay back his medical school debt, but then, not unexpectedly, leaves when his commitment ends so that he can do what he really wants to do. The PSAP, in contrast, selects rural-raised physicians who truly want to practice rural family medicine for their career. The resultant PSAP retention rate for those graduates who entered rural family practice is the highest ever reported—79 percent of those practicing eleven to sixteen years ago, the duration they have so far been followed.

Although students selected for the PSAP must meet all of the academic and other criteria for admission to Jefferson, they are chosen primarily on the basis of their rural background and commitment to practice rural family medicine. By broadening the admission criteria in this way, the PSAP selects a different group of applicants than those admitted through the regular admissions process. However, throughout the history of the PSAP, their admission credentials, attrition rate, and academic performance during medical school and residency training have been similar to their classmates.

More recent research studying more than 3,400 Jefferson graduates over 16 years has now clearly identified those factors that are predictive of practicing rural primary care. These are: growing up in a rural area, entering medical school with plans to become a family doctor, being in the PSAP, having a NHSC scholarship or service commitment, being male, and taking a senior family medicine rural preceptorship. Participation in the PSAP and attending college in a rural area were the only predictors of rural primary care retention. For PSAP graduates, men and women were equally likely to become rural primary care doctors. And, the two main factors used to select PSAP students—rural background and entering medical school with plans for family practice—appear so powerful, that only 1.8 percent of all Jefferson graduates ended up practicing any type of primary care in rural areas if they had neither of these factors!

In addition to Jefferson's PSAP, a small number of other medical schools have developed similar programs that have also had remarkably comparable success in having their graduates practice family medicine in rural areas— proving that the PSAP outcomes are indeed generalizable and true. None of these other programs, however, has yet reported on retention rates for their graduates. These programs include: (1) the WWAMI (Washington, Wyoming, Alaska, Montana, and Idaho) program at the University of Washington; (2) the University of Minnesota, Duluth; (3) the University of Minnesota's Rural Physicians Associate Program (RPAP); (4) the Upper Peninsula Program (UPP) at Michigan State University; (5) the Rural Medical Education Program (RMED) at the University of Illinois, Rockford; and (6) Mercer University. Graduates of these programs are highly likely to be working in a rural area (range 23–79%) and practicing one of the primary care specialties (range 61–74%). Although each of these successful programs differs in its structure, all contain three core features: a strong institutional mission; the targeted selection of students likely to practice in rural areas, predominantly those with rural backgrounds; and a focus on primary care, especially family practice.

• • • • •

Now that the PSAP is more than a quarter century old, it is important to tell the story of this successful program, to share what has been learned over the past 29 years, and to accurately portray what it's like to be a rural family doctor. This is especially important today, considering the continuing shortage of rural physicians and the ongoing disparity in health and health care between people living in rural and metropolitan areas. I felt that the most accurate way to tell the story of this unique program was by capturing the professional and personal lives of the PSAP graduates. So, after contacting and obtaining consent from ten of our PSAP graduates, I visited each where they were living and practicing. It was a kind of reverse *Tuesdays with Morrie*—this time the gray-haired professor visiting his former students. For me, it was truly a wonderful experience. I interviewed each at their home or in their office. For all but one, I followed them for two to four hours, shadowing them as they practiced family medicine—in their office, in the hospital, and in the operating room. I audio-taped each interview and over 100 patient encounters. I spoke with all of their spouses and met many of their children.

These ten PSAP graduates were selected to be representative of all of the graduates of the program who were practicing rural family medicine, based in part on when they graduated medical school, their gender, and where they practiced. They graduated medical school from 1979 to 1996, entering practice from 1982 to 1999. Seven of these doctors are men, three are women. Eight of the graduates are practicing in Pennsylvania, one in a state adjacent to Pennsylvania (New York), and one in a nonadjacent state (North Carolina). Within these parameters, I visited former students who I had known somewhat better when they were in medical school (I had interviewed five of them for admission to Jefferson), or had maintained some contact with since they graduated. They were not specifically selected because of their accomplishments, activities, or any personal or other professional characteristics. Rather, they were chosen to be representative of practicing rural family doctors at the beginning of the twenty-first century. These ten PSAP graduates, the year they graduated from Jefferson Medical College, and the town where they practice family medicine are:

Jim Devlin, MD, Class of 1985, Brockway, Pennsylvania

Mike Tatarko, MD, Class of 1989, Nanty Glo, Pennsylvania

Viola Monaghan, MD, Class of 1995, Ovid, New York

Bill Thompson, MD, Class of 1987, Boswell, Pennsylvania

Christine Dotterer, MD, Class of 1979, Selinsgrove, Pennsylvania

Catherine O'Neil, MD, Class of 1996, Bloomsburg, Pennsylvania

Thane Turner, MD, Class of 1993, Lock Haven, Pennsylvania

Joe Nutz, MD, Class of 1992, Morehead City, North Carolina

Dave Baer, MD, Class of 1979, Bedford, Pennsylvania

Bernie Proy, MD, Class of 1980, Corry, Pennsylvania

During their interviews, each of these physicians was asked about how and why they decided to become a rural family doctor, including open-ended questions related to their background and early experiences, their family, role models, and their education and residency training. They were also asked about their current professional and personal lives, the satisfactions and challenges of a career in rural family practice, and about such issues as the scope of rural practice, autonomy, interdisciplinary medical care, available health care resources, home visits, managed care, rural networks, information technology, telemedicine, rural lifestyle issues, relationships with their patients, relevant financial and economic issues, personal activities, and their spouse and family. While a semistructured interview format was used, the discussion also strayed at times and covered a wide range of issues. Additional information was also obtained while shadowing these doctors as they saw their patients in the hospital and office, from their original admissions applications to Jefferson Medical College, and from publicly available news and Internet sites.

After transcribing these interviews and patient interactions, they were edited for clarity and reorganized to make them easier to read, while making sure not to change any of their meanings. All quotes thus accurately reflect what was said, and were reviewed by each of the physicians. None of the patient names in this book are real, and identifying characteristics and information regarding these patients—such as age, gender, occupation, disease, body parts, family history—have been changed to provide an accurate overall flavor of rural family practice, but so as to not identify any individual patient. To further protect patient privacy, a number of the patient interactions have also been placed in a different chapter (and different doctor) than where they actually occurred.

Each of the ten chapters that focus on one of these physicians alternates between sections addressing their background, their town, their professional life, their personal life, and their interactions with patients. Organizing the chapters in this way accurately reflects the lives of these rural family doctors, with all of these aspects interwoven into part of each day. I also made a conscious effort to let the voices of these rural family doctors come through, so that the reader could hear these doctors—and feel their lives.

· · · · ·

The combined stories of these ten doctors provide a unique view of what it's like to be a family doctor in a small rural town in 2002. Of the ten doctors in this book, four wanted to be doctors since they were young children, three since high school, and three after high school. All wanted to be rural family doctors from the time they decided on medicine. All ten went to college in small towns for at least part of their education, seven for their entire undergraduate education. Nine of the ten grew up in a rural area, the tenth lived rural during college and for a few years afterwards. Half of their spouses grew up in a rural area. Half of the doctors went directly from college to medical school, half took time off to work, do additional course work, or study for the Medical College Admissions Test (MCAT). During medical school, five of the physicians worked in the Department of Family Medicine doing research, and six took a preceptorship in a rural family practice office in their senior year.

Half of these doctors currently practice in their hometown, which for three is also their spouse's hometown. Another practices in her spouse's hometown, and two more are in towns other than where they grew up, but where they or their spouse had prior ties. Five are in private practice, the other five are employed by a hospital or health system. One is fulfilling a service obligation for the NHSC. Half practice in federally designated Health Professional Shortage Areas (HPSAs). Three are in solo practice, one of whom will soon be taking a partner, and all the others practice in a group: two in groups of two doctors, two others in groups of three, and one each in a group of four, five, and six. They care for, on average, three to four patients in the hospital most days (range 2–4 to 5–6 patients; one no longer takes care of patients in the hospital), and 25 patients a day in the office (range 16–20 to 30–40 patients). Three of these family doctors do obstetrics (OB), one of whom also does caesarian sections (C-sections); one assists in surgery and C-sections; one performs esophago-gastro-duodenoscopy (EGD) and colonoscopy. Almost all make house calls. In addition, these doctors work at nursing homes, do occupational health, and work as athletic team, school, and college physicians. Six have one or more nurse practitioners or physician assistants working with them. One of these doctors is on call all the time for her own patients, the others share call with other doctors, ranging from every two to three nights and weekends, to every five to seven nights and weekends. Most indicated that managed care was not as great a problem in small towns, though like doctors everywhere today, they complained about paperwork, and the hassles associated with medical insurance. And most were concerned about the continuing and increasing financial pressures from insurance companies, reimbursement, and the malpractice insurance crisis. Most have a significant leadership role in their hospital or community.

Five of these doctors live less than two miles from their office. Seven live in houses that include between 10 and 60 acres of land. Personal activities are remarkably varied, and ranged from boating, fishing, hunting, skiing, flying, metalwork, carpentry, gardening, raising pheasants, farming, growing bonsai, running marathons, growing American Chestnut trees, growing giant pumpkins, biking, church, and activities with their spouse and kids. Most seemed to have adjusted well to the demands of their profession on their personal life, though some are still struggling with this—much of this seemingly related to their personality and the age of their children, as well as their medical practice per se.

As to what they like best about rural family practice, the consistency of their responses was remarkable: "Getting to know all the families—and the support you get from the families." "Being a part of the lives of and the medical care of a variety of people." "My chance to make a difference, caring for people." "The relationships, the ability to make an impact on a community." "The relationships with people." "I know everybody; I love having that connection with them." "There's a lot of gratitude and reward." "There's an intimacy that develops." "That you are very close to all these people." These doctors also like living in rural areas because: "It's a good place for raising kids." "The biggest plus is raising kids." "I know who my neighbors are." "The openness, the rural setting, the lack of crowds." "People know each other; there's a real sense of community." "Life in general. We're all really close, we all take care of each other. I wouldn't have raised my kids anyplace else."

· · · · ·

Over the years, there has been a notable consistency in how leaders in academic medicine, most medical school faculty, and many urban physicians (some who grew up and left rural areas) have seen, described, and written about the rural physician shortage. As a result, a common wisdom has emerged regarding this issue and its solution. This includes that people who grow up in small towns can't wait to leave, and don't want to return. That most students want to become a family doctor when they begin medical school, but that almost all change their mind. That the advantages of living and practicing in urban areas—personal, professional, economic, and cultural—are so much greater than in rural areas, that no one, even rural-raised doctors, will want to practice in rural locations. And, that no one practices family medicine in small towns and rural areas anymore—it just isn't a realistic career option nowadays. In addition, one frequently hears that you can't provide high-quality medicine in a small town, you can't be professionally satisfied practicing rural family medicine, and you can't make a good living as a rural family doctor. And, that rural family practice is so overwhelming that you can't have a life outside of medicine. There is also a widespread belief that the role of medical schools in addressing the rural physician shortage is very limited, given the powerful forces external to the academic environment that play an important part in physicians' choice of practice location and specialty. And finally, there is long-standing concern that special medical school admissions programs to increase the supply of rural physicians: (1) are not effective; (2) are too small to have a significant impact; and (3) will decrease the quality of physicians.

The stories of these ten PSAP graduates—why they decided to become rural family doctors, why they've stayed, and what it's like—go far toward answering the degree to which this common wisdom is correct and how much represents myth. They also provide a better understanding of why the PSAP has been successful, and why it works. In fact, after reading these stories, it is unlikely that the reader will ever again see rural family practice in the same way.

· · · · ·

Where are you from? What do you do? At one level, each of the people in this book would answer these two questions in a similar way. They are all family doctors, and they all live and practice in small rural towns. But at a deeper level, each lives in a different and distinct small town. Each practices a different type of family medicine. And each has a unique and distinctive life. This book is about these doctors, their family practices, these small towns.

And it is the story of the PSAP, the program that helped them achieve their goals and that ties them all together.

As for me, I learned a lot about rural family medicine when I was actually practicing in Sacaton, Arizona, in the US Indian Health Service more than three decades ago. I learned even more, serving as director of Jefferson's PSAP since 1976, directing the program, and studying its outcomes. But in writing this book over the past two years, I developed an even greater appreciation of this unique program, and the richness and resonance of rural family practice, as I visited these ten PSAP graduates—my former students—and interviewed them about their practice and their lives, and followed them as they went about their daily work of caring for the country.

BROCKWAY, PENNSYLVANIA

Conception, birth, the first steps, growth and development, starting school, puberty, developing gender identity, dating, marriage, giving birth, parenting, striving to succeed, changes such as climacteric and menopause, accepting the ticking of the clock, coping with acute and chronic illness, loss of dear ones—these are the fabric of family medicine, and the elements that bond family physicians and their patients.

—B. Lewis Barnett, Jr., MD

The town below fits in the palm of your hand.

—Tracy Kidder, *Hometown*

Jim Devlin's roots go all the way back to the beginning of Brockway, Pennsylvania. Chancey Brockway, Sr., who settled the area about 150 years ago, and for whom the town was named, was Jim's great-great-grandfather. Prior to the birth of his own children, Jim was the youngest descendent of the Brockway family on his mother's side. His generation was the fifth generation of the family living here, his kids are the sixth.

A small rural community in northwestern Pennsylvania, roughly two and a half hours north of Pittsburgh, Brockway sits in Jefferson County, the same county where Punxsutawney—of Groundhog Day fame—is located. Today, with a population of 2,182, the biggest industry in town is glass. Brockway Glass began in the 1920s as a hometown plant, and grew to become the second largest maker of glass containers in the world. When Jim was growing up, a time when more things were sold in glass bottles, he remembers that you could proudly "pick up a bottle and look at the bottom—and if it had a 'B', then you knew it was from Brockway Glass, made in my hometown." Like many of Brockway's residents, Jim worked as a laborer at the plant during the summer when he was in high school. Having been bought by Owens, the world's largest glass producer, it is now called Owens-Brockway Glass Container, Inc., and remains the largest employer in the county.

· · · · ·

According to Jim, his father was "one of the true old-fashioned family practitioners/GPs. When he finished his internship, they needed a physician in town. And because my mother was from here, he went ahead and set up practice here in 1949. He just hung a shingle. He made house calls, delivered babies, did everything. After following him through the years, watching him, I just decided I wanted to do it. I used to make house calls with him—in the evenings and on the weekends. I sat in the car while he went in. I used to go to deliveries with him too, and either sat in the car over at the hospital or went back into the maternity area. When he went to the hospital, I'd always jump in the car and go with him. He truly was my role model.

"Growing up in Brockway," Jim continues, "I watched my father practice medicine and get to know his patients as people by really getting the opportunity to share in their lives. I knew that I wanted to return to this small town atmosphere and practice medicine in much the same way. The PSAP [Physician Shortage Area Program] helped give me the exposure and training I needed to return home to the place I loved growing up, and to practice medicine." After he completed his residency in family medicine, Jim returned home and joined his father's practice. They practiced together for two years, until his dad retired. "Today," Jim says, "I'm able to care for patients, who are also my friends, practicing family medicine in its purest form."

In a way, the story of Jim and his father—the two Dr. Devlins—mirrors the history of family doctors in America. When Jim Devlin's father first set up practice, general practice was the principal form of medical care in the nation. But with the explosion in medical advances after World War II, specialization became the predominant trend. During the 1950s and 1960s, while Jim's father was caring for the people in Brockway, almost all of the newly trained physicians were becoming subspecialists. From 1930 to 1970, the ratio of general practitioners to specialists had completely reversed, from about 80:20 to about 20:80. Articles were written about the "death of general practice," and considerable concern was voiced throughout the country that the critically important roles of the trusted GP—comprehensively caring for patients and their families for the vast majority of their problems, being available acutely and over time for their problems, serving to coordinate all of their medical care, acting as a medical and personal advisor who focuses on the patient as opposed to their disease—were all being lost. In the early 1960s, four national reports and commissions were released within a 100-day period, all with similar conclusions: that there was a serious shortage of personal physicians in the country, that this would have a negative impact on current and future health care, and that there was a need for each person to have a personal or family doctor who should be well trained in the broad aspects of patient focused medicine.

As a result, general practice was reborn in 1969 as the specialty of family practice. Gaining status as the twentieth official medical specialty, family practice was a specialty of breadth, rather than of narrow focus by disease, organ system, or age group. Family practice provides first contact care, continuous care, competent care, comprehensive care, personal care, and family care. Be-

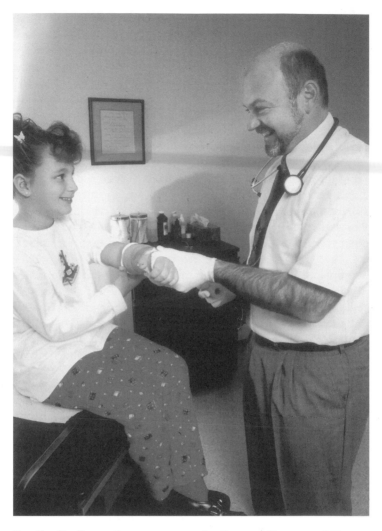

Dr. Jim Devlin casting a young patient's arm. (Courtesy of Thomas Jefferson University)

cause the content of medicine had expanded dramatically, the training required by family physicians needed to be much more extensive and longer
than the single year of internship training that general practitioners like Jim's
father took. The new family practice residency programs were and remain
three years in duration. Also, in recognition that medical knowledge was con-
tinually changing, the newly formed American Board of Family Practice (the
organization responsible for evaluating and certifying all family physicians in
the United States) became the first and only medical specialty board at the
time to require periodic recertification. From its beginning in 1969, being

board certified in family practice was time limited and only valid for seven years. Even today every family doctor in the nation must be reexamined and must be recertified every seven years in order to maintain this status. Since then, almost all of the other medical specialties have followed family practice's lead and adopted this process of time-limited certification and required recertification.

Almost immediately, the specialty of family practice began to grow dramatically. The organization that represented all of the general practitioners in the country, the American Academy of General Practice, was renamed the American Academy of Family Practice (AAFP) in 1970. And, by 1985, when Jim Devlin graduated medical school, there were already more than 350 family practice residency programs and more than 7,000 family practice residents in the country. In recent years, approximately one out of every ten US medical school graduate has become a family physician, and there are currently about 10,000 family practice residents.

· · · · ·

As far back as he can remember, Jim says "my goals were always going into medicine, going into primary care, and coming back to Brockway." Academically talented, he was also an eight-time varsity letter winner in high school—wrestling, football, and golf—and involved in various community activities. He volunteered at his local hospital, and during the summers he worked on a dairy farm, bailing hay. That "was a real education," he remembers. "It was a lot of physical labor. And it's more than ninety degrees in those barns—and no air moving."

When he started college at Penn State, there were more than 300 other premed students, but by the time he graduated, only 26 remained. Jim was president of the Pre-Med Society. "I can still remember the day, when I got my acceptance to medical school," he recalls. "My father and I were working in the back on the tractor, and the mailman came back and said 'There's a registered letter.' We knew you didn't get a rejection in a registered letter."

Jim's wife, Diane, is from "around Reynoldsville," about ten minutes from Brockway. She was born on a dairy farm, "so we're as rural as can be," she says proudly. Her two brothers still operate the farm, which the family has run since as long as anyone can remember. Her mom continues to live in the house where Diane grew up, her brothers less than a half-mile from there, and her sister is about ten miles down the road. "We were high school sweethearts," Jim says. "She was fifteen and I was sixteen when we started dating. She was a grade behind me. We were both valedictorian of our high school classes. She missed being in my class by only four days—so we always kid each other, who would have been valedictorian if she were in my class?"

Married after he graduated from college, Jim and Diane now have two children, a 17-year-old son, and a 15½-year-old daughter. "It's funny, when the kids are little, you think you're tied up—being parents and watching them. But when they start getting older and getting involved, it takes much more time, if you follow them and get involved in what they do, which we do. And that's one thing about living in a small community," he says. "Probably the biggest plus is raising kids."

• • • • •

Discussing his move to "the big city" of Philadelphia for medical school, Jim says, "I'm a country boy, and it was a change going from living in the country, being outside and everything, to city life. It was really the first time I ever had any exposure to city life at all." How was it different? "Just walking down the streets. You're used to making eye contact with people up here. I can remember walking down the street in Philadelphia, and how paranoid people got when they looked out of the corner of their eye and caught you making eye contact with them. And crime. The first week we were in Philadelphia, people got into our apartment building and stole a lot of things. So you learn—coming from an area where you never lock your door, and going to an area where even when you're home, you have to lock yourself in. So, that first week was a big adjustment."

But they adjusted well. Diane got a job in the accounting department at a large law firm in Philadelphia, and it was close enough that she could walk to work every day. And she had a sister living in Bucks County, outside of Philadelphia, who they visited when they wanted to get out of the city. They made friends, and "we got to enjoy the city for what it had," Jim recalls. "We used to take a lot of walks, down to the river, through Independence Mall area, down to the Italian Market—that was our entertainment. And the other thing was, we knew that in four years we were going to be moving out of the city. No way were we going to stay. No, my goal was after the four years to get out of the city."

Like many of the doctors I interviewed, Jim found the first two years of medical school challenging, and he worked very hard in these basic medical science courses—classroom and lab courses that included anatomy, biochemistry, microbiology, and pathology. However, the third and fourth years—the clinical years where medical students work in the hospital and in the outpatient areas seeing patients with residents and faculty physicians— were different. He "finally got to see how to apply things, to integrate things, and I enjoyed it a lot more." As a senior, he took a six-week rural preceptorship, living and working one-on-one with a rural family physician in Bellefonte, Pennsylvania, in the center part of the state. "It was typical of the type of practice that I thought I would have here. Throughout medical school, I was always fixed about family practice, and coming back here and practicing in a rural area. I can't ever remember thinking about doing anything else.

"For residency, I picked a program that would train me for the type of family medicine that I was going to do back here—things like assisting in surgery, doing OB—and I got my first choice, Williamsport Hospital. I had wanted to train in a small town atmosphere, and I'm glad I did. That program gave you a lot of hands-on training. We didn't have any other residents there, so we got to do everything."

Then, after finishing his residency in 1988, Dr. Jim Devlin came back to join his father. "During my last week of residency, my dad gave me a call," Jim remembers. "I had been planning to take two weeks off before I started. But he said, 'Hey, can you start on the following Monday? Brockway Glass just called and they're hiring about 100 kids for the summer, and they need physicals.' And I said, 'Yep, I'll be there.' I had no guaranteed income when I came up here. I remember I had to go to the bank and take out a loan, just to cover things before I got started."

· · · · ·

Practicing family medicine in a rural area means providing a wide range of comprehensive health care for the entire family. "I take care of multiple generations—four generations sometimes. That's enjoyable," Jim says. "You know the whole family. That's family practice. When you're delivering the baby, and you're also taking care of the great-grandma—it's nice when you're seeing them all, and it makes the visit more personal.

"Practicing family medicine in the country differs greatly from providing primary care in the city," he continues. Because there aren't a lot of subspecialists around, Jim has an opportunity to take care of a lot more things than he would otherwise be able to do. He likes doing "hands-on surgical things," like suturing large lacerations, dermatological and minor surgical procedures—such as excisions of large sebaceous cysts and lipomas (fatty tumors)—and orthopedic procedures, like joint injections. Some of the things he used to do, like fracture care, he now refers out, primarily because it no longer pays for him to do it as a result of changing reimbursement rates and malpractice costs. "But, I'm still doing OB," he says. "I used to deliver about fifty babies a year, now I'm probably doing about twenty-five to thirty a year. And, I assist in a lot of surgery. I probably assist in close to two hundred major cases a year." He works with general surgeons, orthopedic surgeons, and gynecologic surgeons, assisting with such operations as gallbladder removals, C-sections, total abdominal hysterectomies, vaginal hysterectomies, colon resections, hip replacements, and knee replacements.

"I have the full gamut of hospital practice," Jim says. "My patients who have a heart attack are on my service, and I consult with cardiology. Our hospital has an Intensive Care Unit (ICU), and we're even doing open heart surgery. With the increased availability of specialists in the past ten years, I do refer more patients. Having a specialist around is usually good, but sometimes it can also make it a little more difficult with continuity and coordination. I also deal with lots of personal issues—divorces, people losing jobs, dealing with sick family members—things that come up in normal life."

Jim loves being in solo private practice, and he enjoys the autonomy—the factor that physicians in general report as being most related to their professional satisfaction. "I have the freedom to make decisions," he explains. "I don't have to check it out with anybody. I don't have to follow the rules; I can make my own. It's enjoyable." But he definitely agrees that it is harder to come out of residency and open a solo practice today. "Back when I started, you could literally make a living on overflow from somebody else's practice. If someone had a sore throat and you were a new doc in town and the other doctor was busy, you had a new patient. Today you couldn't do that because of managed care. I can understand why recent graduates don't want to be independent today—most physicians will need to be employed by someone, or have a guaranteed income."

For a time, Jim's was the only practice in Brockway—just him and his physician assistant. Now, there are two other practices in town, and those practices and the hospital also use nurse practitioners (NPs) and physician assistants (PAs). "My PA has been working for me for almost ten years," Jim says. "Just the two of us, and it's been really good. I'm probably the largest practice in the tri-county area. He goes over to the hospital in the morning. And if I have an admission, I'll see the patient, but he'll help out. But he spends most of his time here in the office, and also helps out at the nursing home. He is busy in the office—he sees twenty-five to thirty patients a day. He sees a lot of the acute problems, like earaches and sore throats, so a lot of my time is scheduled with more chronic problems that take more time. But its nice having him, and from the standpoint of the community, it's nice when people get sick and someone here is always available. Because if somebody needs to be seen, we never have to say, 'I'm sorry we're full and can't see you.' "

• • • • •

Jim Devlin has a lot of hobbies, but his biggest and most unusual hobby is growing giant pumpkins. "Last year my pumpkin was 521 pounds!" he says excitedly. "It was about three to four feet in diameter. The walls were about one-foot thick, and you needed a saw to carve them. We grow the Atlantic Giant. If you go out and take a seed from an Atlantic Giant and just throw it in the ground and water it, you can get a pumpkin that weighs 100 to 150 pounds. Up here, a few of us grow them. We're friends, but we get very competitive. And nationally, there's a competition. In Pennsylvania they have a weigh-off every year in Altoona, and I go down. Last year, we put the pumpkin on a special tarp and lifted it and put it on a palate. You need to get enough people to lift it up. But if they get much larger than that, you have to get a lifting device. I'm having a forklift built for my tractor, so I can lift it up with my tractor. The smaller ones you can put in a pick-up truck, but if you have a big one, you have to rent a truck.

"Two years ago, they had a new world's record in Pennsylvania, down in Spangler, and it was 1,041 pounds. That's a big pumpkin! You usually pollinate them around the end of June. Then, within three weeks, you can tell if it's doing well or not, just by looking at the growth charts from previous pumpkins. These pumpkins can gain up to twenty-five pounds a day when they're growing. You measure them three different ways, and you add the numbers together, and you use a conversion chart to figure how much they weigh, and it's pretty accurate within a few pounds. Usually you end up with one pumpkin on each vine. This year, we're going to have four plants and four pumpkins. Each plant needs an area about thirty feet by thirty feet."

Jim started growing pumpkins because his kids wanted them for jack-o'-lanterns at Halloween. Halloween was a big family holiday, and the entire family would dress up and march in the parade. So Jim started growing normal-sized pumpkins, painting them, and putting them around the house and yard. Then he decided to try and grow bigger ones, then a little bigger, and it just went on from there. "Last year, my buddy and I were crazy enough to drive down to Altoona—which is almost two hours away—once every month for a pumpkin meeting," he says. "It's different, it's just totally different.

"If you're going to grow pumpkins competitively," Jim said, sharing his expertise, "they take a lot of care. You start them inside in the middle of April. I built a little incubator, so I can keep the temperature ninety degrees to get them to germinate, then transplant them and use plant lights inside. When you transplant them outside, you have to make these little greenhouses and try to keep them heated in the cold weather. Then to fertilize them, you use different fertilizers throughout the year. And then you have to be careful with infections. They get a lot of different bugs, like cucumber beetles. That can wipe you out. And then you can get a couple different types of fungus later in the season, when it's wet.

"Even now, my plants are in the ground, but I'll cover them over at night. And after I go to the hospital in the morning, I'll come back home right before I go to the office. I'll run out and uncover my plants and see that they're OK, and then head to the office. And if I can't, I'll have Diane run out and do it. At night, I'll check them out when I get back home from the hospital. So it's an everyday process. And on the weekend sometimes I put in several hours a day. The nice thing is you're right there at the house. You can sit there and enjoy it. If you get called away, you get called away.

"I have two greenhouses up there. One's about 30 × 50 feet, the other's about 30 × 70 feet. The problem with the greenhouse is it gets too warm in the summer, and the pumpkins don't like it. So I'm working on keeping the temperature down. It's just a challenge, a real challenge. I built the greenhouses myself from kits. I like to work with my hands. I do a lot of carpentry work, gardening and things like that. I'm also in the process of building a backstop for my daughter for her softball pitching."

• • • • •

"I just like the diversity," Jim says. "That's why I enjoy family medicine more than I would other specialties. I have a large pediatric practice because I do OB. And that's nice, because as a general rule kids are healthy, and you watch them grow up. I love the diversity—in medicine and everything—that's just my personality."

On this typical morning, Dr. Devlin drives the 12 miles to DuBois Hospital, arriving at 6:30 AM. Once there, he goes to the doctor's lounge where he reviews his patients' lab reports. He rapidly scans, identifies the normals from the abnormals, and signs off on about 50 of these in less than five minutes. He then makes rounds on the patients he has in the hospital today.

The first patient he sees in the hospital is an 81-year-old woman with a history of high blood pressure and osteoporosis. She came into the emergency room (ER) the day before with lower abdominal pain and difficulty urinating. Her pain was so severe that she was admitted for evaluation. His next patient is a 68-year-old woman with a history of colon cancer that has already started to spread, and who was admitted for nausea and abdominal pain. She is also being treated for an ulcer, and is scheduled to get an MRI to see if further spread of her cancer is responsible for her new symptoms. After that, Dr. Devlin sees a 77-year-old man who had heart bypass surgery, and then developed heart failure, kidney failure, and an infection in his arm. He's being treated with antibiotics and is getting better and stronger, and is now on the rehabilitation medicine service, with Dr. Devlin following his progress.

Then, Dr. Devlin sees a 79-year-old man with angina, an irregular heartbeat, aortic stenosis (he had surgery to have his aortic valve replaced last year), and chronic, increasingly severe, heart failure, who has recently had to be admitted to the hospital almost every three to four weeks because of difficulty breathing. He usually gets better fairly quickly after receiving intravenous diuretics to remove some of the fluid that builds up in his lungs, but he knows that he is getting sicker. His wife died last year from lung cancer, and he lives by himself now. The day before yesterday, he was fine when he went to bed. But without warning, he woke up suddenly at 3:00 AM acutely short of breath. Already this morning, after just one day of treatment, he's feeling much better. Dr. Devlin has known this "very nice gentleman since I was a little boy. We go to the same church." As he enters the man's hospital room, he says "Good morning, Mr. G.," and then asks, "How did you sleep last night?"

"Well, with interruptions. It's funny to get weighed at three in the morning." The patient laughs slightly. "You don't go to the hospital to get sleep."

"That's pretty early," Dr. Devlin responds, smiling. Then, after asking a few more questions, he asks the patient to sit up, and bends over and listens to the man's back with his stethoscope. "Your breathing seems to be a little better."

"Yes."

"Well, our game plan is to go ahead and just continue with the medication, and just get things tuned up and get you back home." Dr. Devlin pauses, then looks seriously at the patient and says, "We talked before. I am going to try and keep you home as long as we can."

"Great. Like I said, I had a very good week there."

"Yeah, and with the medication, hopefully we can get you back there."

"I hope so. Sunshine helps too."

"I'll come back and stop in after I'm done in the OR, and if your son's not here, I'll go ahead and give him a call this morning. OK?"

"I'd appreciate that very much."

Next, Dr. Devlin heads to the ICU to see a 91-year-old woman who came into the hospital with worsening of both her chronic lung disease and her heart disease. She's getting a bit better, and Dr. Devlin decides to transfer her to the regular hospital floor today. She has no family around—her one daughter, a teacher, lives about four hours away, and her other daughter is a lawyer who lives in Ohio. So Dr. Devlin talks to her for a little while about her future care, and her support system—she has good friends who come in and keep an eye on her at home. She says she doesn't want to go to a nursing home, but if she gets to that point, she realizes she may need to.

Then, while making rounds, Dr. Devlin is called by his nurse. One of his patients, a 35-year-old woman, is on the phone complaining of chest pain when she breathes, and being short of breath. After asking a few brief questions to assess how critical the problem is, he has her go to the ER for evaluation and a chest X-ray, and he calls the ER to let the doctor there know that his patient is on her way. Although slightly concerned about the possibility of a heart attack, he thinks it's more likely to be a respiratory problem. Later in the morning, when he's in his office, the ER doctor calls him back. The diagnosis is pleurisy, a mild viral respiratory infection. "This way, I'm involved in the decision-making process and what's going on," he explains, "even if I'm not there."

The last of Dr. Devlin's hospitalized patients today is a 78-year-old woman who "just caught me after church a few months ago and said she wasn't feeling good," he says. When he saw her the next day in the office, she didn't have any specific symptoms, and her examination was normal, but some of her initial blood tests were abnormal. Then, after some additional tests, he made a diagnosis of bone cancer. Since then, she's been seeing a cancer specialist and doing well but was admitted a few days ago, just not feeling well again. After a few days in the hospital, she was getting better and about ready to go home, when she developed severe chest pain. "We moved her to the ICU, we had the cardiologist and lung specialist here, but she lost consciousness, and had to be intubated. It looks like she had a large blood clot in her lungs. Now she is developing kidney and liver failure. She's just not turning the curve—she's starting to go into multisystem failure. Now, I'm following her to make sure that everything is being done. And talking to the family. I've known the family all my life. So, when the specialists tell them something, they get on the phone and call me, and ask, 'How's she doing?' They want to hear it from me." The woman's son works in the hospital lab, and her grandson was our waiter at dinner last night. "There are always relationships with everyone around here."

After rounds, Dr. Devlin spends the next hour and a half assisting the surgeon in the operating room, performing a hysterectomy on a 41-year-old woman with uterine fibroids who developed anemia from the recurrent heavy vaginal bleeding. Then he goes home, throws on a pair of boots, and goes out to uncover the pumpkins—the sun is out today—and arrives at the office by 10:00 to see his first patients. He sees patients—usually between 25 and 28 a day—takes a half hour for lunch, and at 4:00 today, he has a hospital board meeting. Later, he goes back to the hospital to make rounds on his patients, then back home to cover the pumpkins, to make sure they don't freeze.

"I still occasionally make a house call," he says. "Most often for an elderly person who's sick and housebound and the family doesn't want them to go to the hospital, or they don't want to go to the hospital. Then, you see what you can do to keep them there, keep them comfortable. Believe it or not, taking care of patients who are dying is a very rewarding part of family practice in a small community. You know these people, you know these families. And sometimes the most rewarding times I've ever had in medicine is taking the stethoscope out of my ears, and sitting down and holding someone's hand and listening to them. I still remember, back when I was in medical school during my first family medicine rotation, I had an elderly patient who had lung cancer. And we all went into her room—a couple junior students, a senior student, a resident and the attending physician. I was her primary person. I didn't know anything about medicine, since it was my first clinical rotation, and I remember her telling me, 'Don't ever change. Sitting here and talking to me, you have so much to offer. And you have more to give to me than anybody else.' And it's true. Sometimes you have to realize that just listening to the patient and consoling the patient is still an important part of medicine. This is an issue that I have trouble with today because it takes time. In a busy practice, you spend time listening to a person who comes in, and you're trying to do the best you can but you know that they really need more time, and you're limited as to what you can do. But it's still a very, very important part of medicine."

Dr. Devlin is "on call" 24 hours a day on Mondays, Tuesdays, and Wednesdays, but has someone cover for him on Thursday afternoon and evening. Then, he rotates weekend call with four other doctors from mornings till 11:00 PM, so he is free for four out of five Saturday and Sunday afternoons and evenings. But he still rounds on his patients that are in the hospital every day, and he still takes call every night from 11:00 PM till morning. For his OB patients he is on call all the time, unless he's out of town, and he is the only family doctor in town who assists in surgery. "So," he says, "if you really want to be off, you need to go out of town. And then there are people who will cover for you. What you do here is very individualized. There are doctors who want to be part of larger call groups, that only want to be on call one night a week—and you can do that. I have chosen not to do that—it's just my personality."

• • • • •

Typical of the vast majority of the landmass of the United States, Brockway is rural. In fact, 2,228 of the nation's counties—more than 70 percent of them—were classified as nonmetropolitan in 1993. They contain 83 percent of the nation's land, an area larger in size than all but five of the world's nations. More than 60 million people live in these rural counties, constituting about 20 percent of the US population—and greater than the total populations of Canada and Australia combined. And despite the overall impression that rural America is disappearing, the population in three-fourths of rural counties is actually growing larger. This predominance of rural areas in the

United States is also reflected in the political make-up of the country, with more than three-fourths of the members of the US Senate and almost one-third of those in the US House of Representatives belonging to the Rural Health Caucus in 1999. Nonetheless, there is oftentimes a bias against rural areas and rural policy, as the majority of the population, and most of the media—and medical schools—are urban.

While demographers have argued for decades over the details of the specific definition of rural, it is clear that rural areas do share a number of common characteristics. They have relatively small populations and low population density with people spread out over a large area. Rural areas are also not very near, nor are they closely connected to a large urban area—either physically, or emotionally—and most people who live there do not work, commute, or do their daily shopping in the city. Transportation into the city is oftentimes a problem, and almost by definition rural areas have a hard time supporting medical subspecialists, who frequently need a large population base.

Most of the official definitions of rural are negative, that is, they are defined by not being urban. One common definition of rural used by demographers is those places outside an "urbanized area," that is, "outside a continuously built-up area with a population of 50,000 or more." Similarly, the federal government uses the term nonmetropolitan to define counties that are outside of metropolitan areas and without a core city of 50,000 people. Using this county-wide designation is problematic, however, as there are oftentimes very rural areas within the outer boundaries of metropolitan counties (usually on the opposite side of a county that has a city located in one corner). As a result, Rural-Urban Commuting Areas (RUCAs) have more recently been developed, combining commuting data with Census Bureau information to identify those zip codes within an urban county that are rural. Yet another definition of rural—this one from the Census Bureau, which first began using the term in 1874—identifies someone as rural if they live in a town of 2,500 people or fewer that is not part of or adjoining an urban area. While none of these definitions is ideal, there is considerable overlap among most of them. That is, most rural areas are rural, irrespective of which definition is used. On the other hand, it is also true that many rural areas and small towns differ from each other in many ways, oftentimes differing from each other in more ways than they are similar.

For Jefferson's PSAP, we have primarily used official nonmetropolitan county designations, and more recently have also begun using zip codes to identify smaller rural areas. Frequently, however, we define a rural area and small town at a more common sense and conceptual level—as a place that is "nonurban, nonsuburban." Of the ten doctors profiled in this book, seven practice in nonmetropolitan counties. The other three practice in small rural towns that, although located within a metropolitan county, have been federally designated as Health Professional Shortage Areas (HPSAs) and are located at some distance from the nearest city. All ten of these doctors practice in towns with populations less than 13,000, nine in towns less than 10,000, and half in towns with fewer than 5,000 people. None of these towns would come close to being considered suburban or urban. And, most important, anyone who found themselves placed in any one of these ten communities would immediately recognize that they were in a small rural town.

But rural towns are not just defined by demographics and populations. They also differ in many other cultural ways from metropolitan areas. There is a different mind-set, a different pace, a different attitude. In fact, while urban individuals often describe rural areas in terms of numbers and populations, people living there describe these small towns more by how they feel. Throughout my visits to the rural doctors in this book, I was continuously struck by how different these rural areas were from urban and suburban areas. Wherever I went with these doctors, people knew them, and the doctors knew the people in town. If we went out to eat, the owner, the waiters and waitresses, the other people in the restaurant, were often patients, or had family members who were patients. The owners of the motel where I stayed were patients. As we drove down the road from the hospital to the office, the doctors knew most of the people we passed in other cars. Each building in town had a story about who owned it, who worked there, who was related to whom. Patients in the office were frequently related to, or had some connection to someone else that I had met that day. Sociologists call these "primary contacts," where people have overlapping and interdependent social roles, relating to each other in many different ways, with family, work, and neighborhood relationships intersecting with each other. Not only do these doctors provide medical care for the people in their towns, but their patients also relate to the doctors as neighbors, their children's teacher, or the person that fixes their car or sells them groceries. The relationship between people in rural areas is therefore very close, and they have emotional ties and a commitment to each other. Those of us who live in urban areas oftentimes try and recreate this "small town feeling," living in neighborhoods and smaller communities, with most of us developing a relatively small circle of people we interact with—usually fewer than 200 people.

While rural areas clearly differ in many ways from urban areas, however, those same characteristics that are viewed by some people as desirable and encourage them to live in rural areas are in many instances the identical variables that dissuade other people from living rural. For example, the rural family doctors in this book see small towns as an ideal place to raise a family and value knowing everyone in town, having lots of space and outdoor activities, lower crime rates, less traffic, short commutes to work, more autonomy in practice, an increased scope of practice, and less managed care. And they seem quite content with having to drive much farther and having fewer options for shopping, restaurants, and professional sporting events, and tolerate having fewer medical resources and more professional isolation. On the other hand, most of my colleagues in the city and suburbs seem to have almost the opposite priorities. They enjoy the anonymity of the city, the separation of work and home, and the diversity of cultural and shopping opportunities nearby, and seem to tolerate the crime, traffic, pollution, commuting, and lesser autonomy, scope, and control in their medical practice.

It is true that many people dream of living in the country at some time in their life. But for most of us this represents a romantic vision of rural. Years of data clearly show that only those with significant rural life experiences, mostly those who grew up in a rural area, are very likely to go there to live and work. For physicians, rural background is, in fact, the strongest predictor by far of rural practice. And while many people who grow up rural do not return, it is even truer that only a very, very small percentage of urban and suburban-raised individuals ever go rural. It appears that where we grew up is an important part of who we are and where we end up.

• • • • •

Driving through town with Jim and Diane, he points out the park. "This is one of my pride and joys here," Jim says. Five years ago someone in town died and left $10,000 to the park. Jim was asked to chair a group to decide what to do with the money. Instead, they decided to try and raise additional money to renovate the entire area, and build a whole new park. And they did. They raised $140,000 from individual and corporate donations, and the community built the park. "I spent every night down there from the first of April through the first of August. We literally built it ourselves," Jim says, with enormous pride. "It's nice for the kids, it's centrally located, and it's where we have all our ball fields, our pool, our park, everything. During the summer, the kids come down and play ball every night, and the younger kids can come down and play in the park if they don't want to watch their brothers and sisters. And on summer nights they go to the pool. And as a parent, you don't worry about the kids—it's safe."

• • • • •

"I would say I know ninety percent of the people in town," Jim says. "I don't know how many people in the area I take care of, but I would say a few thousand. My practice is big—it's one of the things about living in a small town, and being born and raised in it, and having my father practice here." In discussing what he likes about being a rural family doctor, Jim says, "It's the old concept, Do you want to be a big fish in a little pond, or a little fish in a big pond? Honestly, that's what it comes down to. Being in a small community, you are one of the more respected people in the community, because of your professional status. And if that's what you want and you enjoy it, then it's great. Everybody knows you—and everybody knows your business too. If you're willing to accept that, and that's what you want, it's good. But being in a small community, people are going to be watching you all the time. There's a lot of gratitude and reward practicing in a small community, and not just from the standpoint of the practice of medicine, but everything else you do in the community. One of the things that helped the park get built was that I coordinated and chaired the program, and I signed my name to the letter we mailed out to everybody, to industry, and to individuals. And we were able to get money to build the park, and that was very rewarding.

"But, you lose some privacy," he continues. "I mean if you want to go out for dinner, or you don't want people to know what you're doing, or you don't want to be bothered, it's difficult. There's a lot of times when you go out with your family, or go someplace, and somebody stops and asks you a medical question, and you think, "Hey, I'm not on call." But that's the price you're going to pay. I'm very involved with the public, because I'm a public person. The other day I received the Sportsman of the Year Award for all my contributions to sports over the years. I was very honored to get it—I was the youngest person to ever receive it. I go to all the football games and help out. I've been the team physician for fourteen years. And I like that. Sure, sometimes if you're out in public, it can be a problem: If you're out to enjoy yourself, and people come up to you and ask you about their medical problems. I could never figure out why, when the carnival came to town, my father never wanted to take us. But after I was back for a year, I told my wife I found out why. Because you go down there, and you're walking through, and people come up to you and start asking you medical questions—even people you've never seen. But again, that's part of being in a small community. People realize that you have to have time to yourself, but when they're ill, they want you there.

"The hardest part for me," Jim explains, "is trying to give 110 percent all the time. It's part of my personality. Occasionally you get a little sensitive—someone you've known for a number of years may transfer to another physician, and you sometimes take it personally. Was it something I did? Was it something that the office did? Living in a small community, you try and please everybody, but unfortunately you can't. And every once in a while, someone's going to be upset with the way things were handled, even if it wasn't you, but your office. I have a huge practice. And, I'm president of our Preferred Provider Organization [PPO, a group of physicians that jointly contract with insurance companies], vice president of the Physician Hospital Organization [PHO, an organization of physicians and the hospital that jointly contracts with insurance companies], I'm on the hospital board, I'm on the Medical Staff Executive Committee. I'm also the medical director of a nursing home—I have about forty residents there who I take care of. And every once in a while somebody is a little unhappy—maybe it took two weeks to get an appointment for a routine checkup and they don't understand why you couldn't see them tomorrow—and they get upset. And being in a small community and knowing the people, you feel bad. You walk into church on Sunday and they tell you. And that's difficult."

• • • • •

Today, after only three decades as a specialty, there are more than 60,000 board certified family physicians, the second largest medical specialty in the United States. And family doctors take care of a large proportion of the population, accounting for almost one out of every four patient office visits in the nation. As with the other primary care specialties, family practice includes five important components: accessibility, continuity of care, comprehensive care, coordinated care, and accountability. Family doctors offer these services: That patients can see their doctor when they need to; that the doctor will care for them over a long time period; that the doctor will care for the vast majority of their problems (about 94%) by themselves; that the doctor will coordinate their patient's total health care, including those problems they do refer to other providers; and that the doctor will take ongoing responsibility for helping to manage their patients' health and welfare.

In addition, the scope of medical problems that family doctors care for is extremely broad. While some medical students are overwhelmed that family doctors provide comprehensive care for "everything," the reality is that most people most often have the most common problems. In fact, the following 25 most common problems that family doctors care for make up more than half of all office visits, and include: general medical examinations, acute upper respiratory conditions, high blood pressure, minor injuries, sprains and strains, prenatal and postnatal care, depression and anxiety, heart disease, diabetes, rashes, arthritis, urinary infections, obesity, acute lower respiratory infections, skin infections, gastrointestinal infections, vaginal infections, fractures and dislocations, ear infections, emphysema and other chronic lung diseases, post-surgical care, ulcers, headaches, bursitis, and low back pain. But while these problems are common, they are not all easy to care for. As illustrated by this list, family doctors take care of serious medical problems as well as more minor problems.

Family doctors also often see patients as they present with "undifferentiated" problems. For example, they often see a woman when she first develops abdominal pain, and they need to determine at this point whether it is a gastrointestinal problem, a gynecological problem, a urinary problem, or a surgical problem. If the woman is seen by a subspecialist, the problem has oftentimes already been differentiated or categorized, and often a diagnosis has been made. Family doctors also take care of patients who often have multiple problems at the same time. While much of the medical research focuses on individual medical diseases, real patients often have two, three or more medical problems—especially the elderly and chronically ill. And when these multiple problems cross subspecialty boundaries, as with a man who has diabetes and heart disease and prostate problems, his medical care needs to be coordinated to take into consideration all of these problems. Family doctors often find that their patients—say a man with arthritis—has been treated by a subspecialist with a medication that can cause problems because of the patient's other medical problems, for example, an ulcer.

What else do family doctors do? They provide most of the preventive health care in the country, lots of nutrition counseling, and are beginning to become more involved in issues related to genetic diseases. Although not often realized, family doctors also care, in large degree, for the many mental health problems of their patients, including counseling and treatment of anxiety and depression. And with advances in medicine and technology, future family doctors will have an even greater role in coordinating care through the complex health care system providing what most of us would like, quality medical care by someone who knows you. Finally, rural family doctors will play an increasingly important part of the public health care infrastructure, dealing with problems and issues such as bioterrorism, SARS (Severe Acute Respiratory Syndrome), and other emerging infections.

Family practice has also played an important role in improving the medical education of all physicians over the past few decades. Data published in the 1960s showed that of every 1,000 adults in the country, about 250 consulted a doctor in a given month. But, only one of those people was admitted to a major hospital associated with a medical school or medical university. Most medical students and residents, however, were being trained almost entirely in these university hospitals, and their training therefore focused only on the very few people who are cared for in these specialized hospitals—ignoring the vast majority of people (249 out of every 250 people) who seek medical care. Family practice has had a major role in most medical schools since then, expanding student training into the doctor's office and outpatient arena, thereby broadening and improving medical education.

In addition, family physicians disproportionately care for rural America. Research has shown that after rural background, practicing the specialty of family medicine (even planning to do so) is the next strongest predictor of actually practicing in a rural area. In fact, despite the huge number of factors that are obviously involved in deciding whether or not to practice rural primary care, two factors alone—growing up rural, and entering medical school with plans to be a family physician—identified 88 percent of all medical students who eventually became rural primary care physicians.

• • • • •

Jim Devlin's office is located in the same two-story white house on Main Street where his father practiced. The street is lined on both sides with large shade trees, their tops almost meeting overhead. After arriving at his office, Dr. Devlin checks in with his nurse, and then walks into the exam room to see his first patient of the morning, an 82-year-old man with high blood pressure and arthritis.

"How are you today?"

"OK, good."

Then, Dr. Devlin opens the patient's chart, takes out a paper with his latest laboratory test results, and asks, "Any problems?"

"Not unless you have some on that sheet of paper that you're going to show me."

"No, your blood work looks good. Your cholesterol was 192, your LDL was 125. Kidney and liver functions look good. Your blood sugar is 85, which is very good. Your prostate test was good too. Your PSA was 1.1—normal is usually less than 4. And your urinalysis was normal also."

"Yeah."

"Your blood pressure—the top number was a little high today. Now when you were in here a couple weeks ago, it was better. What I want you to do is periodically just stop in and check. If we see that there's persistent elevation, I may need to bump your medicine up a little bit. OK?"

"OK."

"Have you been able to get outside and do any work? Are you cutting any wood?"

"No," the older man replies, "they took my power saw away from me," and both he and Dr. Devlin laugh.

According to Dr. Devlin, "One thing about people around here, their entertainment is not going to the movies or doing things like that. Their entertainment is usually outside, working in the yard, working in the woods. This man's hobby on the side used to be cutting firewood."

The man then adds, laughing, "You forgot my main hobby—that's eating. Last night, there was a pie sitting there, and I had to have two pieces before I went to bed. My wife hit the ceiling."

Dr. Devlin then examines the man, retakes his blood pressure, and listens to his heart and lungs. "Are you going to be able to keep busy this summer? That's important."

"Yeah."

"So your cholesterol's good. Under 200 is super. The LDL of 125 is good. All the other tests are good. And you can keep this paper." Dr. Devlin knows that patients like to keep the results of their blood work, and always gives them a copy of their lab tests. Then, as he often does, he dictates his chart in front of the patient. It's a good opportunity for the patient to hear what the doctor is saying about the visit, allows for the patient to correct anything that might be incorrect, and reiterates the treatment plan—all the while completing the time consuming task of dictating the chart. He then continues, "OK, as I said, stop in here periodically, and if the pressure is still up, we'll titrate up your medicine."

The next patient is a 38-year-old woman with depression and anxiety. Then, he sees an 80-year-old man who is here to get his sutures out. Dr. Devlin removed a skin cancer from his cheek last week in the office and sent it off to the pathologist, who confirmed the diagnosis. Sometimes, depending on the severity and size of the lesion, he refers skin cancers to the dermatologist for removal, sometimes he removes them himself in the office.

"How's it feeling?"

"Well, it feels good today."

"Now, the report did come back that it was a little basal cell—a little skin cancer. It's not a serious type of skin cancer. Basal cells will usually stay in the area they are. Basal cells are very, very common—most commonly you see them on exposed areas, like the face. It isn't like you have a cancer that's going to spread anywhere—they don't do that. So we'll just watch it. OK?"

"OK."

Dr. Devlin looks carefully at the man's cheek. "Are you comfortable sitting there? It's not putting the stitches in that's hard, it's taking them out," he says smiling. Then, after taking out the stitches, he continues, "This seems to be filling in very nicely there. What I want you to do is just put a little topical antibiotic on it for a couple days, and then we'll watch it. It seems like it's healing very nicely here. Let me see this in about two months. OK? And I don't want you to worry about it."

"Will it bleed or anything?"

"No, I don't anticipate it."

"Well, that's my only question." Then as he starts to get down from the examining table, he grimaces due to the pain in his hip from his arthritis and says, "Here's the worst part—getting down. OK, well, thank you. You're quite a guy. Have a wonderful weekend."

Between patients, Dr. Devlin dictates more charts, signs some forms, answers phone calls from patients, and reviews more lab results. All patients are called back with the results of their blood tests within 24 hours of having the test done, even if they are normal. "It's more work, but it works. We tell people if you don't hear back from us in 24 hours, then you call us."

The next patient in the office is a middle-aged man with arthritis of his knees, who also has heart disease and high cholesterol. He is a teacher in town, and a friend of Dr. Devlin. His wife has breast cancer, and she is having increasing problems. He's here for a checkup. He is complaining of increasing knee pain. He had three shots of a synthetic joint fluid injected into his right knee by the orthopedist and also had some fluid removed. The first shot helped a little, the next two seemed to make it worse. The orthopedist feels like he probably should have a knee replacement, but the patient wants to wait, since his wife is sick. His cholesterol is much better now that he is on medication.

Next is a 60-year-old healthy woman in for a routine pap test. Then, a 32-year-old pregnant woman due to deliver her second child tomorrow. Dr. Devlin delivered her first child. He saw her in the ER at 11:00 PM last night with early labor pains, and after checking her, sent her home with an appointment to see her in the office today. She thinks that she had a "bloody show" early this morning, but her labor has not increased. The baby continues to be very active, perhaps a bit less. The Doppler ultrasound that he does in the office shows a strong heart rate of 144 beats per minutes, which is normal. Dr. Devlin tells her to "Call me when you're in full labor. I'll be out of town for a few hours Thursday for my daughter's softball state tournament, but other than that I'm here."

The next patient is an 80-year-old man, a retired glass worker, who's been very active since he retired. He is accompanied by his wife. The man has diabetes, without complications, and also has a high systolic blood pressure and high cholesterol. And he has a benign skin lesion, a seborrheic keratosis, on his scalp that Dr. Devlin removed once before. Dr. Devlin checks that first, and schedules an appointment for him to come back and have it removed again. Today, the man's weight has increased a few pounds, his systolic blood pressure is 180—higher than usual, his blood sugars at home are high—around 200, and his last blood test to measure his sugar over the past three months is high. "I brought my wife this time. I know I need to start watching my diet," the man says. "My sugars are much better when I'm on my diet—usually around 120. But my wife made two peach pies, and I ate one whole one," he says laughing. Dr. Devlin spends some time discussing the fact that his diet is the most important part of the treatment of his diabetes and his blood pressure. Turning very serious, he says, "All joking aside, the mainstay of diabetes is diet."

The following patient is a cute six-year-old little boy with an ear infection. His father works for the local fire department. Then, the last patient of the morning is a baby boy who Dr. Devlin delivered six months ago, here for a well child visit. His four-year-old brother is home with a babysitter. After examining the infant, Dr. Devlin asks his nurse to give him two shots: his second round of DPT (diphtheria, pertussis, and tetanus) and Hemophilus influenzae (which causes bacterial meningitis and other serious infections in children) immunizations.

· · · · ·

The Devlin's house is just up the hill from the house where Jim was born and raised, and where his parents still live. "When I was a little kid, there were no houses up here, this was all fields. I used to come up here and play. So I remembered this piece of land being up here, and I was just walking around one time, and I thought, hey, this is perfect. I knew the gentleman who owned it—he was then living in Florida. And I called him, and I said, 'The piece of ground you have up there, would you be interested in selling it?' And he said 'Sure.' And I said 'How much do you want for it?' and he said, 'You just go and find me what you consider a fair price, and that'll be fine.' So I went ahead and got a couple people to price it. And he said, 'You can have it for that price, as long as you pay for the closing costs.'" So Jim and Diane purchased the entire ten acres of land for less than the cost of a suburban plot in Philadelphia. "It's nice where we live," Jim says. "You're away from things, but with your kids involved, you're only minutes from the school, or from downtown. This is my farm on the right. The house is only a half mile from the office."

The house is beautiful. In back, there is a patio and pool, and the view overlooks the town of Brockway, which sits way down in the valley. "Believe it or not, when we were back in medical school, we started looking at house plans, and designed everything." Jim says. "Then when I came back from residency, we built the house. I found somebody to do the carpentry work, and I subcontracted out everything else myself. I found the stone that we used on the outside of the house in Bucks County, and we had it hauled up here—so we brought a little bit of Philadelphia back with us."

As for the income level of rural family doctors, Jim says, "You can make more money working in a rural community. It all depends on how hard you want to work. Being in a rural community, if you want to work hard, you have the market. I'm in the top income level in the community. People think that being in a rural community they can't make a living, but that's not correct. In some ways there's more opportunity, there really is. Going to a rural community doesn't guarantee you're going to make a lot of money, but if you work hard, you're going to have a busy practice. You have to make sure there are enough patients to support a practice, but mostly it has to do with motivation. Also, expenses are less in a rural area. Housing is a lot less. Reimbursement may be a little less, but our living expenses are less too." Compared to what he thought his standard of living would be when he was in medical school, he says it is "Much better. But, I didn't have any debt—my wife worked so she could support us while I was going to medical school."

Jim feels that "Managed care is definitely putting a burden on primary care that is totally unnecessary. For example, if someone gets hurt at 2:00 in the morning and needs care right then, they have to call me right then and ask for my OK to go to the emergency room or their insurance won't pay for it. That's not necessary. But, one of the nice things about managed care and being in a rural area is that you can kind of control things. You can look over contracts and decide who you're going to contract with. And the nice thing here is that they can't sign up with the doctors across the street and the hospital across the street because there isn't one. So, many of the HMOs haven't come into the area."

· · · · ·

Although he is quite busy, Jim manages to do a lot with his family, and is very involved with his kids. "I coached baseball when my son was smaller, and I also coached softball for my daughter's team. I make sure I get scheduled out of the office. I do things with my family, and then go back to the hospital at 9:30 or 10:00 at night to tie things up if I have to. I enjoy it that way." Jim thinks the best part, by far, of living in a small town is "raising a family in an atmosphere where you still feel good about it. And allowing them to grow up in a school district where they can be involved in a lot of activities and get a good education. And still have a fairly safe environment. I enjoy being part of the community, not just practicing medicine in the community. That's something you have the opportunity to do in a small town. I'm also very involved with the church. Presently I'm an active elder. But mostly what I do revolves around the kids."

Amazingly, Jim Devlin's application to medical school—written more than 20 years ago—not only reflected his long-standing career goals, but also accurately predicted his current role. He wrote, "Because of my exposure to the medical field, I plan a career in family medicine. I choose this particular field because I would like to raise a family in a rural area, be a member of a small community, contributing to it and its citizens, politically and socially, as well as medically. For me, family medicine is a way of life and not just a career."

Nanty Glo, Pennsylvania

It is in these rural areas that a physician has the unique opportunity to become familiar with the life of the patient. The physician may live down the road from the patient, may have purchased produce from his brother's farm, or may have cheered for the patient's son in a soccer game. Relationships have the special ability to create a union that is both professional and personal. It is focused on the betterment of both the physical and social health of the population. Medicine in a rural environment not only heals the community, but is an intricate part of the community as well.

—Jennifer Miller, PSAP student, Class of 2005

If you do all your growing up in the same small place, you don't shed identities. You accumulate them.

—Tracy Kidder, *Hometown*

The Ebandjieff Clinic sits on a small street in the center of Nanty Glo, Pennsylvania. A one-story brick building with white trim, it was built in 1949. The miners in town contributed the money to build the clinic, paying a nickel from each paycheck at the end of every day. Nanty Glo was a small coal-mining town back then, and the mining company did everything. They built the houses, owned the company store, brought in the doctors, and provided health care. Dr. George Ebandjieff, who had arrived in town from the Ukraine a year earlier, had promised the miners that they would have health care forever if they built this clinic. And he kept his promise until he died in 1973.

After that, for almost the next two decades, Nanty Glo didn't have a full-time doctor, until 1992, when Mike Tatarko, who used to be a patient at the clinic when he was a child, came back home to practice family medicine. Mike grew up in Twin Rocks, a small town about two miles away, and went to school in town. "My Dad was a butcher, and Mum raised all of us. They still live next door." Today Dr. Tatarko is not only a family doctor in town, but he is the medical director of the Ebandjieff Clinic and also the president and CEO of Conemaugh Health Initiatives (CHI), a physician group of more than

65 primary care physicians and more than 50 other specialists that provides health care to the people in two and one-half rural counties in this part of the Appalachian Mountains in western Pennsylvania.

· · · · ·

Sitting comfortably at his desk in the clinic, his hair slightly longish and wearing a short-sleeved dress shirt and tie, Mike Tatarko smiles warmly and looks as if he just belongs here. When he begins talking, his sincerity and enthusiasm are almost palpable. "When you move back to a community," he says, "some of the things you do are not just limited to providing medical care. And you don't necessarily know what you're going to be involved in. But you move into a small town, and the town's unofficial leaders—not the elected officials—turn out to be the ministers, the physicians, the school principal, and if you have an attorney in town, which we don't. And if you don't do something, then a lot of stuff doesn't get done.

"So when I came back," he continues, "there was a group of us. . . . The water system in Nanty Glo was dismal. There was no water system in nearby Vintondale and Blacklick Township. In fact, Vintondale had to carry their water in for at least ten years. There were no sanitary sewers out there whatsoever. Nanty Glo had sewers, but they were in desperate need of repair. So I ended up being on the Cambria County Task Force for Industrial Development, the Board of the Blacklick Valley Water and Sewer Authority, the Johnstown Area Regional Industries (the two-county industrial organization), and the Cambria County Business Alliance and Planning Commission. And we put together a master ten-year plan to economically revitalize the area. We needed a blueprint of some kind—we needed road access (which is currently underway), we needed infrastructure, we needed property for industrial development, and we also focused on the environment. So, our Industrial Development Fund secured 1,600 acres between here and Twin Rocks and going up Chickory Mountain, and also 2,000 acres in Indiana County up by the Little Mahoning, and another 1,000 down in Somerset County. We also secured about fifty acres on the top of Route 22 for an Industrial Park, and another sixty acres out in Blacklick Township for another Industrial Park.

"But the real dilemma here was water and sewage. I was treating giardia infections left and right [a form of gastroenteritis caused by the giardia parasite], because we have beaver around here. I never thought I'd ever see giardia. But that turned out to be one of the ways we convinced the state that this area needed priority funding, because I was documenting every case. It was like epidemiology and public health. So we got extra money, and we finished our water project about a year and a half ago. It was the first time that Vintondale had drinkable water that you didn't have to haul in. And all of Blacklick Township got a water system. We're about to dig ground for a $10 million sewage plant that will take care of the rest of Blacklick Township and Vintondale. And Nanty Glo finished upgrading their sewage system— which was originally put in back in the 70s'—so now their system is intact.

"We're also going to upgrade a bony dump—that's a coal refuse pile. You

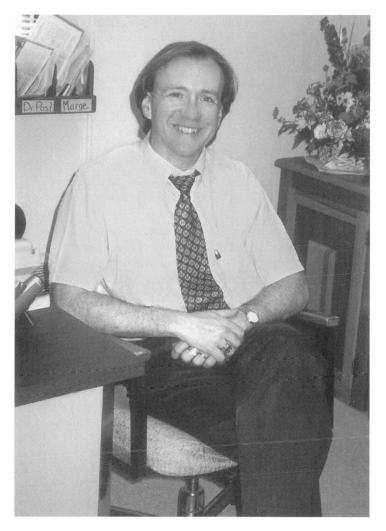

Dr. Mike Tatarko in his office.

know, after they mined the coal, they took the good coal to the steel mills, but the other coal, they just stacked it up—it's just sitting there in big piles now. They're called bony dumps. These piles are huge! I can't even tell you how big, multiple stories high, as big as the surrounding hills. They really create a lot of pollution in the streams. Rain hits them, snow melts off, and lowers the pH in the streams. So now we're going to get rid of one of those piles.

"Also, there was a small acid mine discharge in Vintondale that we got federal money to clean up. The north branch of the Blacklick was fluorescent orange when I was growing up from acid mine pollution. And now it's clean water, it holds trout, all the way down to Vintondale. Here in Nanty Glo, there's one other site, the old Webster mine, which was the original mine in town that was responsible for about ninety-seven percent of the acid load from here, and going downstream about six to seven miles. The Army Corps of Engineers is going to take care of the problem. I've met with the EPA [Environmental Protection Agency] and the DEP [Department of Environmental Protection], and after we get the Webster discharge done, it will only be a year or two till this stream will hold trout also. That was fluorescent orange when I was a kid too. We knew we needed infrastructure and roads, but we also knew that the town couldn't have an orange stream running through it if we were going to entice any business to come back."

As Mike talks at length about these major water, sewage, and environmental projects that he has helped to make successful, he doesn't sound like most rural physicians who talk primarily of practice. "I don't have a clue how I knew all this," he says. "It just kind of happened. As we went along, first there was one bit of information, then you search down another road, and then you pass things through different committees. We also called our congressman's office—you know Jack Murtha has been really great. From the time I came back here as a doctor, the congressman has been really helpful. And so, if I don't know where to go for something, I call one of his staff, and they help."

He then recounts two other examples of improving the community infrastructure. "We just happened to have an old petroleum pipeline, vintage World War II, that ran from Pittsburgh to Philly that wasn't used for oil anymore. And somebody was smart enough to run a fiber optic line through there. It cuts right through this area. And the high school here tapped into it, so we have a huge T1 line for computers, and digital capability. And the Ghost Town Trail is here, one of the national Rails to Trails projects [converting old railroad beds into biking and hiking trails]. We had one of the first ones here. It goes from Nanty Glo down to Dilltown in Indiana County, and the County just received the funds to run it from Ebensburg down to Nanty Glo. The eventual plan is to have it from county seat to county seat, out to Indiana, Pennsylvania.

"I've just finished my ninth year on Johnstown Area Regional Industries," he says, "and I'm no longer on the County Business Alliance, so I've backed off those. I'm still on to the Water and Sewer Authority, and the one industrial group here, since we're not done here yet. I promised my wife I'd back out of those as soon as I finished this—it turned out to be longer than our five-year plan—but . . . it all worked. Of course, I didn't do any of this myself. There was a small group of people—six to twelve people in town—that all worked together. We needed access, which we're getting now, we needed to have sewage and water, and we're in the process of that. One step at a time . . . we're getting there. I can't believe it all worked!"

• • • • •

Mike's family roots go deep into the surrounding area. His mother's family was originally from Twin Rocks, and growing up, Mike's grandparents lived in the house next door. Then, when his grandmother died in 1986, "the family—all my mum's brothers and sisters" as Mike tells it, "decided that my wife, Lori, and I could have my grandmother's house. We thought that we would live there during my residency and save money; that it may be old—you know, an old company house in Twin Rocks—but we could survive in that for a couple years until we got out of debt. Well, right after I graduated from medical school, we had our third child and we had the christening reception at the house. And that was the first time that both of our families—Lori's family and my family—were at the house. And Lori's grandfather—who's one of my patients now, he's ninety now—this was the first time he was at the house, and he's walking around the yard and he said to my wife, 'Oh, did you know, Lori, that this was where *we* lived when we moved here from Hungary?' So, it turns out that this was my wife's great grandparents' homestead when they arrived from Hungary, who sold it to someone, and then when *my* grandparents moved here from Czechoslovakia, they got the house. So, we decided, we've got to fix the house up. We've got to stay here. We can't leave! And so we live in the original house from both families when they moved here from Europe. And so we stayed there."

Mike isn't sure when he first started thinking about medicine. "Probably when I was five or six. I can't really tell you when, but I always knew that's what I wanted to do. I don't know what triggered it. In fact, some of my older patients remind me about it. The old postmaster from Twin Rocks just died a couple of months ago at age 86—I took care of him. And he was telling me the last few times when I was visiting him in the hospital, 'Remember Mike when you used to come to the post office and pick up the mail for your Mum, and you said you were going to be a doctor?' Yeah, all the way back then. And as time went on, everything just reinforced it."

Mike and his family were patients of Dr. Ebandjieff for a while, but when he became sick, they went to another family doctor who was his primary role model: Dr. Martin, of the Colver Clinic. "You know," Mike says, "managed care existed back then too. You paid so much as a family, and no matter how many times you'd go in, that was what you paid. That's what my parents did, they paid him so much per month out of their pocket, and he would see us. The Colver Clinic was more than a clinic. Dr. Martin had a hospital wing beside it, and he would do, not minor surgery, but major surgeries. I have patients, who had appendectomies, hysterectomies, and cholecystectomies at the Colver Clinic!"

Unfortunately, by the time Mike got older and was thinking more seriously about medicine, he never had an opportunity to work with either family doctor. "Both of these doctors had died by the time I was in high school," Mike says. "When I was in college, I did work with some of the pathologists at the hospital. Now, I make it a point to work with any of the high school students around here who are interested in medicine. And every year, I get the high school students down here to see what it's like."

Upon graduating from high school, Mike started college at the University of Pittsburgh. But after his first year, his father lost his job as a meat cutter when the local supermarket went out of business. Unable to afford the tuition,

Mike moved back home and commuted to Indiana University of Pennsylvania (IUP), where he completed college as a pre-med student. He applied to medical school after graduating from college, but was not admitted, and he started to wonder for the first time in his life whether or not he would ever reach his dream of becoming a doctor. Over the next two years he got married, and he and Lori traveled around the country, spending some time in Colorado and Louisiana, working and taking some additional courses, and generally having a good time. Then, he recalls, "Lori became pregnant with our son Mike, and that's when I called my advisor back at IUP and said, 'You know, it's time for me to get serious about going to medical school again. I need to get refocused, because that's what I've always wanted to do.' " So he returned to IUP and completed his MS degree in biology. "And I took the MCATs [Medical College Admission Test] again, and I did tremendous. You know, it's amazing what you can do when you're focused. And how having a little one come into the world can focus you!" And this time, when Mike reapplied to medical school, he was accepted.

Mike's wife, Lori, was from Vintondale, about three miles from Twin Rocks. "We've known each other forever," he says. "She's four years younger than me, but we went to the same church. I went to high school with her sister. I mean I've known her family—and she's known me—since we were small. I can't say since birth, but it was pretty darn close. We started going out when she was a senior in high school and I was back here at IUP. Then we got married a year after I graduated. Lori worked as a secretary and in restaurants before the kids were born. Right now, our four kids are into every-thing, every sport, every activity, and she gets them there, and makes sure that it all works."

Mike first remembers hearing about the PSAP when he attended a talk that I gave at IUP, the first of Jefferson's six PSAP Cooperative Colleges that were selected to help recruit and select PSAP students. And when he heard about the program, he remembers thinking, "Yeah, they're describing me!" "I always wanted to come back home to practice," he recalls. "I never had any doubt in my mind. Even when I went to college, that was what I wanted to do— family medicine and specifically come back here." Mike's personal statement on his medical school application documents that. He wrote: "There are three small communities in the vicinity of where I live, mainly populated by senior citizens. I plan to return to the area from which I grew up, and establish a small clinic."

"The scary part is—when you finally come back and it becomes a reality— you don't know if the town and everyone are going to think that it's OK," he says. "And, I didn't do what most of the other docs do around here—live farther out, and have a farm. I moved right back to my hometown. You know, I occasionally have people who show up at the door at night. I have that typical rural practice—where people occasionally come over cut, bleeding, having a stroke. They sometimes show up at the front door! But overall the community has been *really* good to me. They respect us. It's amazing because we probably have 8,000 to 12,000 people in our area. Even though that stuff happens sometimes, they do try to respect me and Lori and the kids, and know that we have to have time for ourselves. So the community has been really, really good."

· · · · ·

Mike Tatarko was amazed when, as a third year resident, he was told that Nanty Glo wasn't officially designated as a physician shortage area. "How is that possible?" he asked, "There aren't any doctors there!" His lifelong dream had been to return to his hometown area to practice, and he had just heard a talk trying to interest doctors to practice in areas that had a physician shortage. He knew that Nanty Glo needed a doctor—the town hadn't had a doctor in the 20 years since Dr. Ebandjieff had died. But Mike was told that in order to qualify as a federally designated Health Personnel Shortage Area (HPSA), the local community had to fill out the necessary paperwork and apply. So he decided to do it himself. "I asked for the paperwork," he said, "and I got all the data from the courthouse on birth rates and deaths and demographics and the mix of patients on medical assistance and all that stuff, and went through our local congressman, and the area ended up being designated!"

Primary medical care HPSAs are the designations that the federal government gives to areas with a documented shortage of primary care physicians, and is a requirement for eligibility for loan repayment programs and a number of other federal programs that provide additional financial support to these areas. While the criteria to be a HPSA are complex, the government uses a ratio of one primary care physician per 3,500 population or more, as a requirement for HPSA designation, and considers an area as adequately served if they have one primary care physician for every 2,000 people. While not all rural areas of the country are physician shortage areas, two-thirds of the federally designated shortage areas are rural. Overall, more than 30 percent of the people living in rural America live in a HPSA, with people living in rural areas of the United States nearly four times as likely to be in a HPSA as those living in metropolitan areas.

Between 1980 and 1990, the number of federally designated HPSAs remained constant near 2,000. However, during the 1990s, it rose to its current level of more than 3,100 HPSAs, 70 percent of which are in nonmetropolitan areas despite an overall increase in the number of physicians being trained. To eliminate these rural shortages today would require an additional 3,327 primary care physicians, with more than twice that number required to have an adequate physician supply in these areas. Among primary care physicians, family physicians play the largest role by far in providing the infrastructure of rural health care. Of those rural counties that do not currently meet the HPSA criteria, two-thirds (more than 1000 additional entire counties) would qualify for HPSA designation if it were not for the family physicians already practicing there. This compares with only an additional three percent of counties (49) that would qualify as HPSAs if all of the current general internists, pediatricians, and obstetrician-gynecologists combined were to leave.

Even today, it seems obvious that Nanty Glo should be designated as a physician shortage area. "My practice—this office right here," Mike says with enormous personal pride, "we're the only office between Ebensburg and Indiana. That's thirty-five to forty miles from one county seat to the next county seat. That's part of the reason that it's a shortage area. And it's pretty rural—there's nothing in between the two counties—in fact the county line here between Indiana and Cambria Counties is the most indeterminate county line in the state. They don't know exactly where it goes through there. And, this is one of the five poorest school districts in the state of Pennsylvania. We have lots of uninsured and underinsured patients. We also have middle-income patients, but some of them don't have health insurance. The cost of drugs is a big issue. We have a flexible fee schedule for our entire group, based on people's income."

· · · · ·

Moving to Philadelphia was a tremendous culture shock for Mike. "We lived in the student apartments right in downtown center city," he said, "and we were coming from Nanty Glo . . . this area is the lowest crime rate in the country. It's also the lowest cost of living in the whole country. You can buy an acre of ground around my house for about $300 today. My house—I mean it's gorgeous—would probably be ten times as much if I built it in Philadelphia. And we went down to Philly, and it's like, 'You pay how much for rent? You pay that much to park?' "

To try and explain this clash of rural and urban cultures, Mike tells a story that took place when he was taking anatomy during his freshman year. "I would walk back and forth from our apartment to the dissection lab at night. The first couple of nights, I said to my wife, 'People are staring at me!' And she said, 'Nah, its all in your head.' So over the next week, maybe every other night, I said, 'I'm telling you, Lori, they're staring at me as I'm walking by. I don't know why, but they're watching me.' And I think she was starting to worry about me. Then, after one of the anatomy labs, I was walking back with one of the other students, and I said, 'See—that person is looking at me over there!' And he said, 'I'd look at you too with that fluorescent orange hat on!' Nobody in Philadelphia was wearing fluorescent orange hunting hats. And I said 'You're right!' And so I threw that cap into the closet and said to Lori, 'I either need a black, blue, or green hat. I can't wear this orange one down here in Philadelphia.' That's a true story.

"The other thing was," he continues, "when we got to Philadelphia, we were told to lock our doors! We don't lock our doors up here. In fact, when we first moved back from Philadelphia we locked them, and my Mum just chewed me out. She said 'It was raining today. You locked your door. How was I supposed to get in, or Mrs. S. or one of the other neighbors to get in to shut your windows?' So no, we don't lock our doors. But, yeah, it was a hard adjustment. When people from the city come up here, they can't believe how safe it is. Someone I know parked their car at the mall, and left their keys in the ignition, a bunch of CDs on the seat, and the windows rolled down. When they came back a few hours later, the windows were rolled up, the keys were underneath the mat, and the CDs were still on the seat."

Mike's wife did well adjusting to Philadelphia, even though she was nervous for the first few months. "You know there were a lot of 'street people' (i.e., homeless people) down there," Mike says. "She would walk with our two kids, one in the stroller, one walking, up to the mall that's in the middle of town. But the street people were extremely nice to my wife; they would always say hello and would never ask her for money. I would walk out and they were always asking for money, but they never bothered Lori. And then, after we got our wits about us in Philly we moved out to suburban New Jersey, and I commuted to school. And that was actually an easier adjustment for my wife, even though we really liked Center City, because we knew we weren't going to be there long term. I can't say anything bad about Philadelphia. I mean we were members of the zoo, and we did a lot of great stuff, because we figured we'd do it while we were there. But in South Jersey, my wife had a bunch of friends in the apartment complex, their kids were the same ages, Mike was old enough for preschool. So we fit into that community pretty well. And then we moved back here."

Medical school "was really hard in the first two years of the basic sciences," Mike said, echoing Jim Devlin and others. "But once I got to the clinical years, I was golden. I did family medicine at Latrobe and it was excellent. And during my fourth year, I went back out to Latrobe for family medicine. Then, I chose Memorial Hospital in Johnstown for my family practice residency, because I knew I was going to come back here to practice. And I knew that part of learning how to be a doctor was learning who my specialists were going to be. I was really sensitive to the fact that a lot of people in this town would count on me to know who would be the right orthopedist, the right cardiologist, the right surgeon. I also knew I would have lots of hands-on training there, and I had an excellent experience at Memorial. They had multiple residency programs, and—you know there are pros and cons about doing a family practice residency where there are other residency programs. I think it was advantageous for us to have internal medicine and surgery residency programs there. We got to do a lot more surgical techniques, being taught by the surgical residents. And unlike many university programs, where nonsurgeons might be considered second-class citizens, the surgical residents there knew that you were the one who was going to be referring them their patients. So the residents really got along together and counted on each other. And some family doctors do need that training. Two of my graduates are in northern Cambria County now, and I will tell you, they're the ones running the ventilators, they're the ones putting in chest tubes, and they probably got a higher level of training in their residency at Memorial."

• • • • •

Looking down from the top of the surrounding hill, you can see the entire town of Nanty Glo, sitting quietly in the shallow valley. There is one main

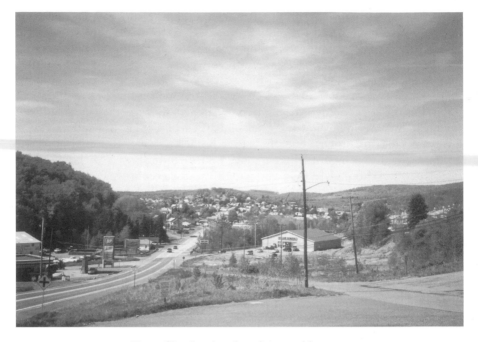

Nanty Glo, the view from just outside town.

road—a two-lane highway running through town, and none of the buildings
are more than two stories high. Surrounding the town are small, green, for-
ested hills. You can see the entire town and the surrounding rolling hills all
in one glance, without having to move your head—or even your eyes.

The borough of Nanty Glo is in the rural Allegheny mountain highlands,
about 60 miles northeast of Pittsburgh. The town dates back to the 1890s,
when it was founded as a coal-mining town along the southern branch of the
Blacklick Creek. Only one-half hour from Johnstown in good weather, it can
take three times that long in bad winter weather when the steep mountain
roads are dangerous and slow. The name Nanty Glo is Welsh, and means
"streams of coal." The original coal baron, John McFadden, owned most of
the land around Nanty Glo, and like many of the Welsh and Scottish immigrants in the area, he was a potato farmer before coal was discovered under
his land. He then opened up some of the coal mines in Nanty Glo and in
Johnstown, while Andrew Carnegie owned the original furnaces there that
made iron ore. Eastern European and Italian immigrants arrived in the early
1900s to work the mines and mills.

Today, Nanty Glo has 3,054 people, and the population is mostly elderly.
But at one time, Nanty Glo had 8,000 to 10,000 people, and was the largest
coal-mining town in western Pennsylvania. "An average coal mine is supposed
to have a life expectancy of about thirty years," Mike explains. "The mine
here in Nanty Glo was into its seventy-second year! The only reason it shut

down was because of the 1977 flood—it filled up with water. But they tell me there's still another thirty years worth of coal there. And that's only in the seam they went after. There are two other seams, above and below, that they haven't even mined." Since the flood, the mines and mills have all shut down. The rest of the industrial base is located in the Johnstown area, and is mostly related to the defense industry. The Nanty Glo's and other small towns that were the original coal-mining towns now provide some of the workforce for the businesses in other nearby larger towns.

"We have a huge problem with people leaving the area," Mike says. "I've tracked our demographics since I came back here. We have a really elderly population. This county is right up there with Dade County in Florida as having one of the oldest populations in the country. I have so many 85-, 90-, 90+-year-old patients in this community, it's unbelievable. The median age of the clinic is probably around seventy-five! But we have a lot of healthy elderly. I mean they are really strong people. They were born before antibiotics or immunizations, and they lived through the depression. I mean they are tough people. If they were going to die of something, they would have died in child-hood. So they're genetically strong. And the problems they have are with their ADLs—Activities of Daily Living. A little bit of decreased hearing, decreased vision, maybe a little diabetes, or systolic hypertension, but most of them are pretty healthy. But then when something does happen, it can be pretty cata-strophic, and at that age it's often hard to bring people back to good health.

"We also have a middle-aged group," he continues. "My age and a little bit older, and their kids have grown up now. They're teachers, own small businesses, work in stores and shops in Ebensburg and Johnstown, and a lot of people are employed by Memorial Hospital." The people who are moving into the area don't tend to move into the small older coal-mining towns, like Nanty Glo, but outside it, like Blacklick Township, where there is more land, and cheaper land. "This area has some of the lowest cost land in the country," Mike says. "Some of the elderly people around here have farm homesteads, and after they die, if their sons and daughters aren't in the area, their land has been sold. I remember one woman who died who had a 110-acre farm— just a gorgeous house, farm machinery, really picturesque—and it sold for $110,000 for the whole shebang, animals included."

• • • • •

Like all family doctors, Mike Tatarko takes care of people of all ages. "We take care of newborns in the nursery, and we work at three nursing homes," he says. "We don't do surgery, we don't do OB, but we do pretty much everything else. I used to do sigmoidoscopes, but I don't them anymore since I've been doing the corporate stuff. Lacerations—you wouldn't believe the stuff we sew together here! We had a snowstorm one year, and I had this guy with a chain saw cut—he wouldn't go down to Johnstown, so we sewed it together here. So we do any lacerations, remove skin tags and moles, joint injections, and those kinds of things. And we're the team physicians for three of the high schools in the area.

"And continuity is way different out here," Mike explains. "Here, you know everybody in town. Our practice probably takes care of ninety to ninety-five percent of the people in Nanty Glo. In Vintondale and Twin Rocks, which is where I live and where Lori's from, I would say we take care of the whole community. I don't know of anyone in either of those communities that see other doctors. In Nanty Glo there's a handful. And we take care of most things there—we do all the firemen's physicals, we're the school physician.

"One big advantage for us here," he continues, "is that you already know how everyone's related. You don't have to write out family trees, you know that this person is related to that person, and that person is related to this other person. I don't know if the word continuity really captures it out here—and I say cradle to grave—but it's not exactly like that either. There aren't enough adjectives to describe all the interrelationships that are going on between families who may have different last names, but you know they're related. And the psychosocial aspects of what we do, which is so important and so common in family medicine. I've been through so many divorces and bankruptcies and tragedies in families here, and people tend not to go to their priests and rabbis and ministers anymore, they come to our office. Placement issues, losing jobs, graduations, weddings—and so you're not just doing medicine.

"Also," he explains, "it really helps to know the local language, the local colloquialisms. People who live around here may say something to me in a slightly different way, and I'll know it's their angina, because that's how my mum and dad would have described it. And you get to know your patients really well. Last night, for example, they called me from my cousin's house, and thought she was hypoglycemic again—she's diabetic and takes insulin shots. But there was something different last night in the way they described it—I don't even know what the words were. And I said, 'No, you have to take her down to the hospital right now.' 'This isn't different than any other time, Mike', they said, and I said, 'No, there's something different. Cousin M. said something different.' And it turned out that she was having a slight stroke."

Mike thinks one of the most difficult things about practice is "trying to make sure that you keep up to date on everything. And getting worn out. I can go eight to ten weeks before I need a couple days or a week off, because the pace is really tough. On the other hand, I'm much more efficient now. You get more efficient after you're out in practice for ten years. I can do the same exam and know exactly what's going on and make the right decision in less time now than when I started. You look at a rash and know exactly what it is—you don't have to go looking through books all the time."

In thinking about the differences between family practice in rural and urban areas, Mike says, "Out here, I think there's more responsibility. In the city, you have a lot more access to a higher level of specialists than we do here, so you may be expected to do more here. Yeah, we manage most things. In fact I teach my residents that the only time you should consult a specialist is when you want a procedure done. We do everything else and we do pretty well.

You know, the definition of 'standard of care' changes depending on where you are, and who's available. Probably if I had some of the same hand fractures and hand problems in Philly, the standard of care would be to refer them to a hand specialist. Well in Johnstown, those normally would go to an orthopedist, not a hand surgeon, because we don't have one. But when you go to northern Cambria County—just fifteen to twenty miles further north—it's either the family doctor or the general surgeon. On the other hand, we have access to Memorial Hospital in Johnstown, and it's pretty sophisticated. They do pretty much everything there other than taking care of major burns, and electrophysiologic heart studies, or some weird esoteric diagnosis that you need a quaternary referral hospital. We have a trauma center, all the specialists, intensivists, and most subspecialty surgeons.

"We manage MI's [myocardial infarctions, or heart attacks]," he says, "sometimes in concert with the cardiologist. If it's an acute MI, we manage it, but if it's going to lead to a catheterization, we get the cardiologist involved pretty soon. The same thing with the Coronary Care Unit. We can manage patients there, and we do it occasionally, but patients who are there are so critical anymore, that we have a full-time intensive care specialist who does a very good job. But we still round there every day. And especially when it comes to dealing with the family, I mean I've had two people this week that we've talked to the family about withdrawing life support. It's not right for a hospital intensivist who doesn't know the family to do that. It's the family doctor's role—who's been with the family and knows multiple generations of the family—to discuss those things."

And like most of the other doctors I interviewed, Mike still does house calls. "You wouldn't believe the number of house calls we do out here—but I mean you don't have a choice. If you don't go see some patients, they just lie in bed. As far as official house calls, we probably average five to seven a week. Some times two to three a day, depending on how many patients are bedbound and their family wants to take care of them at home. But we probably do just as many unofficial ones—it depends on how sick somebody is, so it varies. Like after one older woman's daughter died, I was probably down the house every other night for a while, since she was alone. Also, we had a 16-year-old high school senior die in a car accident a few months ago—and I was at their house a couple nights in a row. Then, last year, I had a 25-year-old patient who had a rare bone tumor, and after the specialists in Pittsburgh did all they could for him, I took care of him for his last four months. And I was over there all the time—they were family friends, and I've known them forever. I was over the house when he died—that's where he wanted to be—and I tried to help get everybody through it. So, yeah, we do a lot of house calls."

That reminds Mike of a story about one of his first house calls. "When I first came back here," he begins, "I got a phone call, 'Can you come out and see our grandpa—we hear you do house calls.' And, I didn't even know this guy existed. You know I was born and raised here, but I never even knew this guy lived back there in the woods. He was ninety-some years old (he's been dead for at least seven years now). So, I got this call, and I said 'What's wrong with him?' And they said 'Well, he's sick, and he won't go see a doctor, but if you come out. . . .' So I said, 'OK,' and they gave me directions to get to the house. Then they said, 'When you're driving down the dirt road, make sure you hold your black doctor's bag out the car window, because he has a gun—but we told him the doctor's coming. If he sees the bag, he'll let you down through there.' So I'm driving out there, and these aren't main roads I'm going on, and I turn off onto this dirt road that goes down through this fill and sure enough this house is down there—like the *Beverly Hillbillies*. And he was looking out the window, through the side of the curtain, and I waved my black bag, and he waved and put down his shotgun, and I pulled down there. The porch had a wood floor, but the next room was just dirt. And I went in, and this guy had UMWA [United Mine Workers of America] insurance—that's the best health insurance there is. That's what we all want—it pays for everything. And he had never used it. Ever! Not one cent of it. He was delivered at home by his aunt. He ate venison that he shot, raised his own bees and had the honey, ate oats and corn bread that he raised in the field. He loved his wine that he made from his own grapes. So I go out there, and this guy was in great shape, his chest muscles were bigger than mine, and he had great big leathery hands. So I took a history and examined him, and it looked like he was having an acute gallbladder attack, and I said, 'Come down to the hospital with me.'

'I'm not gonna do that.'

'OK, how about if you go to the urgent care center, that's closer.' That was only six miles away.

'Nope, I'm not gonna do that.'

'I'll tell you what, I'll call my nurse. We'll go down to my office. We'll do some things there.' I figured that if I could get him here, I could get him to the hospital.

'Not gonna do that.'

'I'll send the nurses out here—home health nurses.'

'Not gonna do that.'

So I said, 'You wanted me to come out here. What can I do for you if you're going to just stay here?'

And he said, 'I'm just a little dizzy. Maybe you can give me something for my ear, 'cause that hurts. I don't care about my gallbladder 'cause I'm old enough to die.'

So, I examined his ear, and maybe, just maybe, there was a little infection in his ear. So I wrote him a prescription for penicillin. His daughter came right over and got it filled and gave him a dose, and wouldn't you know, I just got back to this office, and his daughter called. He had a rotary phone down there, and she said 'He's breaking out.' The guy had an allergic reaction to penicillin! And I had to go back out and give him steroids and epinephrine. And he survived it. He did well, and he loved me to the day he died. I took care of him for two to three more years after that. He survived that gallbladder attack. He broke out in welts, but we reversed that in a couple of hours, although I sweated a lot. And he was fine. And he just thought that was the greatest thing."

• • • • •

During Mike's second year of residency, he began moonlighting at the Ebandjieff Clinic in the evenings. Then, upon completing his residency in 1992, he returned full time to his hometown clinic to practice family medicine, fulfilling his dream of more than two decades. The reality was "amazing," he says. "The practice just took off—and then it got overwhelming pretty fast! And when I looked around, it seemed like—in Cambria and Somerset Counties—I was the only one around here my age. So then I recruited a couple other partners. And then we started to build this network, and I tried to recruit other people into this larger area—younger physicians—and not just in this practice. And the hospital thought that was a good thing. That was back in the days when everybody was theorizing that you had to have this big primary care network. So it fit into both of our strategies. With the hospital backing me, we recruited a lot of docs, everywhere from the Maryland border to up here in Northern Cambria County, and over to Bedford County."

Today, Mike Tatarko is president and CEO of Conemaugh Health Initiatives (CHI), a large organization that owns the Ebandjieff Clinic. CHI is a subsidiary of Conemaugh Health System, the parent corporation, which includes Memorial Hospital in Johnstown, and a few other hospitals. CHI is the employment vehicle for the physicians who work at those facilities. CHI also provides a central billing office for all the practices, does group purchasing, buys group malpractice insurance, negotiates with insurance companies, and contracts together as a group—all of which saves money for the system. The practices also help each other with staffing. "But each practice, each site, and each physician," explains Mike, "has their own profit statement, so I'm cost accounted by my own visits, how I bill, my revenue, and my share of the overhead. Our salaries and our pensions are as good, probably better than if we were in private practice. We have about fifty percent of the physicians in these two and a half small counties. That's not anticompetitive. In a rural area, bring me more doctors! I'd be happy to have them compete against me. The problem is trying to get enough doctors to come out here.

"Our service area is the two and a half rural counties," Mike explains. "Cambria (where Nanty Glo is located), Somerset, and half of Bedford. And some of our patients come from Indiana County, although we don't have an office there. And the very tip of Westmoreland County goes through a very mountainous area that's probably closer to our area, so we have a lot of patients that come from there. In the area, probably one-half to three-fourths of the physicians are employed by a larger organization. The others are in private practice, but most of those doctors are probably fifty years old and older."

For Mike, "it's like having two jobs. I'm the president and CEO of CHI—I'm just blessed with some really good staff support, and I have excellent managers who help me with the hospital finance and operations. And I'm in full time practice at the clinic—myself and my two partners here. We're the largest admitters to Memorial Hospital. We are going to need more doctors at this office. We have a second site in Park Hill, about five miles south of here. We have about 10,000 to 12,000 patient visits a year in this practice, and probably another 7,000 to 8,000 at the other office. We have one nurse practitioner here."

Of the 65 primary care physicians in the area, Dr. Tatarko has recruited about 20 new residency graduates over the past ten years—a remarkable accomplishment considering the fact that when he started, there were no other recent graduates. And he is still actively recruiting. "I'm desperate now," he says. "I could probably hire five or six more primary care doctors without any problem." His latest recruit is a couple from Memorial's family practice residency program. "He had a NHSC scholarship, and we have an office in Confluence in southern Somerset County, that's really isolated—Turkeyfoot, Rockwood—there's no good way to get there. And that practice has been phenomenal since he started there. And he married a woman from northern Cambria County. They met during residency and got married, and she's at Myersdale, which is also extremely difficult to recruit for."

In addition to serving as president and CEO of CHI since 1999, Dr. Tatarko is also the medical director of both the Ebandjieff Clinic and the Park Hill Medical Center. "I was president of the County Medical Society a couple of years ago," he recounts. "I was also president of the county chapter of the Pennsylvania Academy of Family Physicians. I am chairman of Family Practice at Memorial Hospital, and have a faculty appointment in the residency program. I round with the residents down there, and third year family practice residents come up here to this office one day a week—there's a different resident here every day. And one of the three of us supervises them. But I'm a big believer in continuity, and as tough as it is for me, I try to see my own patients. And they want me to see them in the hospital, so I try to do that also." Based on his enormous leadership contributions, Mike was named the 1999 Community Rural Health Care Leader of the Year by the Pennsylvania Office of Rural Health.

When Mike talks about the changes brought about by managed care, he first talks from the point of view of the practicing physician. But then, as he puts on his corporate hat, he also sees things a bit differently. "You know, it's not just the paperwork from managed care. It's someone questioning why you want a CAT scan on your patient, interfering with your care, practicing medicine by protocols, which aren't exactly right for everybody. It's our job to know when it's that one out of the ten patients that has something different. Sure it may work on nine out of the ten, but that's not why we're physicians. It's that interference, it's the decreasing reimbursement, it's knowing which drug is on which insurance company's formulary at which time. So, the managed care stuff is really a pain! But on the other hand, once I started to see the data—and I have the luxury of comparing fifty-some docs—I can see differences between individual practices. I have one practice whose drug costs for antibiotics per day (after adjusting for the practices that have sicker patients) are on average four times another practice. And I'm thinking, what the heck is that about? So we have a couple of initiatives to compare and figure that out. I'm not saying one doctor has better quality than the other, I'm just trying to figure out what they're doing differently."

Like all physicians with administrative responsibilities, Mike worries about things at a regional level in addition to worrying about his own individual patients. The physician workforce in small communities is fragile, even when it is adequate, and the loss of even one physician, through illness or moving, can be a major problem. For Dr. Tatarko, he has "the corporate hat of 'How are we going to do take care of those patients?' " As to how he is able to do all these things—medicine, cleaning up the environment, corporate leadership—Mike answers with his own philosophy, that also captures the philosophy of the specialty of family practice, "You don't have to know all the answers, you just have to know how to get there."

• • • • •

When Mike says that they have a lot of relatives in the area, he isn't kidding. "Lori is one of eight, her mother's one of thirteen, so there's probably at least 200 family on her side that still live within fifteen miles of here. I probably have fifty to sixty relatives around here. I'm one of five, but my dad's one of thirteen. Then, when you get past first cousins once removed or second cousins, you're not even sure anymore, sometimes. Like my nurse Jill is related to me through my aunt and her uncle—but Jill's husband is also Lori's cousin. I mean it really gets close. We joke and say we're all related around here, but even though technically you're not, in practical terms, since everybody is married to someone who's married to somebody else, there is a relationship. And they're really a support system for us, so even though I'm busy with all those other things, Lori's sisters, her mum, my sisters, my mum, everybody's here. So, it fits together pretty well."

As for his own personal activities, Mike says, "I hunt deer. My son Mike hunts too, though Ben doesn't. And Luke and Annie aren't old enough. And my wife, no—she hates guns! When I was growing up, it was rare to see a turkey or a black bear around here. When I was in junior high, you could see the orange smoke bellowing out of the steel mills in Johnstown. Now it is so clean around here that black bear are a nuisance. They are all over the place, and everybody goes hunting for them. I can't get off the first day of bear season or I would. I have to decide between that and buck season, and I take buck season off. And turkeys are everywhere now. It's just amazing. We have bobcats back. We have black bear right behind my house. And turkey behind the house.

"I also fly-fish a lot," he continues. "But my biggest activity is running. I do ultra running—100-mile races. I did the Western States two years ago, I've done Vermont. Actually, I have a stress fracture that should be officially healed as of tomorrow. I probably do six or seven races a year, and three or four of those are regular marathons. I did the Myrtle Beach marathon in February, I'll do Pittsburgh normally, and Johnstown, and maybe Washington, DC, or

Philly's marathons. And then I'll do two fifty-milers, a seventy-miler, and maybe a hundred-miler a year.

"Lori and I have about twenty-some acres of land," Mike explains. "That's not much around here. But where our backyard ends, that's where the Pennsylvania Game Land starts. So I have 10,000 acres of Pennsylvania Game Land right out the back of my house. I mean I can go forever back there, so I don't need to own a lot of land." Then, turning, he points with enormous pride to a group of six or seven trees in the backyard behind his house. "Those are American Chestnut trees. I started them from seed from an original North American Chestnut tree that wasn't blighted. Almost all of the American Chestnuts were blighted during the first half of the twentieth century—somebody brought over a chestnut tree from Asia, and the trees all got this fungus and died out. Before that, chestnuts were a dominant tree in western Pennsylvania—more than oak and maple. It was some of the best wood around, and people fed the nuts to their pigs and other animals. People can eat the nuts too—they're really good.

"They were huge trees," he continues, sharing his extensive knowledge about these trees. "The beams in the old part of my house are two-by-fours from chestnut—from the attic all the way down to the basement—all one piece. But you don't see them anymore. When I came back here, I didn't know that there were any of these trees left. Then, one of my older patients from Vintondale—he's about 85 now—brought me a bag of chestnuts from them, and I said, 'Where did you get these?' And he told me where, and he told me how to start them. He said, 'You keep the nuts in your refrigerator all winter long, because they have to be cold treated. Then in March you take them out and plant them in tubs. And sure enough, they germinated. The ones out here are about eight years old now. They started from nuts right on the back porch. Now they're about thirty to forty feet tall. I'm really proud of them. At the beginning, it was a job keeping the chipmunks out—they tried to come in and dig them out of these big tubs that I had. I've put more of them all through the woods. In the summer, I go out with the kids and dig a hole and put another one in." Later, driving over to where the original tree stands, Mike says "Here it is. This is an original American Chestnut. It's over eighteen inches in diameter, which is impressive."

What else does Mike like to do for fun? "I go to a lot of the Steeler football games in Pittsburgh," he says. "It's only an hour away; and a lot of the Pittsburgh hockey games—although not as many as I'd like to. And we bring the kids. So we probably go down to Pittsburgh once a month or even a little more frequently, or Baltimore and DC, which aren't that far away from us—only 3 hours. We probably go a couple of times a year to DC. Lori has a sister and a brother who live down there. The closest movie theater is about twenty miles, but we still have a drive-in theater in the summer, which is about seven to eight miles away. Mostly, we do the local things in Ebensburg, we hang out with friends, parents of our kids' friends, or our relatives. Our friends are the same friends we've had since we were small. We go out for pizza in Ebensburg, and if we want to go out to have a nice dinner, we go somewhere not far from here.

"When we get away, it normally is a family trip. Last summer, we spent three weeks in California. We go to the beach in the summer, or we'll go up to the mountains in Vermont, or spend a week in South Carolina, where Lori's parents are in the winter. Sometimes I'll just take some time off and stay home—I work in the garden, and we have a pool, and those kinds of things. But I do get called. Patients know that I'm home—I mean my car's in the garage. They'll know I'm in town. But sometimes that's OK, since I'm not physically in the office all day."

• • • • •

Rural communities value their doctors. "They respect you," Mike says, "and you're just so flattered by it, you don't think you deserve it. I don't think my colleagues who practice in suburban areas have that. As far as quality of life, I mean being a physician, no matter what specialty you go into, this is a hard life, no matter where you are. This isn't a nine to five job here or anywhere else. But there are enough people, even in rural areas, that you cross cover with. I have no problem with coverage in my entire group, over the entire two and a half rural counties. Nobody's on call more often than every third week. We do a whole week at a time, seven straight nights, including the weekend. Nobody's doing every night, or every other week. I'm on every fifth week, and then I have the next four weeks off. When we're on call, you may get three to four phone calls, and we have about five to seven hospital admissions during a week. But when we're off, we're off. If we have someplace to go, we're gone. If we want to drive somewhere, nobody knows. So it works out really well. Yeah, its good quality. Now some people choose to be on call one week in three, because there is a financial incentive— the more call you do, the more work you do, and the more money you bring in."

A normal day for Mike is very different than most rural family physicians, because of his major administrative responsibilities—and his running! "I get up at 4:00 AM," he says, anticipating how people react to hearing this. "Then I go to the Johnstown Y, and work out for about an hour, running at the track, and working out on the machines. Then between 6:30 and 7:00 AM, I have my first set of meetings scheduled—management meetings, board meetings, finance committee meetings, whatever. By 8:00 AM, I'll usually start to round on my patients in the hospital with my third-year residents. Then, most mornings I normally meet with one of the physicians from our group, and I'll probably have one to two other meetings a day, either with an insurance company or some other part of our corporation. I probably get up to the office every day about lunchtime, and then see about twenty patients in the office in the afternoon. And I see patients Tuesday evenings up here. The other evenings I usually get home by 6:00 PM and spend time with Lori and the kids, or there's the occasional meeting."

As for practicing family medicine in a small town, Mike says, "The best and the worst are one and the same. It's that you are very close to all these people. I know there are other doctors practicing in their hometowns, but I've known these people since I was a kid. On the other hand, I watch all my friends' family and parents die, and that is really tough! We had a family friend who passed away last Saturday. I ran over to the house, but he had died before I got there. It's not like Philly and Pittsburgh, because everyone here is somebody's family member. You know, that was pretty tough. But on the other hand, I take care of all the kids at the school, and when the babies are born, I'm their doctor—and that's cool stuff. It's strange, I've been out here long enough that I'm doing these kids' driver's license physicals—and I remember giving them their infant shots."

• • • • •

Dr. Tatarko is one of a small number of rural doctors who has had experience working with telemedicine—a technology that many believe will become a major solution to the rural physician shortage. The hope is that with increased technology, a nonphysician can transmit live video of patients to physicians and subspecialists in larger communities. And there have been impressive success stories using telemedicine in a few rural areas of the country. However, there is also serious concern with using an extremely expensive technology, and one that needs costly maintenance and updating, in areas that are among the poorest in the country and least able to afford it. One wonders whether this is yet another example of the urban solution to rural medicine.

Mike has not only used telemedicine, but is also a coauthor of an article in the journal *Family Medicine*, regarding its use in precepting family medicine residents. "Telemedicine has been hot and cold," he says. "It's not one of the most successful things we've done. We still have a telemedicine unit in the back of our office. And maybe we can regroup and start it up again, but there's a learning curve to utilize it. We actually ran a telemedicine dermatology clinic, and the dermatologist was more than fine with the resolution that they had. And it's billable because we're a HPSA. But, it still didn't seem to be extremely practical, except in a handful of cases. We had an elderly man who had a bilateral amputation, and Johnstown's fairly far, especially in the winter. It was easy for him to come in here, so we did the follow-up here with the trauma surgeon in Johnstown using telemedicine. We just called the surgeon up, he ran down to where their telemedicine unit was, and it worked out fine. Even though we thought the wounds looked OK, the surgeon looked with us. So there are some practical uses, but in the regular routine of the day, there are not a lot of practical uses with it."

Mike does say that his group is gearing up for electronic medical records, however, and some of their offices already have them, although the clinic doesn't yet. "All of our offices," he says, "are connected to the hospital now, so I can get labs and X-ray reports. And in a few months we will have computerized prescription ordering, so that if I write a prescription for a patient that interacts with any of their other medicines, it will automatically notify me. But it's hard to connect everybody together out here in this rural area. A lot of those places are in different phone company areas."

· · · · ·

Mike and Lori have four children. The oldest, Mike, is 18, and is about to enter IUP. Their second son, Ben, is 17, and will be a high school senior. Annie is 13, and Lucas is 9. "If the family is home for dinner," Mike says, "if they don't have an activity, I'm normally there. We do pretty well—we make dinner a couple times a week for sure. And I'm there for most of those. And my kids all serve mass, and I lead the folk choir in church for Saturday night masses, and so we're all involved together in church activities too. It works out pretty well. And, in spite of my schedule, with all the patient visits and admissions, I rarely miss a game. The office staff, both here and administratively, really take care of me. And I make it to almost every game. And it doesn't matter if its football or basketball or whatever, they get me there, and I make sure I keep that all together."

Sure, sometimes his personal and professional life blur. "You have to come to terms with it. If you think that you can stop being a doctor, and have a different life at the end of the day, you probably shouldn't have gone into medicine. Even after you leave the office, you're still looked at as a physician. That's the bad side of it. The good side is that out in a rural community like this, people really respect us. Sure, they bother me sometimes when I'm not on call, but they do let us have our personal lives. And when my office calls a patient and says, 'Dr. Tatarko's son is pitching tonight, could you reschedule,' patients usually say 'Oh sure, no problem.' So the community's been great, they've allowed me to keep that separation. But, on the other hand, when I do go to the games, and somebody's having a problem there, they do look at you. You are the physician."

When asked if future physicians should be concerned regarding making a living in a small town, Mike responds quickly, "No. We do really well. In fact if you take into consideration the cost of living out here, you wonder why people aren't running out here, rather than living in Philly or Pittsburgh. I mean, for what you get for your money. . . . Our family physicians in these counties do better than the national average. And we have a lower cost of living, so they actually do way better than their counterparts in the city."

Regarding lifestyle and income options, Mike discusses the trade-offs and options that some of the physicians in CHI take advantage of. "One of the women partners in one of the practices has two little kids and is pregnant, so we restructured things for her so that she has an outpatient practice only, and her hours were reorganized a little different. While some of the women doctors in the group with kids want to work full time, others want to come in earlier in the morning, and be done at 1:00 PM when the kids come home from school. But there are enough of us in the group together that we can pull that off. Some of the doctors want to work in the office early in the morning, while others of us are in the hospital—and that actually works out fine. Then when we get out here in the afternoon, they're done. We get more patients seen that way, using the same space. So we've worked it out. Of course, you have to understand that if you only want to work half-time, you only get paid half as much money. That's just how it is. But you can find a way to meet the lifestyle that you want, and you can make it work for you. You just have to know what you want."

Debt from medical school, however, is a real problem, and one that is getting much worse. As Mike was getting ready to finish his residency and practice, he started to think more seriously about how he was going to pay off his medical school loans. "When I graduated from Jefferson in 1989, I was $120,000 in debt, probably the highest in our class." Today, the average medical student leaves school owing more than $100,000, with 20 percent of graduates owing more than $150,000. And because of the rising levels of debt, many physicians have been choosing higher-paying medical specialties and practice locations that offer more lucrative incomes.

An increasingly important group of options to deal with rising medical school debt has been the federal and state scholarship and loan forgiveness programs. That was how Mike Tatarko had his indebtedness forgiven, as have more than ten other physicians working for CHI in shortage areas. At the federal level, the National Health Service Corps (NHSC) has provided scholarships and loan forgiveness for thousands of physicians over the past three decades, in exchange for practice in underserved areas. In addition to the federal programs, many states, including Pennsylvania, also have their own scholarship and loan forgiveness programs that provide substantial amounts of financial support in exchange for practice in an underserved location. Health systems, like Conemaugh, are also struggling with ways they can help students pay off their loans, especially for practicing in areas that might have a more difficult time supporting a physician financially. However, at the same time that medical student debt is growing, hospitals and health systems are also struggling, especially in rural areas. More rural hospitals are closing, and hospital reimbursement is decreasing because of federal budget cutbacks as well as the impact of managed care. Pennsylvania is also one of a large number of states that is currently facing a medical malpractice crisis, which is having a major negative financial impact on hospitals as well as physicians.

So, Mike says, "It was really hard to recruit when I first came out here, and now it's really getting hard to recruit again. And I'm afraid that if we can't get good quality doctors out here, this will be second-class medicine. The people out here deserve just as good medicine as those in Philly or Pittsburgh. But the situation is getting more desperate. I see a fair number of students from different medical schools who come up here with the residents, and they are so far in debt. I think we're OK right here because we have a strong nucleus of doctors. But, I do think the federal and state governments will have to recognize the burden of indebtedness that medical students have, if they want them to practice quality, cost-effective medicine. And physicians will have to demand a higher reimbursement because they have so much debt. Students may not be so anxious if they had some debt relief."

• • • • •

What does Mike Tatarko like most about living in a small town? "Oh, just life in general," he says. "We're all really close, we all take care of each other. I mean it's small enough that we all know each other, and watch out for each other." Then, quickly, he adds, "And I wouldn't have raised my kids anyplace else—besides the fact that this is home for me, and I grew up here. I mean the community is extremely safe, and the school districts are really good. I don't think we shortchanged them one iota on their education. There are enough activities to keep them out of trouble. And they get a sense of community, they get a sense of civic responsibility that may be missing in some other places. They feel an obligation to the community, and for service, and that's been really good."

As for coming home again, Mike says, "I'll tell you what, they accepted me in this community. It was like I never left. Except something happens in the community's mind—like I was anointed or something at Jefferson, and came back a different person, and they treat me different that way. But no, I couldn't have asked for it to work out any better, really. As hard as it is to see people pass away, I don't think I would want anybody else to do this. I mean these people trust me. They know they're not going to live forever or be cured—they just want to make sure they get their fair shot, and get there gracefully. And they know that I will try to do that because I know them personally. But no, it's been really great to do this. I could pinch myself some mornings—even during the worst days when thing's aren't going right. It's like you really do have it pretty good, Mike."

"So," he says, "I could never see myself leaving Nanty Glo. I couldn't leave here. I'm here to stay. People ask me that all the time. I say 'You've been asking me for ten years now if I'm going to leave.' I have my plot picked out in Twin Rocks. I'm going to be buried up there. Don't worry about it, I'm not going anywhere."

Later, heading home, Mike points to the stream that goes through the center of Nanty Glo, and says, "This is the stream that we're working on cleaning up now. We just finished these flood walls a year or so ago. But this stream has only one more acid mine discharge site to clean up—you can see where the orange comes in over there. And then that stream will be clean."

OVID, NEW YORK

The purpose is to help someone in a deep and personal way.
—Sandy Burstein, MD in *Heirs of General Practice*, John McPhee

Once Viola Monaghan was admitted to Jefferson's PSAP (Physician Shortage Area Program), she was quickly faced with a major problem—how was she going to pay for her medical education? In response, she applied to and was awarded a National Health Service Corps (NHSC) scholarship, which included a future four-year service commitment. "So, when I graduated," she says, "I really felt like I needed to be true to my commitments—both to the PSAP and the NHSC—and that I was going to practice family practice, and that I was going to a rural area."

Today, practicing family medicine in the small rural town of Ovid, New York, as a member of the NHSC, Viola is part of a program that more than 23,000 other health care providers have participated in since its creation in 1970. The NHSC is a federal program that was developed in order to have health professionals, including physicians, nurses, and dentists, practice in underserved rural and urban communities in the United States. These shortage areas are defined primarily by their physician to population ratios, access to primary care, income levels, and infant mortality and low birth weight indices. In 1972, Congress created the NHSC scholarship program, which provided health professional students with substantial scholarships while they were in school, in exchange for future obligations for community service in an underserved area. The NHSC loan repayment program was added in 1987 for clinicians who had already completed their training, and could have their loans repaid in exchange for immediate practice in these shortage areas. Today, more than 2,700 NHSC health care providers—including Dr. Viola Monaghan—are providing primary health care to nearly four million people living in shortage areas, most of which are in rural America.

· · · · ·

Viola June Peachey Monaghan grew up in the small rural farming community of Belleville, Pennsylvania, where her closest neighbors were one-half mile up the road. Located in the Kishacoquillas Valley of central Pennsylvania, the area is about 25 miles from Penn State University, although it takes 40 minutes to get there since you have to cross the mountains. About 1,500 people live in Belleville, including a large Amish and Mennonite population. "My maiden name is Peachey," she says, "and about twenty percent of the Mennonites in that valley are Peacheys. I mean, this is where the Peacheys came from, and still live. The original Peachey family came over in 1762. They were of Swiss origin. There's a book that lists all the Peacheys, and so if I wanted, I could pull out my book and find many of the people that come into my office today, and figure out how I'm related to them, whether it be third, fourth, fifth cousins. And it's pretty amazing to find my own family now in this book. My husband Gerry is from an Irish Catholic family in Westchester, NY, but his name is now in this book, and so is our oldest son Caleb. When it gets updated again, all three of our children's names will be in it. It's pretty neat.

"I'm Mennonite," Viola says. "My parents are Mennonite. They were Amish. But when my mom was eighteen, her family made a conscious decision to leave. And there was a lot of turmoil around their leaving, because all my grandparents' siblings stayed in the Amish church. The story that I heard was that they left because my grandfather went to a revival meeting. They had evangelists back then that came around and set up a tent, typically in the summer, and people would come to these revival services. Well, he decided he was going to go to these services, and he went—something that was not done in the Amish church. So, at the next Sunday Amish church meeting, he was asked to come up in front of the gathering, and he and my grandmother were going to be publicly, I guess, humiliated. And he wasn't going to have it. So, he left. He walked out. And my grandmother walked out, and I guess all the children walked out. And then they received a certified letter, which I think he never picked up. So growing up, if we went to an Amish business, like a greenhouse, the Amish were not allowed to accept money from my mother. She was shunned, which is cruel. So they had to accept it from us children."

Viola's father also grew up in an Amish family but never joined the Amish church. He had done a lot of different kinds of work—he had an excavating business, then he had a pig farm, and later he ended up driving trucks. Then, after all the children left home, Viola says "my parents turned the house into a bed-and-breakfast, and ran that for about fifteen years. In the house I grew up in. They just sold the house last fall to an Amish family, although there was initially a lot of resistance on my mom's part to sell it to an Amish family. I'm sure it had something to do with the way she had been treated by the Amish community. There was a lot of hurt at times associated with the way

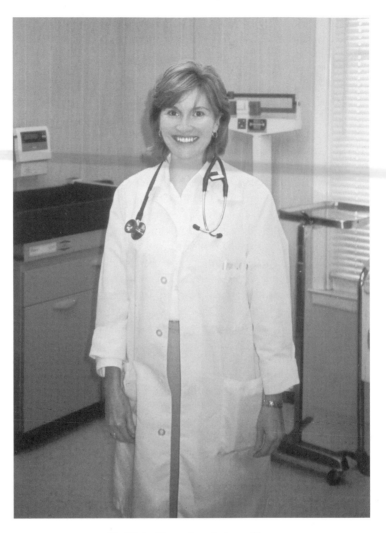

Dr. Viola Monaghan in her office.

they excommunicated her, and the way she's been treated since. But it turns out that this family is so lovely, and we are all so happy that they are in this house."

Then, Viola tells a story about a visit back home about five years ago, when she was still a resident. She and Gerry were out shopping for a quilt, a wedding gift for one of their friends. They ended up at an Amish quilt shop, and the woman who owned the shop wasn't there—she was home with severe back pain from a ruptured disk. Her husband found out that Viola was a doctor, asked her a few questions, and told her that his wife had been bed-ridden for over a month, waiting for an appointment with a neurosurgeon, which was still a few weeks away. "So I went into their home," Viola says. "It was a typical Amish home: It was pretty dark in the house, they had a few lanterns, and she was lying in bed. I did a brief exam, and it was very clear that she had neurologic involvement. And it was clear that she was going to lie in this bed, and hobble out to the bathroom until her appointment in two weeks, because that's often what the Amish will do. They have some very unusual customs and traditions. If somebody tells them to do a certain thing, often they will suffer or put up with something, because they have an appointment on a certain day. And you know, they don't have ready access to communication, they don't have telephones in their homes, they have to go to a neighbor's house to call. And they're not allowed to drive—there are lots of people who drive the Amish around. So I arranged for her to be directly admitted to our hospital. It took a few phone calls and a little work to get that done, and thankfully the neurosurgeon—who was the best—was amenable to having her come to the hospital, instead of making her driver drive her to his office first. And he did the surgery, and I was able to see her in the hospital, and she got better very quickly. She had a great outcome. So there was a really sweet bond that developed because of that. And her family, you know, they opened up to my mom in a way that hadn't happened in the past. And it was her sister that bought my parent's house! And it also turns out that her brother lives up here in this area, so when I came to practice here, word got out that a Peachey from Belleville was a doctor here."

Viola describes herself as being raised in a moderately conservative Mennonite family. Unlike the Amish, there is a wider range in lifestyle choices for Mennonites. She was the third of six children. "Six in eight years," she says laughing. "My mom was busy." Viola went to a Mennonite school from kindergarten through twelfth grade. "It was very small. My senior class had fifteen people. Going to Mennonite school was extremely different than going to public school. The good parts of it were that we respected our teachers, there was a lot of structure in the classroom, and I think the education was good. There weren't a lot of extracurricular activities or educational opportunities that kids who go to public schools or other private schools may have had. I would say that the peer pressure was unbelievably intense, because there was basically one peer group, and if you didn't get along with your peers, forget it. And on top of that, I find that the Mennonite community that I grew up in had very restrictive ideas about many things in life. Many of the people seemed trapped in the Amish lifestyle, where everything is dictated, even their thoughts. What they're allowed to think about, what they're allowed to discuss, their education—all of it is so dictated by the group. There was some of that for me growing up. I'm not sure I was aware of it then. I just had this sort of restlessness, but I really couldn't identify what it was. I was just there. What else did I know?"

But growing up, Viola knew that she wanted to do something in the health care field, although she really didn't have any mentors and didn't know anyone that was going to medical school. The accepted career path for her was nursing, as her sister and some cousins did—but she didn't want to do that.

So she took a year off after high school and worked in a local nursing home as a nurse's aide. Then, she spent two years at Hesston College in Kansas, a Mennonite junior college. "I knew I wanted to get away from home," she remembers, "and some of my friends went there. But I was a terrible student, because I wasn't focused. I still didn't know what I wanted to do."

She had an uncle who was only a few years older than her who was living in Philadelphia, and his fiancée went to physical therapy [PT] school there. "And so," she recounts, "I went to visit, and remember going through the anatomy lab and seeing cadaver parts in boxes, and not being too thrilled with that. It was kind of gross seeing it, but I remember being OK with it. So after Hesston, I decided that I was going to go move to Philadelphia and possibly try to get into PT school. But mostly I just wanted to get out on my own.

"Moving to Philadelphia was unbelievable!" she recalls. "For me, it was exciting. I was how old—nineteen? I was finally getting away—for the first time really getting away, and I couldn't wait. I loved it. It was great. I got a job as a bus person first, then I became a waitress at a restaurant in Center City. I ended up working there for two years, and it was pretty great. I'm sure that my guardian angel was very active, because I did these crazy things that people do. I remember one time, I didn't know which bus to get on to go home, so I got on a bus that said it was going to an area that I thought was close to my apartment. And when it took a right off Broad Street into the worst part of Philadelphia, I said, 'Wait a second, I need to get home, and this is not going in the right direction.' So I got off in the middle of a terrible neighborhood, and walked back to Broad Street, and got a cab and went home. And I did some other things that are much worse that I can't even bear to talk about," she says, laughing. "But I survived."

Having their daughter live in Philadelphia, however, was very difficult for Viola's parents. "My parents took me down to move into my apartment, and when we got into North Philadelphia, my mom just started to cry. Their greatest fears were being realized, that their daughter was going off and doing things they didn't approve of. For example, alcohol was a *huge* issue. And I worked in a restaurant where I served alcohol—and that also brought my mom to tears on one occasion. But, if you look at each of us children, my parents really allowed us to develop an independence that is a little bit atypical for that community. So I credit them with that, even though they haven't always agreed with the decisions and lifestyle choices we have made. But they've always supported us and loved us as their children. But it was hard for my parents."

During that time, Viola also met her husband Gerry on a blind date. "I worked at the restaurant with a woman," she says, "and her husband was Gerry's best friend growing up. And they decided that I should meet Gerry, because they thought I would like him. And I remember not being overly excited about it—I had recently had a blind date that was just miserable. And you know, finally independent and just really not thinking that I wanted to have any kind of serious relationship. I'd never really wanted to have boyfriends, because in my mind it was a way of taking away my independence. And I really thought at the time, I wasn't too interested in getting married. Because, even though my parents have a wonderful relationship and a wonderful marriage, I just could not identify with continuing that lifestyle, especially because I felt that the structure for marriage in that community was so restrictive. But Gerry and I liked each other immediately. It was great. We really hit it off. He was living in White Plains, New York, and I was in Philadelphia. So, we had a long-distance relationship. We'd go for a couple months at a time without seeing each other, but he sent me the most incredible letters and the most incredible packages. He's so creative. And he just won my heart. He was a wonderful boyfriend. He's great! He's amazing."

It was also during this time that Viola realized that she wanted to go to medical school. She feels that "it really took getting away from the whole Mennonite community for me to be able to visualize or even realize that I wanted to go to medical school." Then, pausing for a few seconds as she reflects more about it, almost as if she had never really thought about this before, she continues. "Growing up, there *was* a doctor in our community, about five miles away, and . . . in fact, she was a woman. So, you know what, maybe she was a role model for me. 'Cause here was a female physician, who I liked very much. I thought she was a great doctor, and she was very nice. She did my work physical before I started at the nursing home, so maybe that is all connected. Although I never talked to her about my plans."

So Viola decided to move to Westchester, New York, to be closer to Gerry, and started school at the State University of New York [SUNY] at Purchase. "You know," she says, "it's funny looking back, because you would think with such a clear decision that the path would be straight, but it was really zig-zaggy. I was at SUNY Purchase for four years, and I eventually got my undergraduate degree. And we got married while I was in school. I majored in chemistry, and I was a much better student. And I worked at Cornell/New York Hospital doing research."

When she applied to medical school, "primary care really appealed to me," she said, "because it was what I knew. You know, I never really knew anything else. I was probably thinking that my own family doctor's practice was what family practice was all about." Viola's application to medical school read, "I grew up in a farming community in rural Pennsylvania, and recognize the crucial role of the primary care physician. Looking back I realize that concern for the well-being of others was emphasized in all aspects of my upbringing, and it was this philosophy which initially interested me in the healing arts." "I remember the day I got my acceptance letter from medical school," Viola continues. "I was just . . . so thrilled. And I called my mom, and she said, 'I'm going to cry.' It was great."

• • • • •

During the summer between her first two years of medical school, Viola worked in the Family Medicine Department doing a research study on the Home Visit Program and its impact on the family medicine residency program.

During her clinical years, she remembers her first rotation was in obstetrics and gynecology. "I loved it *sooo* much." she recalls. Then, when she did her family practice rotation at Latrobe, she started to think for the first time that she might be able to do OB as a family practitioner.

Viola also had a number of her own medical problems during medical school. In her second year, she had a miscarriage. "That was tough," she recalls, "that was really difficult. Then, I had Caleb at the beginning of my fourth year. So during many of my rotations in my third year, I was pregnant. Then, when I was in the hospital after he was born, I remember hearing this funny little sound when I breathed at night. But I was so determined that I was going to go home, and I was able to put my bed at a forty-five-degree angle and sleep comfortably with Caleb in bed with me. So I didn't tell anybody. Of course, when I went home and was lying flat, I woke up at 5:00 in the morning gasping for breath, and had to sit up. I couldn't walk up the stairs without becoming short of breath. And my blood pressure was trending up, so I called my doctor and I told her what was going on. And she said, 'Viola, you have to get back to the ER right now!' It turns out I had developed postpartum hypertension and pulmonary edema, and was readmitted to the hospital. That taught me a lot about being a patient. And it gave me a lot of empathy for my patients. And then, everything turned around. They treated me with diuretics, and I was fine, and I went home."

For residency, Viola went to Williamsport Hospital, which she thought was a "fabulous program, with very strong obstetrics training." During her residency, her husband Gerry, who had completed his Bachelor of Fine Arts degree, decided to put his own career on hold, and stay home full time and take care of their children, who now numbered two. Then, after residency, Viola needed to fulfill her four-year commitment to the NHSC. Her husband was the one who started looking into the list of available practice sites, sitting down at the kitchen table with maps from Pennsylvania and New York State. Eventually, Viola chose to practice in the small town of Ovid, New York, which sits on the eastern side of Seneca Lake, one of the famous Finger Lakes in the center of the state. Gerry had originally looked into the area because he had vacationed nearby as a child and loved it—in Penn Yan, on the other side of the lake. And when Viola looked into the practice, it seemed like a unique opportunity for her. Schuyler Hospital, which owned the office in Ovid, had a real need for another physician to provide obstetrical services, since there was only one obstetrician in the area—in fact only one in the entire county. So Viola agreed to spend an additional ten months of fellowship training in Harrisburg, Pennsylvania, focusing entirely on expanding her obstetric skills, including learning how to do such procedures as caesarian sections, tubal ligations, and D&C's, following which she entered practice in Ovid.

Today, Viola has just completed her third year of practice in Ovid. She lives in the small town of Montour Falls, 23 miles south of Ovid, because she needed to live close to the hospital. Gerry has continued to work full time taking care of their three boys, who are now ages seven, four, and one. "I love it," he says. However, he has just started his own photographic restoration company, which he runs out of the house, and they have recently arranged for a woman in the area to watch the children.

• • • • •

Dr. Monaghan's office is located in a renovated old house near the center of town. The building is covered in white siding, and has multiple roof lines, and a central turret. The large dark blue sign outside announces that this is the "Schuyler Hospital Primary Care and Family Health Center." Inside, wearing her long white doctor's lab coat, and with her stethoscope draped around her neck, Dr. Monaghan sees her first patient of the afternoon, a 38-year-old woman, pregnant with her fourth child. Her amniocentesis showed a question of a low fluid level, so she has also been followed by a high-risk perinatologist, with monthly ultrasounds. Entering the room, Dr. Monaghan smiles warmly, as if to an old friend, and says, "How are you doing?"

"OK."

"You look well."

"Thank you."

"How are the girls?"

"They're great. They're outside in the waiting room now."

"How old is Stacy now?"

"She's two."

"She's adorable. She's such a sweet girl."

"You delivered her."

"Yes I did," Dr. Monaghan says with pride. "And you told me that your last ultrasound showed you're going to have a boy this time. Congratulations."

"Yeah, it's great."

"Your due date is getting closer. And you are now thirty-six weeks. How's your baby moving?"

"A lot. I think he's going to have a personality."

"Of course he will. With parents like you and your husband . . ."

"I don't know if that's good or bad," the woman says, laughing.

"It's good, very good. OK, the last test results were good—they were great actually. Are you having any problems at all?"

"No. It's stressful at work, 'cause I have to prepare for maternity leave. This is my last week. But I want to get a lot of things finished there before I leave."

"What are your plans?"

"I'm planning on taking two to three months off."

"What are you going to do about child care?"

"My husband may be staying home for a year."

"He can give my husband a call," Dr. Monaghan responds, referring to her own husband's role in child care. "Anything you want to talk about today?"

"No."

"If you want to do anything different this time, we can. My plan is to pretty much leave you alone. You were amazing last time." After examining her, Dr. Monaghan says, "Your baby is growing appropriately. You look so nice and pregnant. Anything worrying you?"

"Nope."

"OK, I'll see you next week."

Next, an 18-year-old girl comes in with stomach pains, fatigue, and tiredness. The stomach pains have been occurring off and on for the past few years, but are getting worse. Blood tests done last year were negative. There is no pattern to when she gets the pain, and it is not related to eating. She has associated constipation, for which she is taking some alfalfa from the health food store. There is no vomiting or diarrhea. She complains of a fair amount of stress at home—as her father has recently lost his job—and also at school, where she's a freshman in community college.

The next patient is a 16-year-old girl who is there for a school sports physical for field hockey. Then there is a 22-year-old man who cut his thumb in a farming accident. He was fixing his tractor, and got his index finger caught in a piece of the machinery. He had it sewn up in the ER last week, and is in today to have the stitches taken out. Dr. Monaghan examines it and says, "The circulation seems to be fine, and your joint function is fine. OK. I'm going to start taking some of these stitches out, and see, they look like they're ready." But after she takes one stitch out, the two edges of the cut start to pull apart ever so slightly, and she decides to give it more time to heal before she finishes. "I'll have you come back next week and take the rest out."

In the next room, a 17-year-old girl who is graduating from high school is here for a college physical examination. She also needs a routine skin test to check for any possible contact with tuberculosis. Her mother comes into the office with her to talk about some family and behavioral issues that are going on, things that they are both also seeing a counselor about. Her mother does much of the talking early on, saying, "I just wanted to come today because I didn't think she would talk to you about what's going on, and I feel that's part of the doctor getting to know the patient. She does feel very comfortable with you." Later on though, as Dr. Monaghan addresses more and more of these issues directly with the daughter, the girl takes on more and more responsibility for the visit.

Dr. Monaghan asks her, "Do you know what you'll be studying in college?"

"Hotel management."

"How wonderful. How nice. Then you can come back here and open up a nice hotel or restaurant."

"I want to improve this small little town."

"I do too," Dr. Monaghan replies. "Maybe we can work together." Then, in a very soft, gentle, and caring voice, Dr. Monaghan asks her, "What do *you* think's going on?"

"I don't know."

"Are you depressed about graduating from school, about moving on to something different in your life?"

"That was part of it. But now that I'm graduating from school, that's not it. I'm still stressed."

"Are you into any drugs at all? Drinking alcohol or doing anything—often we see major mood changes in kids when that happens."

"No."

"Have you ever thought about depression or anxiety? Do you have trouble going to sleep, or wake up early in the morning worrying about things?"

"No."

"Have you had changes in your appetite? Eating a lot more, or not eating very much?"

"Not really."

"Do you think you have a depressed mood, where you feel down a lot of the time? Do you find yourself crying a lot?"

"Just when I get really stressed. That's the only time."

"Well, I want to do your college physical today. I think what I'd like to do is have you come back and see me next week. Maybe you'd want to come back and see me by yourself?"

"That'd be good."

"And we're going to talk some more about this, because it's really important. You're here at a point in your life, when your future's in front of you and you can do anything you want with your life. You can do anything. And you have a lot of great things set up for you. We'll talk more. And the counseling is a great idea. The exam today is pretty straightforward. They just want to know that you're in good health, and that you can play in all sports activities. Are you having any other problems today at all?"

"No."

Dr. Monaghan then walks over to the girl, who is sitting on the exam table, and takes out her stethoscope. She places it on the girl's back and says, "Just breath in . . ."

The girl startles and exclaims, "Oh, your hands are cold."

"They *are* freezing."

"You forgot to warn me this time."

"I usually don't warn people in the summertime—in the winter time they're like icicles." Then, after completing her examination, which is normal, and after filling out the appropriate forms, Dr. Monaghan says, "OK, I'll see you back in a week. Take care."

The next patient is a six-year-old boy with allergies, who Dr. Monaghan saw one month ago and treated with an antihistamine/decongestant medication. His mother says he's not getting any better. "At nighttime he can't breathe, he breathes out of his mouth, he's so stuffed. And his eyes are real puffy; it looks like he's been crying."

"Has he ever tried a steroid nasal spray?"

His mom says, "I couldn't get him to use them."

"I tried the old one that you sprayed up my nose," the child responds.

Dr. Monaghan then asks him, "Well, will you be willing to try a new one?"

"Yeah."

"If his eyes are itchy, he could try some eye drops for that. The other thing I was thinking with him—has he ever seen an allergist?"

Mom: "No."

"Would you be interested in seeing an allergist?"

Mom: "Yeah, I gotta do something, I've put it off long enough. He was so little, I wanted to avoid the shots. But he's miserable. He tries to go outside and play, and he'll come in—his eyes are itching. So I give him a cold cloth and that makes him feel better, but he can't play outside for very long at a time."

"Well, I would like to refer him to our allergist, if that's OK with you. And what about the inhaler for wheezing?"

Mom: "He hasn't had to use it."

Washing her hands in warm water, Dr. Monaghan laughs gently, saying, "The last patient complained about my cold hands. I'm trying to warm them up." Then, addressing the boy, she asks, "Are your ears bothering you at all?"

"No."

"How are you doing in school?"

"I'm done. Today was the last day."

Then, after examining him, Dr. Monaghan says to his mother and then to the boy, "His lungs are clear. You sound great. I'm going to give you a sample of a nasal steroid spray, and make an appointment for you with the allergist. And I'll give you a prescription for the eye drops."

Mom: "Thank you."

Filling out the referral form for the allergist, Dr. Monaghan replies, "You're welcome."

· · · · ·

Describing her practice in Ovid, Viola says, "It's very much a rural practice. And the area is gorgeous. The Lake is just breathtaking—I love it." In the years before Viola arrived, the office was staffed by part-time physicians and physician assistants. Now that Viola and a new partner who recently joined her in the practice are here, she feels that there are finally enough primary care doctors in town. Schuyler Hospital owns the office, and Viola is employed by the Hospital. After Viola arrived, the hospital put a small addition on the side of the building, so there are currently four exam rooms for the two full-time physicians. But the practice continues to grow, and the building is not big enough to accommodate this growth.

Not surprisingly, Viola says that now that she is a rural family doctor, the part that she loves best is OB. "I love taking care of families!" she exclaims. "That's just the quintessential best part of family medicine, really—taking care of the family. And OB allows me to do that in a way that I find very satisfying. Because I see most of the babies I deliver, and I do their well child checks, and I'm starting to see them growing up, and it's just amazing to see them get through that first year. And they change as quickly as my own children change. I like that a lot."

Overall, the practice cares for more than half of the 2,757 people living in town, and a number from the surrounding areas. About 30 percent of the patients in the practice are uninsured—an unusually high level—and about half are insured by the federal programs of Medicaid (for the poor) and Medicare (for the elderly), both of which reimburse rural providers with lower rates than in urban areas. While Viola's office is the only full-time medical practice in town, some of the people in the community obtain their medical care elsewhere. And since the office did not provide care for children prior to Viola's arrival, the pediatric population is still growing and represents the fastest growing part of the practice. Unlike Jim Devlin and Mike Tatarko, Viola did not choose to return to her hometown to practice—similar to half of the doctors in this book. And because she has only been in Ovid for three years, she is still figuring out all of the family relationships in the area. "Sometimes, I don't even know that I'm taking care of multiple generations," she says. "I don't always know who somebody's mom is—they might not have the same last name—until somebody in my office tells me. It takes a while to figure out who belongs to whom."

Schuyler Hospital, in Montour Falls, is a small hospital, with only about 40 to 50 beds and an ICU, along with a long-term care facility. Here, Viola does inpatient OB and pediatrics, but because OB makes up a large portion of her practice, she refers her adult patients that need hospitalization to other physicians in the area. In discussing the other physicians in the area that she consults with, she says, "For the most part, the other specialists have been wonderful." As for managed care, Viola says, "It's starting to come in. This community has been isolated, but managed care is finally starting. But right now it's not been a problem." Viola likes that she doesn't have to deal with the business side of medicine. She finds it "overwhelming and oppressive. The hospital takes care of all our billing. We have a computer in my office, but I don't have Internet access, and our scheduling is still not computerized. That's supposed to change."

Differing from most of the other doctors in this book, Viola expressed concern about the ability of family physicians to do well financially, unless they do OB or a number of procedures, which are reimbursed by insurance companies at much higher rates than seeing patients in the office for their medical problems. On the other hand, she acknowledges that she isn't very experienced about reimbursement. And she admits that compared to the community, her income is "much higher—yeah, it's really quite good." Because of her NHSC scholarship, her loans at graduation were limited to about $50,000. And even though she feels that without the NHSC she would have owed four times that much, she still feels the burden of paying off her loans.

· · · · ·

Viola is one of three female physicians of the ten doctors in this book, roughly proportionate to the overall percentage of women throughout the history of the PSAP. As with women physicians in general, this has increased substantially over time. Today, only slightly more than one-fourth of practicing family doctors are women, although this will increase significantly in the future since almost one-half of current family practice residents are women.

The role of women physicians in rural areas has become increasingly important in recent years. Traditionally, women physicians have been less likely than men to practice in rural areas. A number of policy analysts have pointed out that if this trend continues, and is coupled with the dramatically increasing number of women physicians—with women now representing almost half of all medical students—the result will be a substantial decrease in the total number of rural physicians. While overall data appear to support this potentially very serious concern, outcomes of the PSAP, as well as from the rural family practice program at the University of Minnesota Duluth tell a different story. These results indicate that women who enter medical school highly likely to practice rural family medicine—based on their rural background and commitment to become rural family doctors—are equally likely as men to enter rural family practice. Nevertheless, because fewer women currently practice in rural areas, there is less opportunity for female medical students to encounter a woman physician as a role model. And for both men and women, their spouse's background and preferences for where to live are critically important factors in where physicians decide to practice. Likewise, balancing their profession and parenthood is a critically important issue for all physicians with children, but because of the traditionally more dominant role of women in child rearing, this has frequently raised more challenges for women physicians.

Women physicians in all areas and all specialties also continue to face different expectations and biases, more often from male patients and from female staff. Viola smiles when she recounts that "One of my favorite patients said to me, 'You know, I didn't know if I'd like having a girl doctor, but you're great.' " Then she continues, "Sometimes there's some resistance in the male population, between ages fifty and seventy, but that's been pretty easy to overcome. And that's pretty similar in the city. And every once in a while a patient will initially assume that I'm a nurse because I'm a woman. But as soon as they realize it, they're often upset with their mistake."

• • • • •

Although many people assume that obstetricians are the only physicians who deliver babies nowadays, fewer than 10 percent of all obstetricians practice in rural America, and family doctors therefore play a critically important role in these areas. About one-third of all family physicians deliver babies in the United States, with an even greater proportion (42%) of rural family doctors providing these services. And, like Viola, 14 percent of rural family doctors also do C-sections. However, even with both obstetricians and family physicians delivering babies, many rural areas continue to lack an adequate supply of providers. As a result, there is a continuing access problem in the provision of obstetrical services, and many rural women have difficulty finding any doctor available to deliver their babies. Both Viola and the obstetrician in the area support many of the local midwives. Viola says, "They give great care," although their own malpractice rates are also going up, which could force some to leave the area.

"The OB experience that I have here is very different than anywhere else I have ever practiced," Viola explains. "In other places, most of my patients were very medically managed. And I learned what I could from that. Then in residency, I started to become exposed to different styles of obstetrics, and I also worked with midwives. But it wasn't until I got up here that I saw obstetrics practiced in a completely different way that really honored the body's natural ability to have a baby without intervention. But on the other hand, we were able to safely deliver babies if we needed to intervene in any way. There's something incredible about practicing obstetrics here. That doesn't mean I don't value my prior experiences. I loved my obstetrical training. I loved the surgical experience. I loved all the interventions that I learned, and all the tools that I was given. I like to be able to have those if I need them, as a backup, but to really go with what nature has essentially intended. And there's a trust relationship that develops. I don't do it perfectly, but for me it's such a powerful experience. I love the practice of obstetrics. I really really love it."

In addition to her wide scope of practice in obstetrics, Viola also does a number of dermatological procedures such as skin biopsies, removal of small lesions, joint injections, and laceration repairs. "Because we're in the middle of this rural community, a lot of patients appreciate coming in to have things taken care of here—having a joint injected or a mole removed. And I have people that come in and just want me to sew them up, and don't want to go to the ER. I also do colposcopy [microscopic examination of a woman's cervix to look for infections and malignancies]."

Partly because of her own background and partly because there are a large number of Mennonite and Amish in the area, about 20 percent of Viola's practice consists of patients from these groups. "But they don't come in for well child checks—they only come in when they're ill, for the most part. A few that have hypertension or diabetes or thyroid conditions will come in sporadically. I do home visits for some Amish, especially ones that have requested it. One family—we're related—his wife will ask about my grandmother, it's pretty sweet. I took a skin cancer off of her cheek. But periodically he becomes quite ill, and will not necessarily want to come into the office. One of his sons will show up in the office and tell me that he's ill and wants to see me, and they think he might be in heart failure. So I've gone out and visited him. I take my nurse along, and we take a pulse oximeter to measure his oxygen level, and a blood pressure cuff, and stethoscope. I take samples of antibiotics—in the past he's had pneumonia. It's great, I go out to his house and we spend a little time together. Then there have been other times, when I've been really concerned about an Amish patient, maybe they had a really bad laceration, and I know they're not going to come back in to have me check it. Or, I did a circumcision in the office that I was really worried about, so I went out and checked this baby a few times. I think the Amish patients here are very glad to have me here. I get the sense that they trust me, that they think I'm going to take care of them in a way that I think is most appropriate. They're the ones that I have to negotiate the most for their care because they do not follow the same rules."

One of the biggest differences Viola sees between rural and urban family practice is that "there's an intimacy that develops in a rural practice. Taking care of people in a small community is more rewarding, but I also think more about the impact of my care on a patient and on the community. So it's not something I can just cut off and go home, because I see my patients and their relatives back in the office, or I see them in the post office. So I think about it. I do take it home with me." Also, Viola definitely feels that she has more professional autonomy and independence than she would in a larger city.

Transportation is another real problem in the area. Some people have to drive one-half hour for care. And even worse, many people have to walk miles for medical care. "I have a pregnant patient," Viola says with disbelief, "that had to walk three miles for her prenatal visit. And so I see things here that I haven't seen anywhere else. You know, in the city, you take public transportation. You can at least get on the bus or the subway. But here people walk, or try to get a ride from somebody else. And so they miss their appointments, or they only show up when they're really sick. And that's a challenge."

Overall, Viola feels that her present practice is "pretty close" to her original vision of rural family practice. "Because," she says, "I found that family practice is flexible, and you really can meet the needs of your community—if you've gone through a good family practice residency program. I knew that I was going to practice in a rural area, so I wanted to be able to do a lot of procedures. And I wanted to be able to really offer a broad range of services and patient care, and I feel like family practice has prepared me very well."

• • • • •

Dr. Monaghan has a remarkable way of interacting with her patients, working with them in a collaborative fashion to help them make medical decisions. Discussing this, she says, "I love my patients. I really do like them. And I guess I found that if I'm too heavy-handed, they're not going to do what I suggest anyway. So I guess that's my way of teasing out how they want to go with it."

Entering the next room, Viola says hi to a patient who she seems to know very well, and who is obviously very pregnant. The young woman is 26 years old and her baby is due very soon. This is her second pregnancy, and she has a two-year-old daughter at home. Unlike her first pregnancy, which went smoothly, this one has been more difficult, and she has had a lot of pelvic and abdominal discomfort for much of the pregnancy. Because of this, and because tests showed that the baby was fully mature, Dr. Monaghan had tried to induce labor last week, but it was unsuccessful. So, she's scheduled for another induction this Tuesday, four days from now. But the woman is back in the office today, Friday, complaining of much more pain.

"What's going on?"

"I'm having a lot more discomfort. Mainly when I walk. It really hurts. It feels like there's something pushing down so hard, it's hard to walk."

"How's your baby moving?"

"Slow, not as active as he was. He's a lot slower."

"Are you doing movement counts?"

"No, but like I was telling my husband last night, I didn't feel him move for quite a while." Then, laughing nervously, the patient continues, "So I was poking him, trying to get him to move. And he moved, but it wasn't like . . ."

Sensing that the woman is concerned about her baby's health, but not yet convinced that this is serious, Dr. Monaghan asks, "Do you think he was in a sleep cycle? . . . Well, let me ask you this, are you concerned about how he's doing? Has it dropped off that much?"

"No, it's dropped off, but I don't know if I'd say concerned. He still gets the hiccups two or three times, so I know he's got that, but . . ."

Still trying to quantify whether this is normal or not, Dr. Monaghan asks her, "When you do your movement counts, are you getting at least ten movements in about a half hour or so?"

"Uh-huh."

"OK. I would like you to do that every twelve hours, two times a day. And if you're not getting it, I want you to go to the hospital again, and get another checkup." Then, reassured that the movement counts are normal, Dr. Monaghan tries to reassure the patient, continuing in a very calm, slow, and comforting tone of voice, "Your baby looked beautiful last week. He was really very active, and everything looked fine. But I would be very happy to get another nonstress test if you're not getting the numbers, or if you're really concerned and feel like something's wrong with your baby. OK?"

"Uh-huh."

"All right." Then, Dr. Monaghan checks her pocket OB calculator to see when the baby is due. "Your due date is in ten days, so you're thirty-eight weeks and five days. Your measurements had fallen last time, but you don't feel like you've dropped? I'm just going to measure you again, and then I'm going to listen to the baby's heartbeat, and then I'm going to see if you're dilating."

"The day that I came home, this mucous-y stuff had come out, but it had some white streaks in it."

"Oh, OK . . ."

"But I didn't know, I mean there wasn't a lot of blood or anything, so I didn't call that night."

"Yeah, it sounds like that was your mucous plug. And it doesn't really mean that you're going into labor, unless it comes with contractions. Some women will lose their mucous plug a week or two before they actually go into labor." As Dr. Monaghan measures the woman's pregnant abdomen and pushes gently in a number of areas, she says, "Your baby's head is here. Is that where you're having your pain?"

"Yeah."

"OK, the baby's head is *really* snug against your pubic bones." Then, she takes out the Doppler ultrasound machine, squeezes some gel on the woman's belly, and gently pushes the microphone into the gel. The baby's heartbeat sounds like a beating whoosh under water, or like the ticking of a loud clock with a bad head cold—whoosh, whoosh, whoosh. Dr. Monaghan says,

"150—that sounds great. Your strip in the hospital looked great. I haven't seen one like that in a while, it looked so good. Is it hard to get comfortable?"

"Yeah."

Dr. Monaghan then does an internal examination, and says, "Your cervix is a little more thinned out, but it's still pretty thick. This is the baby's head, are you feeling that?"

"Yes."

"Unfortunately, I think you're having the discomfort of the baby moving down and settling in your pelvis. I think when you start to go into labor, I don't think it's going to take a lot. I don't think you're going to have any problems delivering, but . . . we'll try to move it along next week. Certainly I'm here all weekend if you need me."

"I am just so stressed out . . . and so sore . . ."

Appreciating that the woman is having difficulty coping, Dr. Monaghan says, "I know, that's why I want to try to induce you again. Unless you change your mind and want to try and do something sooner."

"No, unless I have an emotional breakdown . . ."

"If you really want me to, I'll rupture your membranes, and I'll make sure you have a baby, but we have to really think of the risk-benefit here. I don't want to do a C-section if I don't have to. But I know that you're at the end of the rope. I know that it's been rough for you. On Tuesday, if you really want me to, we can talk about breaking your water 'cause I know you've had it. Do you think you can make it through the weekend?"

"It's hard, but I'll try." Then, starting to get teary-eyed, she says, "It's really hard."

"Are you sleeping at night?"

"Not well."

"Do you want something to help you sleep, or something for the pain? Either one?"

"No, I want to try and go natural, but it's just the emotional stuff too," the woman says, and then starts to cry.

"What can I do to help you right now?"

"I don't think anything. It's just . . ."

"Do you want to come in on Monday instead of Tuesday? We can do an induction on Monday."

"Yeah. . . ."

"OK, let's move it up a day. Let's hope you go over the weekend. You can try castor oil again if you like."

"No, that makes me really . . . I've done everything else," the patient continues, and starts to cry harder. "I don't understand why . . ."

"We don't understand either. We don't completely understand what causes women to go into labor. I don't know."

"With the first one, it was so simple, you know. The week or two before, you just stripped the membranes, and . . . I just went into labor. This time I'm just not doing it."

"Well, if you want me to try strip the membranes [separating a small portion of the membranes surrounding the baby from the edge of the uterine wall, thought by some to occasionally help precipitate labor], I will do that today."

"Before you said it wasn't . . ."

"It was too posterior last time, but I can try today. You're a little bit more effaced, a little bit more thinned out. If you want me to try, I will. But I just don't want you to have the expectation that it's absolutely going to make you go into labor this time. Do you want me to try?"

"Will it hurt?"

"A little uncomfortable, especially with the head being up so high. If it's really bothering you, I'll stop. Want to try it?"

The patient shakes her head yes.

"OK. Here's what I want you to do. Lay back, same position as before." As she does another internal examination, Dr. Monaghan talks constantly, in a soothing, calm, voice, almost like a hypnotist, talking slowly and continuously. "Take some deep breaths. You're going to feel my hand. If you have discomfort, I want you to breathe it away. Are you doing OK? A little more pressure . . . I'm almost done, I can feel the membranes right there. . . . OK?"

"OK."

"OK. We'll see. Hopefully it'll do something. In the meantime I'll call down to OB and have them schedule the induction for Monday. And if you feel like you're not getting appropriate baby movements, call the hospital. Are you going to be all right?"

"I don't mean to be a bother . . ."

"You're not a bother, you're in a really tough spot right now. You're going to have your baby soon [her voice is *very* comforting and reassuring]. You just have to hang in for a couple more days, and if you feel like you can't, please call. The nurses in the hospital will get in touch with me. OK? We can do it this weekend if we have to."

"OK."

"I'll see you soon."

"Thank you so much."

"You're welcome."

Three days later, after a successful induction, the woman delivered a beautiful and healthy baby boy. The delivery was quick and without complications. And both mother and baby are doing fine.

· · · · ·

Describing the area, Viola says, "It's beautiful up here. It's so peaceful. Montour Falls is a small town. It has about 1,700 people. Our house is one of the older homes in town. It's on a really nice street in a nice part of town. It's on a piece of property that's a little bit less than one acre, and is less than one mile from the hospital." Their large house has a wonderful wraparound porch that spans the entire front and side, and is located just down the street from the "falls"—Montour Falls, which is located right on the main street in town, and is the eighth highest waterfall in New York state. The falls are beautiful, and there is a one-acre park at the base of the waterfall. Grocery shopping is one-half mile away, but Viola and Gerry have to drive 15 miles to buy things like clothing. Like many rural communities, they're getting a Wal-Mart in Watkins Glen, which is five miles away.

On the drive up to Ovid, "there are beautiful wineries that go all the way down to the lake," she continues. "It's magic." Seneca Lake is over 600 feet deep. It's two miles wide, and 36 miles long. The major industry is tourism, and it's seasonal. There are a lot of farmers in the area. Also, people in Ovid work at the local drug and alcohol rehabilitation center, or at the state prison in the area. A lot of people also drive up to Geneva, or over to Cayuga, or down toward Montour Falls for jobs as well. Viola's husband Gerry, who grew up in the suburbs of New York City, says that his idea of poverty growing up was "vertical—all housing projects. Here poverty is horizontal. There's so much poverty in the hills around here."

Because Viola is practicing in a rural area that wasn't her own hometown, moving to a new place where she and her husband didn't know anyone was difficult at first, and it took a while to settle in. "We felt very welcomed into this community as a family. But it still takes a while to get to know people." But what she likes most about living in a small town is that "people know each other. There really is a sense of community. That can be an advantage and a disadvantage, but I really like it." Viola also feels that this is a good area for raising her children, but does have concern regarding the public school system, especially when Caleb goes into third grade next year. She and Gerry have been thinking about private and parochial schools, and also about home schooling, which is a "really big movement here."

• • • • •

Viola finds that there are a number of real challenges in her practice. "There's desperate poverty in the area," she says, "and all the sequelae of poverty. There's a higher incidence of anxiety and depression, and probably drug abuse and alcoholism. It's a difficult practice. It's hard taking care of some patients with chronic problems that don't always want to take care of themselves. They want me to fix something that I can't always fix. I think that's something hard for all physicians. And I know that some patients have difficulty paying to see me, and I can't do anything about it, really. So there are a lot of things in my office that are out of my control. But, some of this is getting better. I've recently been elected vice president of the medical staff for the hospital. So, I'm becoming much more involved in what's going on at the hospital, and I've decided to take a much more active role. And so that feels good."

Also, having come out of a residency program with lots of support, she feels somewhat professionally isolated practicing in Ovid, a HPSA, with only one other colleague in her office. This can be a real shock for all physicians, as they leave the security of the medical school and residency teaching environment where there are always a large number of more experienced physicians with whom they can discuss almost every medical case and decision. Then, when they enter practice, although other physicians are available for formal consultation, the constant support of having someone around to ask questions and review things with no longer exists. So many physicians feel this professional isolation in their early practice years, though it is clearly a bigger problem when there are fewer physicians in one's office and area. For Viola, this is compounded by the fact that the office is not yet connected to the Internet. "So," she says, "there are times that I have questions, or I just want to discuss something with someone. For example, I have a large Amish, nonimmunized community, and sometimes they come in with something I've never seen before. Sometimes I call my colleagues from medical school and residency." This has improved significantly in the past year, since Viola now has a colleague, a woman physician—a general internist who also has subspecialty training in infectious diseases, and who has a three-year commitment to practice in Ovid. "I'm thrilled that she's here," Viola says. "It's really helpful to have another full-time physician here. She's wonderful, although she's an internist and not comfortable seeing kids. The advantage of being up in Ovid is that I can really practice the way I want. But it's also kind of hard sometime—I really kind of miss the support I had during my training."

· · · · ·

Viola also continues to struggle with the border between her professional and personal areas of her life. "It's one of the problems that bothers me the most," she says, "because I would like it to be a little bit more defined." Outside of her profession, Viola spends most of her time at home with her family. And she and Gerry enjoy going out to dinner. With wineries up and down the road between Montour Falls and Ovid, there are a number of very nice restaurants in the area. They've also been out on the lake sailing, and plan to do more of that.

Viola delivers about 40 to 50 babies a year. She's on call about every third night, including covering the nurse midwives in the area in case of problems or the need for a C-section. And she takes call all the time for her own OB patients unless she's out of town, and then she signs out to the obstetrician in town. But compared with residency, where she found being on call a burden, she says that call here is "just different. It doesn't bother me. I don't mind it in the same way. And I don't tend to get called for anything other than a delivery when I'm off call." She spends Mondays through Thursdays in the office from nine to five, and usually sees between 16 and 20 patients a day. Some days, she goes biking along the lake at lunchtime. And on Friday, she's off.

· · · · ·

The next patients are an Amish family—a husband, wife, and their ten-year-old child. They are dressed in traditional Amish clothes, the father with a long black beard. They are related in some way to Viola's grandfather. The father is here because of hypothyroidism, the daughter because she is having headaches. Dr. Monaghan had seen the father recently, found that his thyroid level was very low, and prescribed thyroid hormone for him.

"Hi. How are you feeling?"

"Oh, I'm still tired."

His wife interjects, "Oh, don't let him scare you. He was really working hard, that's why he's tired. Putting the hay away. I can't believe the difference."

Then, turning back to the husband, Dr. Monaghan says, "I was going to say, you look so much better today. You look like you have much more energy. What do you think? How are you feeling?"

"Oh, the only thing is my energy still isn't where it should be. But that's improving every day."

Wife: "I don't think you realize how tired you were before. He has much more energy compared to what he was."

Dr. Monaghan asks the man, "And so, you're up doing your usual work at this point?"

"Yeah. Pretty much so. As long as it keeps improving, or it doesn't get worse, then I think we're happy."

"You know, it takes some time to get the maximum benefit of the medicine, so if you've made this much improvement in two weeks, I would expect that you will continue to get better."

"I have a lot of work that has to be done right now. If we weren't going to be doing that, I wouldn't be pushing."

Wife: "I kind of figure after the hay's done, he's going to be kind of tired. But right now, it's something that he likes to do, and it has to be done."

Dr. Monaghan continues, "OK, we're going to keep you on the same dose for now, and then get another blood test in a few weeks. Normally, I would see my patients back in another four weeks, and then in another month. How does that fit into your schedule? Is that OK?"

"I'd be happy with the least often we can, since we're getting a discount. I don't like to have people do things without . . ."

"Well, why don't you just come back in four weeks, 'cause I'd really just like to see you again. And then we can spread the visits out if you're doing well. Because last time you were in, things were pretty bad."

Wife: "Yes, they were. I just can't believe how fast he's improved."

Then, the husband asks Dr. Monaghan, "Who pays for you when you have a card like this?"

"The hospital has set this program up. I think they get some government funds to help. I'm not exactly sure. But I know that's something they did in response to our request, since a lot of people don't have insurance, and because the fees in offices tend to be high. So I'm hoping that you'll just accept it," she says, smiling warmly. "And just come in to see me. It has nothing to do with my salary—I'm still getting paid."

The patient returns the smile, and says, "Maybe when things go better, we can give them a donation, but things are pretty rough right now."

"Yeah, I don't want you to feel burdened by this at all."

"We're really lucky to have you as a doctor in this town."

Then Dr. Monaghan and the husband and wife briefly discuss their common relatives and a new baby that was just born in the community. Addressing the daughter, Dr. Monaghan says, "OK, you're in today because of headaches?"

Wife/girl's mother: "Well, she's had them for a couple years already, off and on. But, I thought it was getting to be a little bit more serious, or more often."

"Has she ever had a doctor check this out?"

Mother: "She did once. The doctor took some blood tests, but he didn't find anything. That was about two to three years ago."

"So would you say in the last few weeks, or couple months, it's gotten worse?"

Mother: "In the last half year or so."

"Does there seem to be any pattern to it?"

Mother: "More in the morning, when she gets up. The other morning we were planning to take her to the emergency room, we ended up with a natural healer—she uses herbs. She was having so much pain, we were trying to get a driver to take her down to the emergency room, and called one of our neighbors, and they took her down there, and she gave her a packet of six different herbs. It kind of helped at the time, but it only lasted a few days."

Turning to the girl, Dr. Monaghan asks, "How many times a week do you get this pain?"

"I haven't had it in the past couple days."

"How old are you?"

"Ten."

"How many brothers and sisters do you have?"

"I'm the oldest. I have four brothers, and two sisters."

Mother: "You missed one."

"Five brothers."

"Does she have vomiting?" Dr. Monaghan asks her mother.

"No."

Then, after examining the child and finding everything normal, Dr. Monaghan says, "I want to get some blood tests again. And why don't you come back with your dad in four weeks. Here's some lollipops to take with you for your brothers and sisters. Bye."

Dr. Monaghan then enters the adjoining room to see her next patient, and asks the middle-aged woman sitting in the chair, "How are you doing?"

"Like a cat on a hot tin roof! I don't know if I've seen you since my husband had his cancer surgery?"

"No, he was getting ready to go."

"So that's been a month. Since then, I've been doubling the dose of the pills you gave me for anxiety."

Concerned about her taking an increased dose, but never judgmental, Dr.

Monaghan always asks patients how they think things are going for them-selves. "How do you feel on that?"

"I don't feel any different. I don't think it's working. And, I don't want to take this much."

"And you're not sleeping well?"

"Oh, no. I am fatigued, but I'm not sleeping good at all."

Thinking that she should switch to a different medicine, Dr. Monaghan asks the patient what she thinks first, "OK. Are you thinking we should try a medicine change?"

"Gotta do something."

"Yeah, if you're not getting the benefit of the medicine you're on, we should change to another. You've been on it long enough, and the dose is high enough that you should be getting some benefit. And I know that your life has been very challenging recently. Now what is bothering you the most?"

"My nerves."

"Your nerves? Anxiety?"

"And just being exhausted when I wake up."

"When is the last time you really felt rested?"

"Oh, probably before my husband got sick."

"How is your husband doing right now? Is he recovering?"

"He started driving yesterday."

"And how about your relationship with your mother? How's that going?"

"We're still having the same problems."

"How's your counseling going?"

The woman sighs, and says "I don't know. . . ."

"Well, we certainly can try a different type of medicine, and see if you can get some benefit. I think that it's wonderful that you're going for counseling. And, what I'm feeling is, if this isn't a benefit, I'm thinking about how you would feel about seeing a psychiatrist?"

"What do you think would help by seeing a psychiatrist?"

"I see a lot of patients with anxiety and depression, and I've seen some tremendous benefits, but when I get to the point that the medicines that I'm accustomed to using aren't getting the benefits I expect, then I think of refer-ring to a specialist. In the same way if I have somebody with indigestion, and there's something beyond what I'm used to treating, then I refer to a gastro-enterologist. The same with anxiety and depression. Because they're really comfortable using medications I'm not."

"Can I try one of these medicines first?"

"Of course. And if that's not working, then we can talk about it again. OK. I'll see you in four weeks."

The next patient is a 35-year-old man who had an operation to remove a small brain tumor. He is doing fine now, but began having seizures after sur-gery, and takes medicine to control them. Then, Dr. Monaghan sees a 36-year-old woman who is having irregular menstrual periods. Reviewing her chart before entering the room, she notes that she last saw the patient six months ago for bronchitis, which resolved. Married with three children, the patient had her tubes tied after her last child was born five years ago. Dr. Monaghan enters the room, smiles, and says, "Hi. What's going on?"

"My last period started on time, but it continued for nine to ten days. That's not normal. And then it started again in less then three weeks."

"Are you having any pain?"

"I was, a little, on my right side here. But today I'm OK."

"Any abnormal discharge?"

"Um, no. But my breasts have been very tender. That usually happens five days before my period."

"Well, this is very, very unlikely," Dr. Monaghan says, "but one of the things we need to do today is to do a pregnancy test."

"Uh-huh. I'm glad you mentioned it, 'cause I was thinking about it."

After the patient gives Dr. Monaghan a urine specimen, the nurse does a pregnancy test, which is positive. Dr. Monaghan goes back into the room and tells her the news. The woman begins to cry.

"I'm sorry. I know this is not what you're expecting."

Dr. Monaghan and the patient spend the next ten minutes quietly discussing the situation, and as the shock wears off a bit, the woman becomes much calmer. Then, Dr. Monaghan examines the patient, but because the pregnancy is early, she is unable to feel the location of the baby. So, she explains to the patient her concern that this could be an ectopic pregnancy—a pregnancy which is lodged in the tubes, rather than the uterus—a common problem with women who get pregnant after having their tubes tied. And she explains that tubal pregnancies can have serious consequences: As the pregnancy grows, there is no room to go, and they rupture the tube, leading to very heavy bleeding, and even possibly death. So Dr. Monaghan arranges for the woman to go down to the hospital to have an ultrasound test to try and find the location of the pregnancy. "You're going to be OK. Do you want somebody to come up here to the office? You'll probably want to take somebody with you."

"I knew something was not right."

"I'm going to call the ER and tell them you're coming down, and they will do an ultrasound. I'm really glad you came in today."

"Thank you."

Later, Dr. Monaghan is paged by the hospital. The ultrasound is not definitive. It doesn't look like there is a pregnancy in the uterus, and there is something in her right tube, but it might be a cyst. By the time Dr. Monaghan goes down to the ER to see the patient, she and her husband had gotten over the initial shock, and were even starting to hope that this might be a normal pregnancy and they would have another child. Then, after making sure that the woman was not bleeding, and that her condition was stable, Dr. Monaghan admits her to the hospital overnight to watch her closely and to follow her blood pregnancy test levels and her blood count. The patient did well, but as Dr. Monaghan suspected, tests the next morning did confirm that she had an ectopic pregnancy in her right tube, and Dr. Monaghan assisted the obstetrician in her successful surgery.

• • • • •

"I think that programs like the PSAP and the NHSC are critical," Viola says, "because many physicians, unless they've had that experience, unless they've grown up in rural areas, won't practice there. So, I think if you have programs like this, it will happen, otherwise only rarely." As to her own future after her four-year NHSC commitment is over, she says, "I don't know for sure. I really think about what I want my practice to be after next year." While she is seriously considering remaining in Ovid, she would also like to have more control over her office and her practice. So while part of her would like to open a private practice, she is also concerned about the business and financial side of things, and worried about reimbursement levels from Medicare and Medicaid, as well as malpractice premiums for doing obstetrics and C-sections. "I could practice in another nearby community. But there's something very special about this place for us. So I would enjoy staying in Ovid if it were the right circumstances." One of Viola's dreams is to open a health center there—to have primary medical care, social services, mental health, and public health services all under one roof.

Viola "loves being able to come back from the hospital and have dinner with my family and tuck my boys into bed, and go back up again. Or, on a weekend, I can spend time around the house, and know that I can be in the hospital in a minute. And, now that we've been here for three years, we're really starting to become connected to this community. And I love the lake. I love being out here in the country as long as I have access to things that I find to be satisfying, and there's lots of that around here." But one thing seems clear. She says she does not want to practice in the city or suburbs, because there are so many subspecialists there. "So, I don't really see that happening. We like it here."

Boswell, Pennsylvania

When I arrive at the office in the morning, I greet Dr. Thompson and am received with a warm "hello"; that's all. I've realized Dr. Thompson wastes no words. I consider this a notable characteristic. He rarely speaks when unnecessary; when he does speak, he chooses his words carefully and takes his time doing so. A private man, Dr. Thompson is serious about his family, his Christian faith and his work.

Dr. Thompson lightly taps on the exam room door prior to entering. He greets his patients, introduces me as the medical student and begins to wash his hands—all in one fluid movement. All of Dr. Thompson's patients are devoted to him. The pledge he made years ago to serve the rural poor was not made lightly or forgotten.

It's sometimes hard to believe small towns like Boswell, Stoystown, Somerset still exist; where the simple relaxed life is not an exception but the everyday standard. People sincerely greet you at the store, remember how to pronounce your name and are truly grateful for your time.

—Vera Limcuando, PSAP student, class of 2002

When Bill Thompson was a senior medical student, he took a six-week rural preceptorship working with Dr. Jan deVries, a family doctor in Boswell, Pennsylvania. Bill remembers that this experience "really showed me what a rural family doctor does for the first time. Before that, I had only seen patients in the hospital, or a family practice center. So it was different being in a rural area and seeing patients in the office. I remember going with Jan to the hospital one night to deliver a baby. And we went to the Lions Club one evening, so it gave me an idea what it meant to be a part of the community and take care of rural patients. I could tell the relationship he had with his patients and with other doctors, and that seemed to be a special kind of thing. And that was attractive to me." So, in 1990, after completing his residency, Bill Thompson returned to join Jan deVries in the Medical Associates of Boswell. There, in addition to practicing family medicine, he too now serves as a teaching preceptor for senior medical students, continuing the cycle and carrying on the tradition of practicing doctors teaching—and serving as role models— for the next generation of physicians.

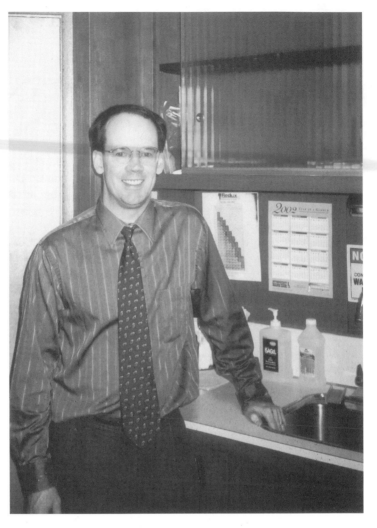

Dr. Bill Thompson in his office.

Even before he had taken his own preceptorship in Boswell, Bill was very familiar with the area. He had spent every summer since he was a kid—until his second year of medical school—at a Christian summer camp a few miles down the road, first as a camper, then as a counselor. So, "when I was finishing up my residency, I knew Jan was looking for someone to join him. I was looking for a rural practice in Pennsylvania, and this particular area was certainly in need of a doctor. It was an area that I liked, as far as being rural and out in the country, and having the mountains and forests. And also I had friends here. My good friend growing up had become the director at the camp, and one of the guys that was a camp counselor with me was living here—he was the pastor of a church right here in Boswell. So those things were very attractive to me—having friends in the area, a kind of a support group—and it seemed that this was a good area to come to. And it was also not far from where I had grown up."

· · · · ·

During the last two years of medical school, students spend almost all of their time in hospitals and medical offices, working under the supervision of faculty and resident physicians. This on-the-job training is referred to as the "clinical years" of medical school, separating it very clearly from the first two years, or "pre-clinical" years, where medical students spend almost all of their time in classrooms and labs. The third year at almost every medical school is structured in a very similar format, composed of a series of six clerkships, each usually six weeks long, in the major specialties of family medicine, pediatrics, internal medicine, surgery, obstetrics and gynecology, and psychiatry. For most of these third year clerkship experiences, students are primarily assigned to the inpatient floors of a hospital; for family medicine the clerkship almost always takes place in an outpatient (ambulatory) office or doctor's office. The fourth, or senior year in most medical schools, has a less defined structure, with a combination of some required, and many elective clinical experiences. The senior preceptorship, most often available in family medicine, consists of working one-on-one with a physician or group of physicians in a private practice or outpatient office. This clinical experience provides students with a real-life role model practicing family practice. In addition, it oftentimes provides students with more responsibility and supervision than occurs in the medical school or university hospital environment, by virtue of the fact that they are the only student in the practice.

The role that preceptorships and other clinical experiences play in the career choices of physicians has been studied for many years, but without definitive results. Most of the literature related to preceptorship programs has not found them to have a decisive role by themselves in increasing the number of physicians that practice primary care or in underserved areas. Initial research did show that those medical schools that had rural and family medicine clerkships and preceptorships graduated more rural doctors and more family physicians. However it is difficult to sort out many of the other confounding factors involved. That is, was it the clinical experiences that were having an impact? Or was it the fact that those schools that early on provided rural family practice clinical experiences were also state schools that were supported by public funding, were in states with larger rural populations, and already had more students entering with rural backgrounds and primary care interests? Clearly, clinical experiences do have an important role in career choice, shown most impressively by the Rural Primary Associate Program (RPAP) at the University of Minnesota, where students take their entire nine-month third year at a rural location, including their core clinical rotations in all specialties. Their outcomes show that a large proportion of their graduates practice primary care in rural areas. Here again, however, most of the students in the program grew up in a rural area, and all had to be selected for the program during their second year of medical school, where they first had to demonstrate a strong preference for a rural career even before their rural curriculum began.

Our own experience with the PSAP has shown that fourth year preceptorship experiences—like the one that Bill Thompson took—are independently associated with practicing rural primary care, while third year rural clerkships are not. However, almost all of the students who decided to take the rural preceptorship were already likely to become rural primary care doctors, either having grown up rural or planning to do family practice. And since the preceptorship doesn't occur until the senior year of medical school, when most students have already decided on their specialty choice, it seems more likely that its most important role is confirmatory. As with many of the doctors interviewed in this book, Bill Thompson's senior rural preceptorship seemed to solidify his already clear leanings, showing him that you really could practice rural family medicine, and that you could be satisfied and happy doing it, both professionally and personally.

So, clinical experiences in rural family medicine are important. For those students who are already most likely to become rural family doctors, such as those in the PSAP, it is very important to give them a real life experience to allow them to confirm that this is what they want. It is difficult for most of us to make a final definite career decision without actually having a relevant life experience and role model. And we do know that even "high likely" individuals are less likely to end up in rural family practice without this experience. On the other hand, most non-rural students—especially those uninterested in rural practice and those planning to become subspecialists— are very unlikely to ever practice rural primary care, whether or not they participate in a rural clinical experience. For these students, the rural experience itself will almost never change their mind. In fact, it usually reinforces their plans not to practice rural. Then, there is a group of students in the middle, those who are not highly likely based on their background and initial career plans, but who are open to the possibility of rural primary care. For these students, it is very important to provide them with the opportunity for a rural clinical experience that allows them to "try it on for size," to see how it feels, and see how they like it.

• • • • •

The headline from the July 12, 1962 issue of the *Boswell News* read "Lions Medical Clinic Dedication." Next to it was a large picture of Dr. Jan deVries, who had just been recruited to staff the new office. The Boswell practice that Jan deVries began more than 40 years ago has a unique history, having been started as part of a national program of the Sears Roebuck Foundation. Since the Sears Roebuck Company had made much of its fortune in rural America, the Foundation decided in the 1950s to help rural communities with their most pressing health care need—recruiting general practice physicians. The Foundation helped rural communities determine whether they could support a physician, provided them with free blueprints for building an office building, and made available pre-fabricated interiors. The community, however, was required to raise the money to build the office building itself. In Boswell, as in many other small towns, the GP who had been practicing there was getting older and sicker. The town had tried for some time to help recruit another doctor, but had been unsuccessful. So with the help of the Sears Roebuck Foundation, an office building was planned, and the Lions Club in town raised the funds to build the structure.

The building was completed in 1962, just as Dr. deVries was completing his internship in Washington DC. He had graduated medical school in the Netherlands and had spent four years in missionary work in Indonesia before coming to the United States. Then, after his internship, Jan, his wife, and three children moved to Boswell, where he has been in practice for more than four decades. And he and Bill Thompson still practice in that same one-story red brick building with its gently sloping roof, and the words "Lions Medical Clinic" clearly posted on the outside wall.

· · · · ·

Bill Thompson was born in the suburbs of Cincinnati, Ohio. His father was a chemical engineer who worked for Proctor and Gamble. When Bill was ten, the family moved to Westmoreland County in western Pennsylvania when his father took a position as an administrator and manager of a Christian study center that was starting at the time. Along with his parents and three younger siblings, Bill grew up here, at the Ligonier Valley Study Center, about two miles outside the very small town of Stahlstown, until he went to college. The center provided adult education, lectures, and college-level credit. Bill's mom helped cook dinners for some of the students who were staying at the Center, so that two or three students would have dinner with the family a few nights each week.

Bill remembers being very excited about moving to the country. "I was at a stage in my life where I didn't feel too tied down to where we were— although I enjoyed living in the suburbs, and had friends there. But it seemed kind of exciting to move out into the country and be in a rural area. I really enjoyed being out in the woods. I liked the spread out land. When I was twelve, my parents bought me a motorcycle—a dirt bike—and I could ride that all over, which was a lot of fun. There was a little pond there for fishing, and I liked camping—we could just camp out in the backyard. And we had a horse that I rode." Today, the center no longer exists. It became a drug and alcohol treatment center for a while, and then a bed-and-breakfast. Only 30 minutes from where he now lives and practices in Boswell, Bill and his wife Kathy went back there two years ago to stay the night at the B&B—the place where he had grown up. In his typically understated manner, Bill uses few words, saying, "It was fun."

During high school, Bill took a series of vocational tests to help him think about a future career and was told that he should become either a teacher or a doctor. "I had done well at school, and I enjoyed science and liked people.

[He laughs, as this is a classic interview response of medical school applicants.] And for some reason, I felt that doctoring was what I would like to do more than teaching. I do remember being a little concerned about being a doctor because I didn't want the responsibility of people's lives in my hands. But somehow I got over that. So I decided I wanted to be a doctor, and never thought otherwise." He also remembers "talking to my own family doctor about things that he liked about being a doctor. And at some point, I spent some time at Latrobe Area Hospital, observing different areas of the hospital, which confirmed and strengthened my desire to be a doctor."

Bill was a pre-med student at Hamilton College in Clinton, New York, which he chose because "my grandfather went there, and because I thought a small liberal arts college environment was where I would do best." Then, when he was applying to medical school, he read about the PSAP. "I liked rural areas, and lived in a rural area, and thought that's probably where I would want to be. That was my idea of what a doctor was—being a family doctor in a rural area. I'm not sure that I was aware of all the different specialties. So I thought that would be a good thing to do. The rural part fit who I was, and what I wanted to do, and where I wanted to be." This is clearly reflected in Bill's application to medical school 20 years ago, which read, "I hope to be a family practice physician so that I can care for people of all ages. I hope to settle down and practice in a rural area such as the Jenner Township area" (three miles from where he currently practices). "So I'm grateful for the PSAP being in existence and for choosing me."

· · · · ·

The first thing this morning, Dr. Thompson begins making rounds at Somerset Hospital, where his practice has ten patients. The first patient he sees is a 50-year-old man who has been in the hospital for three weeks. He has bad asthma and smokes, and came in with a severe asthma attack. He had to be intubated (have a breathing tube inserted into his airway and put on a ventilation machine), and because the only lung specialist in the area was out of town, he was transferred to Pittsburgh. Then, as soon as he was starting to improve and was taken off the ventilator, he decided he wanted to be closer to home. So he was transferred back to Somerset Hospital. Then, Dr. Thompson sees a 28-year-old woman without health insurance who just had a baby; a 72-year-old man—who is wheelchair bound from severe arthritis and who Dr. Thompson usually sees at home on house calls—who is in the hospital to have a bleeding polyp removed from his colon; and a 91-year-old woman with severe chronic lung disease, heart disease, and dementia. She had been living at home with her husband, but about nine months ago it became too hard for him to care for her, so she's now in a nursing home. She's in the hospital today because of difficulty breathing from her lung disease.

Dr. Thompson then goes into the next room to see a 75-year-old man who had a heart attack three days ago. The man's daughter was the first grade teacher of Dr. Thompson's son. This is the first time Dr. Thompson has seen him in the hospital, as one of his partners has been caring for him during the past two days.

"Dr. B. told me you had a heart attack. What did it feel like for you?"

"It just struck all of a sudden. It was just a pressure here, a pressure pain. I felt all right that day. My wife said, 'What did you do?' I said, 'I was just going down to sit at the table, and all of a sudden this pressure pain'—that's just what it felt like." Then, pushing on his chest, he continues, "Some horrible pressure right in there."

"How long did it last?"

"Well, till after we got into the hospital—I don't know. They gave me something." His wife, who is sitting next to the bed adds, "I don't think it lasted over two hours."

"How are you feeling today?" Dr. Thompson asks.

"Pretty tired. I just tried to take a bath myself over in the bathroom. It didn't go that good."

"Having had a heart attack will make you weak," Dr. Thompson explains. "When you have a heart attack, we like you to rest and take it easy for the first few days, so there's not a lot of strain on your heart. But then after that, resting and taking it easy means you're not exercising your muscles much, and then that can make you weak. So we think it's now time to start increasing your activity again. Did you have any pain in your chest last night or today?"

"No, I don't have any pain now."

"Are you eating OK?"

"Yes."

"How about your breathing?"

"It was all right."

Dr. Thompson examines the man's heart while he is lying down, then asks him to sit up, and listens to his lungs in the back. "Take a big breath. . . . OK. The cardiologist has ordered for you to start on some rehabilitation, to do some strengthening exercises, to gradually increase what you can do. And I'll be back to see you tomorrow."

"All right. I'll be here. Thank you for coming."

• • • • •

The town of Boswell was named after Thomas Taylor Boswell, builder of the world's largest coal tipple. In 1900, he bought a small farm in the area in order to mine the coal underneath his land. To get the coal from the mine to the railroad, he built a ten-story high tipple, a steel viaduct that took the coal from the mouth of the mine and dropped it down a 1,200-foot slide to where the train was waiting to load it. Incorporated in 1904, the borough is laid out in a one-mile square. Bill's office is in the center of town, and standing in front of the office and looking in all four directions, you can almost see the entire town—all 11 streets, none with sidewalks, each stretching only three to four blocks long.

Boswell was a company town, with a company store for the miners. Their

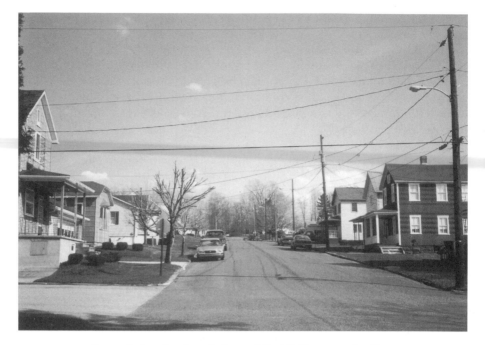

Boswell, the view from in front of Dr. Bill Thompson's office.

pay—company store money, not legal tender—could only be used there. The miners also rented their houses from the company, so if they went on strike, they couldn't get food or pay rent. A unique thing about the town is how the coal company built the houses for the miners. They alternated brick or stone houses with the wood houses, so as to decrease the chances that a large fire would spread. Because of this feature, Boswell was placed on the National Register of Historic Places in 1994.

Today, the population of Boswell is 1,364. In its heyday, it was a larger and somewhat rowdy town—it had an opera house, a bowling alley, and three movie theaters. And the railroad from Somerset to Johnstown ran through the town. By 1940, most of the coal mines had closed, and were replaced by garment factories, but by 1970 these also closed due to overseas competition. It was then that the local economy was at its worst—when it was the poorest in Pennsylvania. Today, the economy is doing somewhat better. There is still some farming in the area. And the hospital and school districts employ a number of people, as do some small industries. But it is sports, recreation, and tourism that have really helped the area. Close to Seven Springs Resort, it is known as the first place in Pennsylvania where it snows each year, and the last place for the snow to leave.

The area also made the news on September 11, 2001, when one of the terrorist hijacked planes heading for Washington, DC, crashed in a field in Shanksville—only five miles from Bill's second office in the nearby town of

Stoystown. Bill was in that office seeing patients at the time of the crash, although he didn't hear it, and the local hospital in Somerset had been placed on emergency standby.

• • • • •

"Medical school was very intense and academically challenging," Bill remembers, "but it was interesting and I enjoyed it. I especially enjoyed it when I started to have clinical contact with patients. I felt somewhat intimidated by it, but I definitely enjoyed practicing medicine more than just learning about it. I had my third year family medicine rotation at Latrobe," which is where he had also spent time as a high school student testing his initial interest in medicine. "During my third and fourth years, family practice was still what I wanted to do. I never really considered anything else—I just felt that was the right thing for me. It had the things that were most attractive to me—taking care of the whole family, babies and adults, and a wide variety of different problems, rather than just focusing on a particular organ system."

Bill also met his wife Kathy at Jefferson. They were in the same year there—Bill in medical school, and Kathy in a PhD program in developmental biology. They took some of the same basic science classes together and lived in the same dormitory. What started out as a dinner rotation, where Bill, his three roommates and Kathy, who lived two doors down, would take turns cooking for each other, developed into being running partners, and then dating. Bill and Kathy were engaged when he was a senior, and they got married during his first year of residency. Bill remained at Jefferson for his family medicine residency, in part because Kathy had not yet finished her PhD program. He was extremely happy with his training at Jefferson, and although it meant three more years in Philadelphia and training at an urban program, he already knew he was going to go to a rural area to practice.

When Bill first decided to come to Boswell, Kathy was somewhat unsure about how she would do there. "She grew up in the suburbs of Philadelphia," Bill explains, "and is the only one in her family that's moved this far away—five and a half hours. But, she spent some time out here when I did my preceptorship, and she was here when we came back to look around. Now, she's doing very well in Boswell. She likes being here in this rural area, and likes being part of the community. She does youth ministry for the North Star Youth Outreach, a nonprofit organization, and enjoys trying to help out the high school kids who are in trouble. She also connects with people in our church. She's considering getting a more official type of counseling degree. She does voluntary teaching in elementary school and high school, and is planning to teach a college-level biology course at the high school in the near future. Our three children—Zachary is twelve, Conor is ten, and Kristen is six—are all doing very well. We live three blocks from the office and right across the street from the high school. When we came here we wanted to get involved with the community, have a positive influence on the community, and feel that being involved in the school system is a way to do that—and to get to know people better."

• • • • •

What Bill Thompson likes most about being a family doctor in a small town is "being a part of the lives of and the medical care of a variety of people. I like being able to interact with people and help them with their problems on a long-term basis. I like to establish relationships with people over time. I don't know if the people here are that much different than those in an urban or suburban area, but there's more of a sense of community. And, I know lots of people from different generations in the same family. A lot of the patients are related to each other. Also, I see my patients when I go grocery shopping, at school functions with my children, at sporting events—I'm the team doctor at football games. I enjoy being able to see patients outside of the office. I don't feel that they impinge much upon my private life, or that I want to keep that separate. Sure, on a few occasions, patients come to me when I'm not on call. But I want to be accessible and available, and most of the time I enjoy that."

When he first started out in practice, there were not many doctors in the area. "I felt good to be able to meet a need. That's less now, since there are more family doctors than when I first came. But we are still the only doctors in town and take care of about half of the people here." And Bill says that the area, which remains a HPSA, continues to need more doctors. "Being a family doctor is a prestigious thing in the local community and in the medical community. The quality of family doctors is very good here, not only in our practice. They're well trained, highly respected, and looked up to as providing good care. And they are well respected in the hospital—the past chairperson of the hospital medical staff and the next one are both family doctors."

• • • • •

The hardest thing for Bill is to try and "maintain relationships with my family—my wife and my kids. I constantly try to work on that. I have chosen on at least three occasions in the last twelve years to decrease the number of hours that I work, with a resultant decrease in income each time. I've done so because it allows me to have more time with my family than when I first started. For me, it is more important to have more time than to make more money.

"I'm on call one out of every four nights. Usually that's not very busy—it averages about five calls a night. I'm usually home by 6:30 for three nights a week. One night I have office hours in the evening, and one night I usually have a meeting. And then, I'm home for two out of every three weekends. So, I usually get to about half of my kids activities.

"I think it's nice to be in an area where there are mountains close by—we can get to a ski slope in fifteen minutes—and where there are lakes, and woods, and camping close by. When we were in Philadelphia, we thought it was OK to be there, but we didn't like the traffic, the buildings, the crime, and things like that. Now, we're an hour and a half from Pittsburgh, and we probably go there once every two months or so. My mom and dad and my brother are all there. So it's not too far. We can do day trips, or they can come out here. And there are shopping malls within a half hour from here, food stores twenty minutes away, Home Depot and Lowe's are twenty-five minutes away, the closest movie theater is twenty minutes.

"I'm not sure why more doctors don't practice in a rural area. But my sense is that most people, even if they grew up rural, go to college, are around other people, go to medical school—usually in cities. And they become accustomed to that lifestyle, enjoy it, meet and marry people who are also from more urban and suburban areas, and feel like that's the way life should be. And some may be concerned that they can't have the kind of life they want, the amenities of suburban living. Some may feel like it may be hard to make enough money. But this is a good place to raise kids. It's a friendly community, and having the outdoors close by is also nice for the kids."

· · · · ·

Inside the exam room in Dr. Thompson's office, the wall is covered with patient education posters ranging from such problems as high cholesterol to osteoporosis. His first patient this afternoon is a 12-year-old boy who is having school problems. He comes in with his mother.

His mother begins. "He failed sixth grade last year, and he's still failing science and English this year. The teachers say he is having trouble staying focused. We can see it when he's with us. First he's fine, and then the next thing, he's gone. I'm at my end of the rope—with his failing. This is going to be the second year. All I get from him is 'I don't know.' He's doing fine in math. Reading and history are OK this year. But the science—he says he just doesn't understand. He had a tutor this year, and when the tutor was there he was doing better."

Turning to the boy, Dr. Thompson asks, "What grade are you in?"

"Sixth."

"So you're at the middle school this year. Do you like school? Your teachers?"

"Most of them."

"There's some you don't like?"

"Some are mean, some don't teach well, some give us too much work. In science, I just don't get all the little symbols. I stay pretty focused in the other classes."

"Do you have friends in school?"

"Yeah, a lot of them."

"Are you involved in sports?"

"No." His mother interjects, explaining, "He was involved in soccer, but we stopped that when his grades fell. He doesn't miss a day. I just want to rule out everything. I just don't know what to do. He doesn't see his friends because of the grades. The phone is the biggest problem now, because he's constantly on it. I just don't know if he doesn't care or if it's a problem."

Dr. Thompson listens very attentively to each answer. He pauses and thinks for a few seconds before asking the next question. He is very deliberate in his approach and his comments. "How are things at home? Do you get along with your brother?"

"Yes."

His mother then asks, "I also wanted to ask you about his legs—while we're here. He has pain every night when he goes to bed."

Acknowledging her concern, Dr. Thompson turns back to the boy and says, "I'm going to check your blood pressure and listen to your heart and lungs. How are you eating?"

"OK." His mother adds, "He eats well, it's the other one who doesn't eat well. But he doesn't eat breakfast in the morning."

"It's a good idea to eat breakfast in the morning. It might help you focus better." As Dr. Thompson begins to examine the boy, he asks, "What time do you go to bed?"

"Ten. And I get up at seven."

Dr. Thompson examines the boy's legs. "How long has this been going on?"

Mom: "At least two years. I brought him in before, and they thought it was growing pains."

"Does activity make it worse?"

Mom: "Not really."

Dr. Thompson then asks the boy, "Where do your legs hurt?"

"The front—here."

After examining his legs and not finding any abnormalities, Dr. Thompson says, "Hmm. OK, sit back up." Then, switching back to the school problem, Dr. Thompson does a neurological exam, which is also normal, and asks, "Have the teachers filled out any questionnaire forms on his behavior?"

Mom: "I get biweekly grades on him, because he has been doing so poorly. One of his teachers wrote that he didn't turn in four of seven homework assignments. I called the guidance counselor. They don't feel like he has a learning problem. They said that he's just lazy. He's not a dumb child. I don't know. I don't know!"

"Have they done any testing?"

Mom: "I'm told there's nobody available to give him help at school. I was not great in science myself. I was lousy at it. I could never get the important stuff."

"Well," says Dr. Thompson, as he tries to put all of this information together and develop a plan, "it sounds to me that he should have some formal testing to see if there's any evidence of a learning disability, assess his intelligence, and whether or not he has attention deficit disorder. I would try and see if they can do that through the school. You could do it on your own through a place in Johnstown that might be able to get it done faster. But I think there's a mechanism through the schools to see if he's eligible for an individual program. So those are two options. I can even write a note to the school to see if they can do it. There are people who have attention deficit disorder, inattentive types. What are your thoughts on that?"

Mom: "That's good."

"So is there a time set aside for homework?"

Mom: "Well I'm not home when they get home from school. My husband is. Usually, they're right out the door playing with the kids. Then when I get home at 6:00 they have all this homework to do, and then we have to get their showers, and all of that. So it's rushed, and I'm upset. And I'm the bad guy all the time. And I'm harping on him, and sometime I feel like that maybe he's trying to push mom's button."

"Is it hard to find out whether there was homework?"

Mom: "It was, but now I can go on the computer and download their work."

"Well one suggestion is maybe they need a brief time when they come home from school to have a snack and play a little. But then from say 4:30 to 6:30 it should be set aside as time to do homework. And not watch TV and talk on the phone during that time. And get that set up everyday. Then after 6:30, they can eat, and then watch TV and talk on the phone."

Hearing this, the mother turns toward her son and says, "See, I'm not the only bad guy."

"I'd keep that time for homework only."

Looking again at her son, the boy's mother says, "Doctors orders." Then, she turns back to Dr. Thompson, and says, "He says I'm just the worst mom in the world. And I tell him that when I was little, I had two brothers to look after. And my mom, if she found out you were on the phone, you were spanked. He's not a bad kid, I just can't get it in his head that school's very important."

Dr. Thompson then hands a note to the mother and says, "Here, give this to the school, if it's helpful. If that doesn't help, get back with me. As far as his legs go, we should do an X-ray, and get some blood tests to do a blood count and a thyroid test. What does he take for the pain?"

"Tylenol usually helps," the mother answers.

"Does he get tired easily?"

"Not really."

"The nurse will give you the papers to get these things done," Dr. Thompson continues, "and I'll get you the name of the place in Johnstown to get him tested. And I would check in regarding a tutor. Saying he's lazy isn't real helpful. And let's talk in a week."

Mom: "Thank you."

Next, Dr. Thompson sees a 58-year-old woman with a rash under her breasts and prescribes an antifungal cream. The next patient is a 61-year-old woman who works at the local ski resort as a cashier. She has arthritis and high blood pressure, and was recently in the hospital for her gallbladder. Then, a 46-year-old woman with a history of alcoholism and depression comes in for a checkup. She is in counseling and on medication, and is doing a little better. Following that, two twin infant girls are brought in by their mother and grandmother for well child checkups. Both babies are doing well, and there are no problems reported. Dr. Thompson discusses their diet, their development (and did a Denver Development Screening Test, which was normal), and plots their height, weight, and head circumference on the preprinted growth charts for normal children. He does a 'lap exam,' examining one baby on her mother's lap, the other on her grandmom's. Then, after declaring them both in excellent health, his nurse gives each their third (and last) hepatitis B immunization.

The next patient is a 42-year-old man from a neighboring town who hurt his leg in a skiing accident a year ago. He has chronic pain and hasn't been able to work, and now has become depressed. The orthopedist doesn't think an operation will help, and physical therapy hasn't helped much. The man's sister just had a baby, who Dr. Thompson cares for. Then he sees a healthy 11-year-old boy who is here for a summer camp physical.

The patient in the next room is an 88-year-old woman with a long list of medical problems on her chart. With gray, thinning hair and glasses, she has a small green oxygen tank on wheels sitting next to her, connected to plastic tubing that fits around her ears and into her nostrils.

"The nurse told me that you're having chest pain," Dr. Thompson begins.

"It's over on the side."

"When did you start noticing it?"

"This morning."

"Have you been having more trouble with your breathing?"

"Not anymore than I usually do."

Dr. Thompson listens to her heart with his stethoscope, then says, "Your heart rate is good."

Pointing to a small black and blue mark on the back of her hand, she asks him, "Why do I get so many of these?"

Dr. Thompson examines the small bruise, and says, "As you get older, your skin gets thinner and easy to bruise."

She smiles and says, "Yeah, but I'm not that old."

"Not yet . . ."

"My brother's older."

Dr. Thompson takes her blood pressure. "Your blood pressure is perfect— 130 over 80."

"Yeah, my brother will be ninety soon," the woman continues.

"I know. He goes to my church. He and his son like to travel a lot. Show me where it hurts."

Pointing to an area to the left of her breast, near the corner of her under-arm, she says, "In here."

Dr. Thompson listens to her back. "Take a big breath." Then he pushes in the center of her chest. "If I push there is it sore?"

"No, it doesn't seem sore."

Examining her ankles, Dr. Thompson says, "Your legs haven't had much swelling."

"Yeah, they've been pretty good."

"OK, I want to have you lie back. How are your bowel movements?"

"Well, they're pretty good since I took that stuff you prescribed."

"What does this pain feel like to you?"

"Like a muscle stretch."

"Does it make you short of breath?"

"No, it hurts mostly when I move."

"OK, I'm going to ask the nurse to come in and do an EKG."

After the nurse completes the EKG, Dr. Thompson comes back in the room and says, "Has the pain been pretty constant today, or does it come and go?"

"Well it just depends what I do. It hurts if I twist or something. Sitting here right now, I don't have any."

Looking at the EKG, Dr. Thompson says, "Well, the EKG looks about the same for you, but it's hard to know for sure. Your pacemaker kind of interferes with it. It sounds to me very much that this pain is not from your heart. It sounds, like you said, like muscle strain or cartilage pain. Have you done any pushing, pulling, or heavy lifting lately?"

"No, but maybe it's the way I lay in bed, too. It wouldn't be a collapsed lung would it? One time I did have a collapsed lung."

"No. But I think we should get a chest X-ray and get some blood tests just to check your heart enzymes. Would you be able to go to the hospital to get these tests today?"

"OK."

"OK. Do you have a heating pad?"

"Yes."

"What do you take for pain?"

"Tylenol. I take two every night."

"Well, try the heating pad, and take two Tylenol when you get home and again tonight. If this isn't getting better, let me know. We should have results on your tests within a day. If there is a problem, they'll let me know right away."

• • • • •

Bill sees patients in the office four days most weeks. Unless he's on call for the hospital, he takes Wednesdays off. Usually, he sees about 20 people a day in the office. In addition to their office in Boswell, Bill and his partners also have an office in Stoystown, another small town nearby, though a totally separate community. They have two PA's in their practice, one in each office. All the physicians in the group practice in each office, with Bill spending more time in the Boswell office, since he lives there.

To keep up with the changes in medicine, Bill listens regularly to audio tapes of medical lectures and also goes to formal conferences periodically. This year, he is going to go through the family practice recertification process, and therefore must have completed at least 300 hours of formal continuing medical education over the past seven years, as well as passing the written examination from the American Board of Family Practice in order to continue to be a Board Certified Family Physician.

Recently, Dr. deVries—who had also served as a past president of the Pennsylvania Academy of Family Physicians a number of years ago—decided to cut back and work part time. So Bill and one other physician are now half owners of Medical Associates of Boswell, and have two other physicians that also work in the practice. Like many physicians, Bill feels that the business aspects of practice are the least enjoyable. Nevertheless, "I could have joined a larger group from the start, or been bought by the hospital or others, but we've chosen to remain independent and be our own bosses, so we can do things the way we want to do them. But that also means we're the people responsible for personnel and other business decisions. We do have an office manager and she's very helpful. The cost of malpractice insurance is a big problem, and there are times when managed care won't cover tests or hospitalization."

• • • • •

As far as income, Bill says, "Compensation is slightly less than in a suburban or urban area, but the cost of living is considerably less here. So those things probably balance out." Then, discussing his own situation, Bill says, "I also need to add a caveat: I'm slower than most doctors and so my productivity is below average, and my income is related to that. Considering that, we're still comfortable. We're certainly in the upper ten percent of people living in town. And we're a one-income family, as Kathy is not currently getting a significant salary for her work. So family doctors in rural areas can certainly make an adequate living."

As for his nonmedical interests, Bill says, "This year, I've been able to do a lot of skiing. I'm a physician advisor for the Laurel Mountain Ski Patrol and I'm also on the Ski Patrol, so I get a family season pass. Skiing is something I've enjoyed ever since we moved out here when I was 10, and started taking lessons. And I've gotten back into it after we moved back and now that the kids are old enough to do it. The boys are snowboarding, our daughter is skiing, and my wife has also learned to ski recently. So it's a family event that we all can do, and that's been fun. We also like to go tent camping in the summers. We're involved with the church. And, my sons wanted a halfpipe for skateboarding, so we've just started to build that in our garage."

SELINSGROVE, PENNSYLVANIA

> It's the humdrum, day-in, day-out, everyday work that is the real
> satisfaction of the practice of medicine; the million and a half
> patients a man has seen on his daily visits over a forty-year pe-
> riod of weekdays and Sundays that make up his life. I have never
> had a money practice; it would have been impossible for me. But
> the actual calling on people, at all times and all conditions, the
> coming to grips with the intimate conditions of their lives, when
> they were born, when they were dying, watching them die,
> watching them get well when they were ill, has always absorbed
> me.
>
> —William Carlos Williams, MD

When Christine Dotterer talks about how rural family medicine differs from
practice in a city, she says, "I live with the people that I have my professional
relationships with. I see my patients when I go to Wal-Mart. You walk down
the street and you see them. Anywhere you go, you see your patients. When
we walked into the restaurant last night, that couple we said hello to—I know
both of them thought, 'What's on my plate?' because I know they're both
trying to watch their weight, and I've talked about lipids with them. You go
to the grocery store and you run into your patients, and either they turn in
the other direction, or they walk up to you and say 'Look what I have in my
cart.' And, there's just this honor, that people let you into the most important—either painful, deeply felt, or sometimes the happiest—parts of their
lives. To be allowed into that is really something. And when you have that,
and you see these people on a nonprofessional basis every day—it's just a
wholeness. I don't know how else to say it.

"You know, I really like Lowe's—you can see my construction projects at
home. So you go and are trying to decide which piece of lumber you're going
to get, and you see your patient. And they ask you what you're up to, and
you tell them about your project, and they tell you about their project. Actually, when I was buying some heavy lumber to put up a trellis right by the
deck for the vines to go up, I had stopped on my way home from work, and
had on a dress and all that. And I'm about ready to get a guy from the store

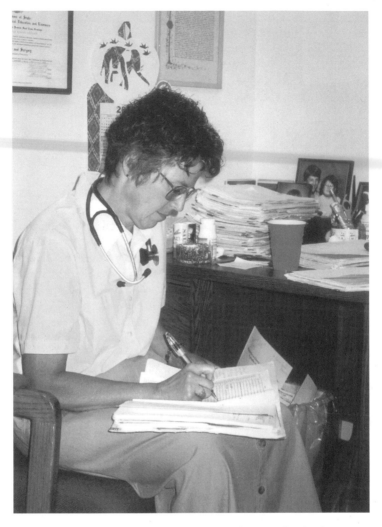

Dr. Chris Dotterer in her office, completing a patient's chart.

to help me load it, and one of my patients comes up and says, 'Hey, can I lift that for you?' I mean these are just little interactions, but it just . . . makes you feel like you're living in a world with people you know.

"So, in a small town, the connections—they get tighter and tighter, in a pretty nice way. And I've been practicing here for twenty years now. You know who's related to whom, and honestly taking a family history usually isn't necessary. I frequently know more about their family history than they do! A patient may say 'There's something wrong with my mother's heart.' But I often know the details, the exact diagnosis.

"And not only do I see patients in restaurants and the grocery store, but there's often a kind of 'mutuality,' for want of a better word. When I take my dog to the vet, one of the vets is my patient, and the family of another vet are patients. When I go to Lowe's, often one of my patients is at the checkout. When I had knee surgery, many of the nurses who took care of me are my patients. A couple of my kids' teachers were patients. So, not only do I take care of all these people in my job, but they take care of me in their jobs. I walk down the street, and I can't walk a block without seeing at least one and probably several people I know. It's just nice. There's just a real connectedness."

· · · · ·

Chris Dotterer was born in Cleveland, Ohio, and moved to Belgium when she was two years old. "We lived there for a year because my dad was a consultant in electrical engineering," she explains. "My enduring childhood regret was that my parents shielded me from learning French because they didn't want to confuse my language development. I was so annoyed—I'm sure that was why I became a French major in college. I really have no memories of being in Belgium, alas." Chris really grew up in a suburb of Pittsburgh, where she lived from the time she was three until she went to college. Before her mother had married, she had worked in one of the labs that Dr. Jonas Salk (of polio fame) was associated with, and her mother's older brother was a rural GP. But Chris's uncle "practiced an hour and a half away, so we didn't see him for medical care, although we went to visit a lot. After I graduated from medical school, my brother told me that Mom had wanted to be a doctor, and her brother had told her that she couldn't because women didn't do that. She never told me that. When I decided to go to medical school, she was not very happy about it. You know, I had a three-year-old and she was concerned about whether it would be fair to him. But she's proud of me now.

"Growing up," Chris continues, "I loved being in the country. I spent my summers at the family cabin along the Delaware River in northern New Jersey. My grandmother's father bought a lot of land in 1920 for a hunting camp, and they spent their whole summers there when my dad was growing up. It was a big farm and really rural, and you didn't wear shoes all summer. I loved it. I loved just checking stuff out. You know, like going in the river and getting mussel shells, and opening them up and seeing what's inside. And walking in the cornfields, looking at corn smut, figuring out what it is. When corn stalks are growing," Chris explains, "there's a fungus that gets big and black and yucky, usually on the base of the ear. And helping my grandmother in the garden. And looking at birds—my grandmother was a great birder. She taught me a lot about birds."

When she was a child, it never occurred to Chris that a woman could be a doctor. "It's really funny when you think back over these things," she recalls. "I have this vivid memory in first grade—we were supposed to draw a picture of what we wanted to be when we grew up. And the boys had all these choices, and the girls had—like, Jeez, I can be a nurse or a teacher. What if I don't want to be either one of those? I'm thinking, well, I guess I better pick one of them."

Chris went to college at Bucknell University, where her grandparents had met, and where her father, his brothers, all their wives, and some cousins all went. "I didn't have a choice, honestly," she says, laughing. "But Lewisburg was nice—and rural." She started out as a French major, possibly thinking she might be a teacher. Then, she ended up as a psychology major. "I think probably, like a lot of people who become psych majors, they do it because they wanted to figure out what makes themselves tick. And, I had some vague thoughts about going to graduate school and becoming a psychologist. Then, I got married my senior year. My first husband went to Bucknell, and he went to graduate school at Columbia University, so pretty much I was going to go where he went. We were in New York for two years, and I worked as a social work aide for the Brooklyn Bureau of Community Services. It was a private agency, and I coordinated services for sixteen foster children, and provided counseling for the kids and their families."

It was there that Chris encountered a woman physician for the first time in her life. "It was when I first took one of the foster kids to the doctor," she says. "I took a four-year-old child for a neurological exam at Long Island College Hospital. The physician asked me all these questions, you know, 'How old was he?', 'When he walked?', 'How old was he when he talked?' And I said, 'I don't know, I'm his case worker. I've only known him for about three months.' She was clearly frustrated, and so I said, 'Look, I'm sure there's a lot of stuff we clearly should be bringing to you, but we don't know what it is. Tell me what it is.' So, she and I sat down, and she told me what she wanted to know for his developmental history. And I went back, and talked it over with my supervisor. And I made up a form that, before we took any kids for neurological exams, we had to get the answers from the foster parents, or whoever—answer as many of these things that we could. And in the process, I started to get excited about medicine. I thought, 'This is what I want to do!' I wanted to take care of people, help them get better. And the intellectual stimulation was a real big thing, you know, figuring out how to get information and come up with answers. It's really cool."

But Chris didn't have any of the required courses for medical school, since she was a liberal arts major in college. "I studiously avoided sciences. So I went to talk to the people at Columbia and told them what I wanted to do. And they told me, 'OK, the first year you need to take physics and organic chemistry and math, and continue working full time, and get straight A's—and then you can get into medical school.' And I was just so overwhelmed, I said to my husband, 'Let's have a baby!' " Laughing, she continues, "So we did. But even during the pregnancy I thought, 'You know, we're going to be moving out of New York, and I'm not giving up on this dream. I don't think that having a baby is going to make it impossible to do.' "

When her husband got a job at Susquehanna University and they moved to the Selinsgrove area, Chris took her pre-medical courses at Bucknell and

Susquehanna. She also got a job as a social worker at the Selinsgrove Center for the Retarded, a residential unit, working with the highest functioning women, and doing group counseling. And, she applied to medical school.

"I was generalist oriented even then," she says. "I was not interested in being narrowly focused. You know my uncle, even though I don't remember if I talked to him, I saw what he did. He was really a revered person in his town. And, you could tell he loved what he did." What Chris wrote on her medical school application was "I anticipate that as a physician, I will concentrate in a primary care area." And she remembers her interview at another medical school. "When I told the interviewer that I was interested in primary care, he said, 'So you'll see people and decide which specialist they need to see?' And I said, 'NO! I'll see people and take care of them, and *if* they need a specialist, then I'll send them.'"

As far as where she planned to practice, Chris says that "at that point it was, 'I'll follow my husband.' I hated New York the first couple of months—it was just horrible. And then, I got to like living there. But I couldn't imagine raising a kid there or living there forever. And we liked small universities. We liked living in this area a lot." So, although Chris had grown up in a suburban area—the only one of the ten doctors in this book (and one of the few in the PSAP) who did not grow up rural—she qualified for the PSAP because she had lived in the small rural town of Selinsgrove for three years. She knew what it was like to live there as an adult, and wanted to live and practice family medicine there. And she did. "Although I grew up in the suburbs," she says, "my family is from the area around here. My fifth great grandfather settled in Snyder County (where Selinsgrove is located) in the mid 1700s. They were all from around here. My grandfather grew up here, and graduated from a one-room schoolhouse, and then the next year he taught at that schoolhouse. Then he decided to walk from Milton to Bucknell with fifty dollars in his pocket, and said he wanted to go to college—and he became an electrical engineer. So, I kind of felt like I was coming back home. I still have a lot of relatives around here."

● ● ● ● ●

Chris entered Jefferson in 1975, the second class of PSAP students. But she describes medical school as being a very different experience than most of her peers. During her first two years, she lived in Philadelphia with her preschool-aged son, Seth, while her husband stayed in Selinsgrove. "Seth was at the Salvation Army Day Care Center," she remembers fondly. "They were wonderful. It was really funny, within two weeks I went from *being* a social worker to *having* a social worker. Because everybody there had to have a social worker. That was really bizarre. I'd talk to my social worker some about Seth, and then we'd talk social work. But they were just wonderful to us. I'd take him down there in the morning and pick him up around 5:00 PM. And I made a rule that from when I picked him up till when he went to bed, around 8:30 PM or so, that was his time. And it didn't matter if I had two tests the next day, or whatever, that was the time for him. And it was really good for me to be able to do that and have that time together. Then I'd put him to bed, and—you know my classmates would go out to Doc Watson's and have a couple beers. But you don't do that when you have a kid in bed at home—so I'd study hard then. It really disciplined my study habits. People would say 'How can you do that with a kid?' But in a lot of ways, I had more time."

During her freshman year, she and Seth usually went home to Selinsgrove three weekends out of four. "Coming back, we'd take the bus to Harrisburg, and the train from Harrisburg to Philly—which was just a big ordeal. I'd get into the train station at midnight with a sleeping three-year-old and a suitcase." As for medical school itself, "I realized the importance of the first two years—that it was laying groundwork. But I was anxious to get to the clinical work. When I was doing my rotations as a third and fourth year student, I loved everything I did. At one point I was really thinking about doing ob-gyn. It was in my third year and I was having a wonderful time delivering babies. Boy, I'm glad I didn't do that. But really, after every rotation, I'd think 'I can't give this up.' 'I can't give up dermatology,' 'I can't give up pediatrics,' 'I can't give up OB,' 'I can't give up seeing old people.' So, there was only one way to get all that—family practice! During my fourth year, I spent three months at Geisinger [the Geisinger Health System, in Danville, Pennsylvania, a large rural hospital and health care system originally modeled after the Mayo Clinic], which is about a half hour away from Selinsgrove. So I was living up here, which helped a lot, because during the last two years of med school, Seth was living up here with his dad."

Chris also took her family practice residency at Geisinger, which was the only hospital she applied to. "When I was an intern, I had a patient who helped break ground for Geisinger Hospital using a horse and plow. Now, you can get there by helicopter. It was exciting, but it was difficult. During residency, you felt like you were really learning something, getting somewhere—but there were some real rough moments. Through residency, my plans were to stay around here. I got pregnant with Kate in my second year, and she was born during the middle of my third year." Chris took night call twice as often during the first half of the year, so that she wouldn't have to work any nights after Kate was born. "That was really hard. During the day, I took her to a babysitter, and the days I was in clinic and could take a half hour or forty-five minutes for lunch, I'd go over and nurse her."

• • • • •

After residency, Chris joined a local family practitioner who practiced in Sunbury, the town just across the Susquehanna River from Selinsgrove—and where the hospital is located. She started out working half-time. "That was really nice," she recalls. "You feel like you're raising your own kids *and* you've got intellectual stimulation." Over the next few years, she gradually increased the amount of time she worked, and then in 1986, she decided to open up her own office in Selinsgrove, where she still practices. "I was tired of being employed by anybody, honestly. I wanted to do things my way." Just recently, when her own parents decided to move into a smaller place and get rid of things from their house, "my mother had a book about my grandfather: the official history of the 315th regimen in World War I. So I was reading it. Some of the narratives were interesting, and I took a look down at the list of names—I don't know why—and I saw that the chief medical officer was Dr. Elliott Griffen. That was my first partner's grandfather—and he was also my patient for the last couple years of his life. And I thought, my God, here he was in the same regimen as my own grandfather, who was a second lieutenant. What a small world! And both grandchildren were in practice together."

When she started her own practice, "I came in with a fair number of patients from Sunbury. But soon after I opened up, two local doctors had died and one had a stroke. So, six months after I was here, I wasn't accepting new patients, which is pretty amazing. At first I said I'll take new family members, but pretty soon you realize that everybody's related to somebody. So then I narrowed it down to 'family members living in the same household.' The way I looked at it, there's two ways to make sure you have a life. One of them is to get partners, join a group, whatever. The other is to limit how many people you see. But when I was on call with the other family doctor I was in practice with, I'd get phone calls from his patients, people I didn't know, which is standard on call procedure for everybody. But with my own patients, I knew them. My more seriously ill patients, I know their medicines. Now, if I get paged at home, I don't need to look it up on the computer, I know what medicines they take. I mean that's just the way it is. And I just decided I would much rather be on call all the time for my own patients. One of the real nice things about having a closed practice is you know everybody pretty well."

• • • • •

Chris's office is on the first floor of a three-story blue building on the wide, tree-lined main street in Selinsgrove. Her first patient of the day is a 62-year-old man with hip pain. He also has high blood pressure, diabetes, and recently had surgery for his gallbladder. As Chris enters the room, she greets him, and says, "The nurse said your hip's hurting you."

"Well, I don't know about my hip. I think a Mack Truck run over me!"

Exuding warmth and caring when she speaks, Dr. Dotterer quietly asks, "How's that?"

"Well the pain just goes from one spot to another. It's mostly in this hip, and I was using a cane, but I forgot to bring it. It just came on all of a sudden—I just couldn't get out of bed. I tried to roll around, and carried on, till I got myself out. Boy it was terrible pain."

"And this was about a week ago?"

"Uh-huh. Thursday, and I knew you weren't in."

"You know we're in on the evening Thursday."

"Yeah, but I didn't want to bother you in the evening. I almost called because . . ."

"You know you can come here in the evening."

"Yeah, but that's for people who can't get here in the daytime."

"Or people who get sick that day."

"Well, I was sick, I'm telling you."

"I know you were. Yes. Is it any better?"

"Well, I got up yesterday morning and I could walk. Today I can walk, but I still have that pain."

"Stand up and show me where it is."

Getting up slowly, the man grimaces, saying "Ooh!"

"It looks like you're hurting."

Pointing to his hip, he says, "Well, it was mostly right here."

"Did it go down your leg?"

"No."

"Good. Why don't you get up here on the table?"

"I'll try."

"Here, lean on me."

"I don't want to hurt you."

After the patient gets up on the table, Dr. Dotterer takes out her rubber tipped reflex hammer and says, "Let me check your reflexes."

"You gonna hammer me?"

Laughing, Dr. Dotterer replies, "Yeah, I'm gonna hammer you." Then, moving the man's leg, she asks, "Does that hurt?"

"No, not now. But I couldn't have done that the other day though."

"You're getting better then?"

"Yeah, I'm getting better, but I didn't know what to do the other day. I rubbed some cream on it, and then I felt worse. So then I had some—what is it called—it's green and it's a gel. It's for something like that—my neighbor told me. And I put that on. It helped before, but boy, it didn't help this time. So I didn't put anything on, and I didn't put any heat on it—or cold."

"Did you take any Advil or Tylenol or anything?"

"I did take Advil. Then I found those pills I got when I was operated on. You know, that . . ."

"Darvocet? Or Percocet?"

"So I've been taking them."

"Which ones? Darvocet?"

"Yeah, but it has both names on it. I got it back when I had the operation. I didn't know anything about pain then, but boy I know it this time. I tell you I almost came down, but I wasn't sure I could make it."

"OK," Dr. Dotterer continues. "How's the rest of you? How's your breathing?"

"It's all right. I don't bother about that, as long as I can get going." Then, the man laughs and says, "And I jammed the paring knife in my bad hand, but it's almost healed over—where my dog had bitten me."

When the patient mentions his dog, it reminds Chris of their common interest in animals, so she says, "I have a story to tell you about Will, my youngest dog. He got in a fight with something over the weekend."

"A skunk?"

"I don't know what it was."

"Will?"

"Yeah, Will, the baby."

"That's the little one. Up at the barber shop where I go, they have one like your other one. Yeah, I'd really like to take him home with me." Then he laughs again, and says, "I don't know what my other dog at home would do though."

"Is your dog behaving himself?"

"Pretty good. He gets a wild streak every now and then."

"Has he bit you again?"

"No."

"Good." Then Dr. Dotterer listens to the man's back and says, "OK, breathe."

"He better not, he'll get his block knocked off."

Listening to his heart, Dr. Dotterer continues, "Breathe normally now."

Looking at the wall of the office, the man says, "I love that picture there on the wall, that little boy and girl."

"That picture? Do you know the story of that? Did you know John Louis?"

"Yes."

"His wife painted that. She was a pretty good artist. She had cancer. And when she was dying, I was making house calls on her. And after she died, John came down and brought this. He said that she lined up all her pictures, and told him which ones she wanted to go to whom."

"He was a nice fellow. I worked with him a long time. He died now, too."

"Yep. He was in his nineties."

"When I first started working, he was one of my bosses. Nice guy. What was his wife's name? Blanche?"

"Betty. Are you watching your sweets?"

"Yeah, watching them go down," he answers, laughing.

"You've lost what, ten to fifteen pounds over the past couple of . . ."

"Almost thirty there for a while."

"That's good."

"I see you got a new scale in the office."

"Well, my nurse isn't sure she likes it," Chris responds. "She thinks it weighs a pound heavier than the other one."

"Oh well, what's a pound."

"That's a good attitude."

Then, after examining his hip, and finding no indication of a more serious problem, Dr. Dotterer says, "For your hip . . . are you using the cane?"

"The cane? Yeah, most of the time. But I didn't bring it along today, I forgot it. I put it by the sofa, and I walked out without it. 'Cause I could walk pretty good."

"Well, I want you to take it easy. OK?"

"What should I take for the pain?"

"Is the pain pill you have from your surgery a capsule or a tablet?"

"It's white. No, it's not filled with anything. It's solid."

"Listen, if you need more of it when you get home, call in and tell us what the name of it is . . ."

"Well, I probably do need more. I didn't take any today yet, 'cause I was coming down here."

"Well, it depends what it is. I need to see if it's safe for you to take for very long."

"Well, I told you it's one of those . . . what were those names? I think it was Darvocet N."

"Percocet was the other. But those are two different things."

"It was the one with an N, and it had 100."

"Darvocet N-100. OK. Do you want some more of that?"

"Yeah."

"OK. That I can give you. I just didn't want to give you something that might make you unsteady."

"Well, there are times that I get unsteady, staggering around like I was drinking. I think I'm going to start drinking and enjoy life." Then laughing, he continues, "Or I could pass out over there and die and nobody'd know it."

"Your sister would."

"When I call her sometime, she can't hear me on the telephone."

"Really?"

"But she comes over every day to check on me. Yep, she does. She said, 'You ought to leave your door open at night.' And I said, 'No, I might get a bill that I don't want.'" The patient laughs as he tells this joke.

"Does she have a key?"

"Well, she does. She said the neighbor next door said he'd come over and help me. I should have taken him up on it."

"Well, give him a key."

"I've been thinking about it. I said to her, 'I think I'll get a key made and give it to them, because they're such nice people.' And I know he would help me. You never know when you're going to fall or something."

Then, getting off the table he grimaces again and says, "Right now my pain is flying back there."

"Well, I think it's getting better now. You know, I would try using a heating pad on that."

"I didn't know whether to use heat or cold."

"Try using the heat."

"After the creams didn't help, I thought I'm not putting that on yet."

"Just don't put the heating pad on top of the cream."

"No, I know that."

"Alrighty."

"Well, have a good day. Thank you."

After seeing each patient, Chris circles around the back of the office and settles into the open space on the other side, where her desk is. She sits at her desk, stethoscope draped around her neck, and writes a note in the patient's chart.

The next patient is an older man in his 90s who is here to get his diabetes and arthritis checked. "He's the last surviving member of his group of friends," Chris explains. "And he's been a good friend and almost caretaker for several of them, all of whom have been patients of mine. And it's really sort of sad watching. Some of them worked for the university, so I knew all of these people, even before I went to medical school. I have a number of patients that I've known for thirty years. So it's just . . . sort of sad watching him. A couple of them have had cancer, one died from a heart attack, the last one died from a stroke. And I go to those funerals. The people that I knew before I went to med school, I go to their funerals, because you know, I know them in so many different ways. I always feel a little bit funny. Not guilty, because I felt I took great care of him. I made house calls, everything. I went to the funeral, but sometimes I wonder if people are looking at me, thinking 'Well, you were his doctor, and he died.' "

The next patient is a six-year-old boy with asthma, who is here for a checkup with his mother.

Mom: "Hello, there."

Dr. Dotterer first asks the child, "How are you doing?" Then she turns to his mother and asks, "OK, so you're here today to talk about his breathing. So how's it been?"

Mom: "It's been a lot better. He hasn't been sick."

"Has he been sick at all?"

Mom: "He had a cold. Whenever he starts to get sick at all, we've done the nebulizer. And he does do the spacer thing at least once a day."

The boy interrupts and also answers, "Well, I haven't been sick. Usually when I get sick, I stop breathing."

Dr. Dotterer continues, explaining, "I'm just going to plot him on the growth chart here. He's perfect."

Mom: "What height and weight range is he?"

"Fortieth percent for weight and twenty-fifth percent for height." Then, noting a raw area on the boy's knees, Dr. Dotterer asks him, "How did you get your brush burns?"

"I fell at the playground."

"I'm going to check your ears now. The bad news is you need a flu shot again this year. The good news is you just need one."

Mom: "When do we get that?"

"Whenever we get them in. October is usually when you're supposed to get them."

The boy asks, "Do I have to get a flu shot again?"

"Yeah. You know what they're working on, though? They're trying to make a flu shot that's not a shot. It goes into your nose."

"So you just sniff it?"

"Yes."

"Will it hurt?"

"No, it doesn't hurt. It's just a nose spray."

"So all you have to do is go like that [sniffs]?"

"Yeah. They're working on it. They didn't get it made yet. But they're working on it."

"OK, I want to take that."

His mother and Dr. Dotterer both laugh. Then Chris says, "OK. Do you want to go out and play for a little? Or stay with mom?"

"Do I have to take a flu shot?"

"Not today."

Mom: "OK, so we can stop doing the spacer thing. And we'll start up again when he turns seven. And get a flu shot."

"Or, if in a few weeks he's wheezing again, then start it up again—and call and let me know."

"OK."

"Anything else?"

The boy responds, "Yes, I don't want to get a flu shot!"

"OK, you don't need one today. I'm going to see your sister in the other room now."

Then the mother turns to her son and says, "Why don't you go out in the waiting room and play now."

And Chris then goes to the next room with the mother to see the patient's ten-year-old sister, who is here for her yearly checkup.

• • • • •

Chris was divorced from her first husband in 1988. Becoming more serious and pensive when talking about it, she says, "Actually he was an abusive husband, and I was a battered wife. It took me a while before I could even acknowledge it and do something about it. One of the things I did after the divorce, as I was learning to deal with it—there's a woman's health fair in Bloomsburg—was to present something on domestic violence for that. So I had to sit down and write something out. The main focus of it was just to say that there are battered women where you don't see them. They're not all poor, uneducated people. In fact, sometimes it's even a little more invisible in people with means. You know, police don't come to their house, and nobody expects it. And I tried to address some of the issues. People say, 'Why doesn't she just leave?' Well, there are lots of real important reasons why. And, I just wanted people to know, so they could see it from the other side. Around the same time, the AMA [American Medical Association] also started to publicize the problem. So I contacted them and said I had an article, and they published it in the *AMA News*. And then they asked me to come out to Chicago to speak at the national AMA convention. There were about 500 people in the audience, and it ended up being picked up by the *Washington Post*. I also spoke at the American Academy of Family Physicians meeting, and the Pennsylvania Medical Society made a video." As to whether it was appropriate to share this information, Chris said, "You can. It was in the *Washington Post*, and I mean, I made a video that the Pennsylvania Medical Society distributed to every county in Pennsylvania, and to other people who asked for it. So at this point I've been real public."

The issue of domestic violence also came up in my interview with Dr. Viola Monaghan. She told me about one of her patients, who is now divorced. "Her experiences helped me to become much more sympathetic to the whole issue of domestic violence," she said, "because I never could understand how somebody could get stuck in a relationship and not just leave it. And then I saw this person—a very beautiful, intelligent, educated woman, who married this man. And he was able to undermine her self-confidence, isolate her from her family, do a lot of things that made it very difficult for her to leave. And as things were escalating—you know it doesn't start off that way—if the behavior was evident the first time you met someone, of course you'd never become involved with them. But that experience made me much more sympathetic, and I could understand it in a way that I had never thought I would be able to. It was a really scary thing for her family—they didn't know what to do. But she's in a really great situation now."

• • • • •

After the divorce, Chris and her children lived in Selinsgrove for five years. She remembers days bringing Kate with her to the hospital when she made rounds. "She would sit at the nurses' station and color, and would have a wonderful time. I would take her back to see a couple of my patients to say hello to them, after I was done with the medical stuff—and they loved it. And she did some nursing home rounds with me. From the word go, she was there. And that was really pretty cool, and you couldn't do that in a big city."

Chris was also on the Selinsgrove Borough Council for five years. "I was a town father! I was only the second woman ever to be elected to the Borough Council. It was fascinating. I learned a whole lot about local government, and how things run. You know, most of the people on council didn't have a college degree, but they knew *Robert's Rules of Order* and followed them very appropriately. As a contrast, at the medical staff meetings nobody had a clue, and everybody was yelling. I thought, 'That is really interesting.' But I helped to get fluoride into Selinsgrove's water. My dentist is the one who suggested it. He said, 'You know you're in a position to do something about this.' So I did. I resigned from council when I got remarried and moved out of the borough."

• • • • •

Chris and her nurses continue to make house calls every so often. "We also drive patients home sometimes," Chris adds. "A few years ago, a woman who I know—she's Mennonite, but she learned how to drive—showed up at my front door at 11:30 at night. Her grandfather was a patient of mine, and she said, 'Would it be all right if I gave my grandfather another water pill?' So I said to myself, 'There's something going on here.' So I asked her some questions, and it sounded to me like he was in pulmonary edema. So I went with her to his trailer—there was no electricity, just a gasoline lamp on the wall. His bedroom was tiny, and he's sitting propped up in bed absolutely gasping! I said, 'You really need to go to the hospital.' And he said, 'No, I'm not worth the money. I'm an old man.' And so I gave him some IV diuretic. I had stopped by the office and grabbed some nitroglycerin patches, and put a couple of them on, and I took an inhaler with me. I thought I'm going to do everything I can, because I had a sense that he wasn't going to go to the hospital. That's what I did, and I gave them some instructions, and he pulled through and lived another couple years. I went to his funeral."

Chris often makes house calls when someone is bedridden or dying. "Once, I took care of a young woman who was dying from breast cancer," she recounts, "and the family asked me if I would come out to the house after she died and pronounce her. She had died at 5:30 in the morning. She lived about five miles down the road, and so I drove out there to pronounce her. I had made a few house calls to see her before, when she was very sick. Those are some of the moments of being let into people's lives that are just irreplaceable."

Chris doesn't do obstetrics, but she does do prenatal care for a few of the Mennonite patients who are delivered by midwives. "I do very limited prenatal care, because they don't want much," she explains. "They come in for that, although they decide how many times they come in. One of the midwives delivers at home. Another one has what is essentially a little maternity hospital in her home. She has a three-bedroom addition to her home. She delivers them, they stay overnight, and she cooks for them. That doesn't happen in Philadelphia.

"I did OB when I first came here and worked with the other family doctor," Chris continues. "After each delivery, I would think, 'This is fantastic, I'm going to do more of this.' But it was a huge time commitment. I remember one of the last deliveries I did: A young woman came into the office, and she was having a headache, her ankles were swollen, her blood pressure was really high. I said 'You really need to be in the hospital.' So she called her husband and her father to come into the office to have me explain to them why she needed to be in the hospital, and she had a seizure right there in front of me. That was really horrible. But, she did well, she's still a patient. And the baby did well. Yeah, he's graduating from high school."

• • • • •

The next patient in the office is a 38-year-old woman with depression. As she enters the room, Dr. Dotterer asks, "So, the antidepressant didn't agree with you?"

"No, it didn't. I should have called you and told you, but I didn't want to waste your time."

"That's OK. How are you doing as far as coping with all this stuff?"

"I'm OK."

"Are you?"

"Getting better."

"You don't sound quite better yet."

"Well, I mean I do a lot of crying all the time, but that's all right. That goes with the territory, I guess."

"Well, a certain amount does, you know, but . . . Are you sleeping?"

"Yes, I did start sleeping pretty good. I wasn't for a long time, but I am now. Yeah, I'm doing pretty good."

"How's your energy?"

"It picked up a lot. I got out in the yard all day yesterday, working and shoveling and planting. I am doing much better."

"So you took this medicine for about three weeks then?"

"I didn't take all of them. I took them for four to five days, and that's when I started getting nauseated, sick to my stomach."

"Oh? Well, it sure sounds like that's not the medicine for you."

"No, but I'm doing good. I am now, I got some energy back."

"Well, that and sleep are pretty important. Well, let's leave you off the medicine for now."

"OK."

"If you feel things are slipping, if you think things are going back to where they were, and you just don't have energy to do anything, just call up."

"OK. I will."

"Looks like when you were here two months ago, that was your regular asthma check."

"Uh-huh."

"And we didn't set up another one, so I'll set you up for a regular asthma checkup."

"OK. I'm sorry to take up your time like this."

"Well, you know what, don't be sorry. Because it's important to see how you're doing."

"I'm glad. You're a good doctor. I love you."

The next patient is a 94-year-old woman with chronic lung disease, diabetes, and most recently severe back pain. She has bad osteoporosis, and has a compression fracture of her vertebrae. "There's not a lot to do for her," Dr. Dotterer explains, "except to try heat and pain medicine." Then, she sees a 28-year-old woman who is in for a repeat pap test. Her last pap test three months ago had some minor abnormalities. Following her is a 24-year-old woman whose face and eyes are extremely swollen and red. She had been picking strawberries yesterday, and there was a man spraying his plants nearby—a likely culprit for her allergic rash.

"This is impressive," Dr. Dotterer exclaims after looking at the woman.

"But this is better than this morning," the woman responds, laughing. "I mean my nose was clear out here."

"Any trouble breathing?"

"No, if I had started with that, I would have gone to the emergency room."

"Good. I'm going to give you some steroid pills."

"OK."

"And cold helps. Use cool compresses."

"I put ice on it last night, and it did help."

"And call that guy and see if you can find out what he was spraying—and call and tell me."

"OK, thanks a lot."

· · · · ·

Before heading to the office each day, Chris stops off at the hospital to pick up her lab reports. She sees about 18 to 20 patients a day in the office, working from 9:00 AM to 5:30 PM for four days a week, and from 4:30 to 8:00 PM on Thursday evenings. "I have about 2,000 active patients," she says. "Most days, about a quarter to a third of our patients are 'same-day' appointments. Anybody who calls up and needs to be seen is seen that day, even if we end up going home at 7:00 PM, which usually doesn't happen. To not do that is just insane to me. Some of the days go longer, some of them end earlier." With weekends off, Chris works about 45 hours a week, all told. "I tell people that's part-time for medicine."

Chris stopped admitting her own patients to Sunbury Hospital in 1993, and today refers all her inpatients to other physicians in the area, something that only 18 percent of family doctors do today. "For two years," she explains, "I was chief of medicine at Sunbury Hospital. But when Dick and I got married nine and a half years ago, we had five teenagers in our house, and only one person getting up and going out at night was enough. [Her husband is also a physician—a cardiologist.] There are some people, especially older people with chronic diseases, or people who are dying, that I wish I was taking care of in the hospital, doing it just my way. I do miss being able to take care of those people in the hospital—although I have more and more people now dying at home in hospice. I make rounds in the nursing home once a month."

Chris chooses to be on call for her patients all the time, but says that this never feels like a burden. "It isn't to me. I'm on call twenty-four hours a day, seven days a week, except when I leave town. And even then, if I'm anywhere in Pennsylvania, I get calls. It's funny, but I don't feel like I'm being harassed. If I go to Philadelphia and have my pager with me, it does *not* feel like a burden. My patients are truly pretty respectful. Some Saturday mornings I get two or three calls, and some I don't get any. You know when patients are calling, it's almost always sensible, or they need to go to the ER and it's clear they need to call and get my authorization. Which is a pain, but I don't need to go in at all."

Chris's office building is owned by the hospital, and there are lab and X-ray facilities on the first floor. There's another family practice group on the second floor, and a parking lot in back. The office has a small waiting room, with a fish tank and paintings on the wall. "I've been here since they opened it up as an office building in 1986," she says as she shows me around the office. "And I was really lucky because they let me design the space. I wanted three exam rooms, a nice bathroom for the patients, and I really like this sort of circular arrangement—I walk around in circles all day long." The three exam rooms are on one side, and on the other side are Chris's open office area—with pictures of her own kids partially hidden by the small stacks of patient charts piled on her desk—and the shelves of charts, the fax, and Xerox machine. Chris runs the office with nurses only—one full-time RN (registered nurse) and one LPN (licensed practical nurse) who are both originally from central Pennsylvania. She likes having highly trained people with good medical knowledge at the front desk, answering the phones, and assessing people in the waiting room.

Walking around the office, Chris points out a picture in the waiting room. "This is a painting of the train station in Sunbury. A local painter did this." Then, pointing to the tiny figures in the painting she continues, "Here's the nurse who works in my office on Thursday night—she's a train buff. There are a lot of people in this picture that we know, they were the models for it. These two people were patients of mine. That's cool—the connections."

"I have more women patients than average," she continues. "But you know, a lot of men have searched me out because I'm a woman. They say they find it easier to talk to a woman doctor, which is sort of interesting. And I take care of some Mennonite families—they don't have insurance. Did you see the hitching post out back? We have a lot of horse and buggy traffic around here. Shortly after I opened up here, I wanted to put a hitching post in the back, but the hospital said 'Oh no, we couldn't possibly do that.' It wasn't even paved in the back, it was dirt. So I had a Mennonite baby in the hospital, and after I discharged him, his parents built a hitching post for me and put it in the back. Then, five years ago, when the hospital paved the back parking lot, they just replaced the hitching post. They didn't even realize the whole story, what had happened." Today, the simple hitching post out back has a sign over it that reads "Horse and Buggy Parking Only."

Throughout the day, the two nurses interrupt Chris with questions about patients who have called, usually already pretty sure of what needs to be done, or providing important information and perspective of their own. A patient with a cough, a child with a fever, a man with high cholesterol who Chris wants to come in for blood tests. Chris says her biggest challenge is keeping up to date, more so in solo practice than in a group where you can consult with your colleagues. "When you're solo," she says, "you learn from the people you refer to. Sometime I'll call up the specialist and talk something over, ask them 'Do you think I need to send this person to you?' or ask them what they would suggest."

Chris has been in practice in this community for more than 20 years—the longest of any of the doctors in this book. And, like all of the doctors I interviewed, she has practiced in the same community for her entire professional career. "When I saw a patient yesterday," she says, "I decided I really needed to take his childhood growth chart and put it somewhere else. He's a father now, his growth chart really doesn't need to be there any longer. And there's a family that lives in Shamokin that I started taking care of [the mother] when I was an intern—her kids come here, and now her grandchildren come here. Makes you feel old sometimes. They travel quite a distance to get here—about thirty-five to forty minutes."

Chris thinks that her practice today is pretty much what she expected she'd be doing when she first decided to be a doctor, and without hesitation, says she'd do it again. She loves the autonomy and independence in her practice. "That's what I want. If I had to either join a group or retire, I'd retire! The reason why I went into solo practice and why I really am dedicated to solo practice, is that I didn't like having to fight to do things in a way that made sense and was caring." Then, reflecting that it might not be as easy to open up a solo practice today as it was 15 years ago, Chris continues, "The big problem would be the billing issues, I think. And coding. Although the kids coming out of residency now know a lot more about coding than I certainly did—or than I probably still do. I mean, you'd have to have somebody do billing for you right from the word go. You'd have to have figured out your coverage arrangements. Mine sort of evolved. But, I love this kind of a life. In 1986, the first four to five months I was in practice I had to get a line of credit from the bank. So for people who already have a lot of debt, that's tricky. And I was also in a situation where I knew I was going to have a lot of patients. So I wasn't worried about sitting there and not having a practice. But, it's doable."

In 1996, Chris was featured on a front page article of the *New York Times*, which focused on graduates of Bucknell University. It told her story: a third-generation Bucknell grad who decided to practice in Selinsgrove because of her family and her roots in central Pennsylvania. She wanted the autonomy of a small town practice, and "wanted to run it with what she thought of as a woman's sensibility." In that article, Chris says, "I talked about being a mother hen to my patients—and I really am. I think for some doctors, this is more of a business. For me, this is what I do, and that's also why it doesn't bother me to be on call 24 hours a day. Because it just feels like these peoples' well being and their lives and their medical issues are my responsibility. And that takes 24 hours a day."

Listening to Chris, it struck me that she is providing a kind of primary care that is very similar to what has recently been called "boutique medicine," one of the newest phenomenon taking place in major metropolitan areas. Here, a small number of primary care physicians, frustrated with feeling that they need to see increasing numbers of patients in less and less time, have decided to provide more personal and time-intensive care to a small number of patients for a large surcharge. These physicians have been reported to charge a yearly fee of a few thousand dollars per person—in addition to their regular fees from insurance and co-pays—in return for total availability to their patients. But unlike these boutique doctors in the city, Chris has made an active decision to practice this more personal brand of medicine at significant reduction in her own income. This also raises the question that if primary care is so important that wealthier individuals are willing to pay a large surcharge for it, why is it that primary care isn't valued more, and why isn't it reimbursed at a higher level?

• • • • •

"Getting a patient seen by specialists around here," explains Chris, "can sometimes be really hard. I pick and choose specialists. Some of it depends on insurance, but some of it just depends on who does a good job. Williamsport's about an hour away, Hershey's about an hour and a half, Lewisburg is a half hour, Sunbury's about 20 minutes, and Danville's about a half hour. Most of the time, I'm able to send people to a specialist that I have a good relationship with, someone I know. I refer about one or two patients a day. Psychiatry is a real problem. I probably see three or four people a day for psych issues. I mean people with depression, schizophrenia, people who are suicidal. And sometimes the soonest appointment you can get for them with a psychiatrist is six weeks or more. I had additional psych training when I spent a year as a registrar [similar to a resident] in London, so I'm able to do a little bit more than some other family doctors."

As regards income, Chris says, "Yeah, you can make a living in a small town. I'm definitely on the lower end of the income scale for physicians, but a lot of that is choices that I made. There are colleagues of mine in this town who make a very good living doing family practice. They may see people faster than I do, charge more, not give cash discounts—but people make choices like that. And I'm on the high end of the nonmedical community. But, oh my God, you can live on a much lower amount in a small town. And a lot of entertainment is either free or inexpensive—like outdoor things. And housing is a whole lot less, and property taxes."

In discussing managed care, Chris says, "The paper work is a problem—it adds about two hours a day to my front desk's day. It ties up our phones, making it harder for people to call in. If my nurse is on hold with an HMO for fifteen minutes to get an authorization for something—which happens—that's fifteen minutes that patients can't get through to us if they need to. You end up writing letters because there's a good reason why somebody can't be on the medicine that's on the formulary, and maybe it works and maybe it doesn't. At times people have to drive down to Hershey to see a specialist in their plan—and for older people, that's a long drive. And they may not drive, which is a big deal.

"Our office and the office upstairs are the only family doctors in the Borough of Selinsgrove," Chris says. "So we take care of a fair proportion of the population of the town, and lots of patients from Sunbury. I think there's probably a family doc shortage, just hearing how long it takes people to get appointments in other places. And, we have people coming up from Liverpool, down along this side of the river. That's about a half hour drive. For a lot of them, it's either coming up here, or going down to Harrisburg. There have been doctors in Liverpool over the years, but they never last."

• • • • •

The next patient in the office is a 64-year-old man with abdominal pain, who had been seen in the hospital ER the night before last. As Dr. Dotterer enters the room, the patient is sitting in a chair, bending slightly to the right with his right hand holding the side of his abdomen.

"Well, Lou. So, you're hurting?"

Grimacing, he says, "Well, I am. But they say there's no real pain."

Looking over the ER report that has just been faxed over to her, Dr. Dotterer says, "Well, let's go back over that. Actually, they didn't say there's nothing wrong with you. They just don't know what's wrong with you. So, why don't you just start and tell me when this started and how it's behaved."

"Well, it started on Friday already of last week. I had a belly ache across the whole lower side. And it would be harder at times than other, and Monday afternoon my wife went up to that sale in Sunbury, and it still hurt me across here. But then till we got home, it was more or less around here, and around my back. And that's where it still is—maybe not quite as hard as it had been, but it's very uncomfortable. I can't cough, it hurts. I can't sneeze, I can, but it hurts."

Very concerned as she listens to what he says, Dr. Dotterer asks, "Does anything else make it worse?"

"Not really."

"Does eating do anything to it?"

"Well, I haven't eaten much. I haven't been very hungry."

"Are you sick to your stomach?"

"I was. And I thought I had to throw up, but then it went away and I didn't have to. That was on Monday. Then we went to bed on Monday night, and I just couldn't lay still at all. Then around 10:00, my wife said we better go to the hospital. And I said 'No.' But by 12:00, I was ready to go."

"And they gave you a shot. Did that help at all?"

"Yeah. They gave me a shot of a pain reliever."

"And I heard you had a CAT scan. That's what I don't have back yet. Did they tell you anything about it? Did it show anything?"

"No, they said everything was normal."

"Were they looking for—a kidney stone?"

"They didn't say. They took blood work, and said everything was normal, so, I asked them a few figures, and all I got was 'It's normal.' "

"Your blood count's OK. Were there other particular ones you wanted to know?"

"Well, I wondered how my good cholesterol was."

"They wouldn't check that. That's not done when you're sick like this. And your kidney tests looked OK. And they didn't see any sign of infection."

"Yeah, well."

"There was some blood in your urine. I think they were probably looking for a kidney stone. And they checked some liver tests. And checked your pancreas. OK. Let me see if I can summarize, and if I have it right. You started with some belly pain here, and then it gets worse, but doesn't go away, and coughing hurts. Now it's just on that side and round the back. Did you ever have your appendix out?"

"No."

"Did you have a fever with this at home at all?"

"Nope. Not that I know of."

"All right, let's see what we come up with. Have a seat."

As the patient slowly gets up onto the exam table, his face reflects the intense pain he is experiencing as he moves. Choking back tears, he says, "You know, you're just the best doctor in the East!"

"Well, thank you. Are you coughing more than usual?"

"No. Just like, you know, in the morning."

Listening to his lungs, Dr. Dotterer asks him to "Breathe."

"Now that's hard to do too."

"So, it hurts when you take a deep breath?"

"Yeah."

Then, tapping on his back with her fist to check the area where his right kidney is, she asks, "Does that hurt?"

Lou jumps, exclaiming, "Whoa—that does!" Then wincing, he says, "Ohhhhh!" Then, he reflects, "You know I went back through my mind—when I was young, before I was married, I had a dose of shingles around there."

"Yeah, this isn't shingles, though."

"It isn't?"

"No. Does it hurt when you pee at all?"

"No." Then, after lying down, Dr. Dotterer pushes on his abdomen and he responds, "Yeah, that's where it hurts."

"OK, I'm going to push down and then let go, and I want you to tell me which one hurts the worst."

"About the same." Then, when she pushes again on his belly, he grimaces. "There. That's the sore spot. Right in there."

"So this was Monday night when you were in the ER? Are you feeling worse now than you were? Or about the same?"

"About the same." Then, his voice wavers and he says, "You know, the compassion you have, Dr. Dotterer. Excuse me. I guess maybe I just strained a muscle. What do you think?"

"I think that's probably unlikely. Let me go out and see if we have the CAT scan report faxed to us yet."

Outside of the exam room, Dr. Dotterer quickly goes and calls up a local surgeon and says, "Hey, I've got somebody I need you to see. He's a 64-year-old man who has a five-day history of abdominal pain, started in the left lower quadrant, but moved to the right. Anorexia. He hasn't vomited, no dysuria, and it's getting worse. No real bowel symptoms except he was at the ER about a day and a half ago, and he had a CAT scan. Loose stools this morning, but he thinks it's probably from his oral contrast. I'm having the CT results faxed over, but it was apparently normal. I think they were looking for a kidney stone—he had some blood in his urine. And he's got some right CVA tenderness. But, he's got very quiet bowel sounds, and pretty significant right lower quadrant tenderness. He's not lost his appendix. His white count was five—a day and a half ago. No fever. No shift. I really don't know what's going on. Except he's really uncomfortable. He's had heart surgery before, but that's been stabile for a while. His name is Lou G. Listen I'll fax some stuff over to you. . . . OK, good. Thanks a lot."

Back in the room, Dr. Dotterer says, "We got your CAT scan report, which doesn't show a whole lot. But there's something going on—it's just not clear what it is. I called Dr. J., the surgeon. Do you know him? We usually have surgeons look at belly pain. So he's going to look at you. I'm copying your stuff. I know you've been all over. But what I'm worried is that sometimes when people have appendicitis, it doesn't act exactly the way you think it should. And that's something that really has to be thought about. OK?"

"Yeah, well. Maybe it'll be better till tomorrow."

"No, he's going to look at you right now. He's going to see you now. Is your wife with you?"

"No."

"Did you drive yourself?"

"Yeah."

"Can you get over there OK?"

"Yeah. Very good—I'll go over. You're the MD."

"Well, I hope he can find out what's wrong, and I hope you feel better."

"Thank you."

Later, after seeing the surgeon, the patient was admitted to the hospital overnight. All the tests for appendicitis, kidney stones, and other problems were normal. Over the next two days, his pain slowly improved, and he went home entirely better, without the doctors ever finding out why he had been sick. Family doctors often find that this happens—that when they can't figure out what the problem is, subspecialists often don't come up with a diagnosis either. As Chris says later, "It just goes to show, you don't always get an answer."

The next patient is a seven-year-old girl, whose left ear has been draining for the past two days. She had a similar problem last month, and went swimming last week against Dr. Dotterer's advice. She also had recurrent ear infections and tubes temporarily placed in her ears as a young child. Dr. Dotterer examines her, and finds a ruptured ear drum with pus draining out. She prescribes antibiotic pills for ten days, as well as antibiotic ear drops. In between patients, Dr. Dotterer receives a phone call about an 86-year-old woman who she used to work with when she was a social worker in town, before she went to medical school. The woman now has dementia and Parkinson's disease, and she is becoming increasingly agitated and needs a change in her medications. She has been in a personal care home for five years, but will likely need to be moved into a nursing home soon.

Then, a 16-year-old boy arrives for a camp physical. After reviewing the form she needs to fill out, Dr. Dotterer remarks, "A ranch camp. That's great. When do you go?"

"July 20."

"OK. Your mom said she's not sure how to fill out this question. How often do you use your allergy medicine?"

"When I need it."

"Any other problems?"

"No."

"Do you do any sports?"

"Soccer."

"You haven't had sports injuries have you?"

"No."

"Are you training this summer?"

"Yeah, I guess. I'm doing some stuff."

"Do you have hiking boots that are broken in?"

"Yeah. The hiking is way back, not that far though. The longest hike is only twelve miles."

"Lie down. Are your knees OK?"

"Tired, but OK. When you work full time on the chicken farm . . ."

"Catching chickens?"

"It's not catching chickens. It's the 'layers.' The chickens lay eggs, and then a machine packs them into a flat (6 × 5, so you get 30 eggs) and then you stack them six high, then you lift them onto a skid. So you're lifting twenty-five pounds—I don't know—300 times a day. So you get a bit of a workout."

"Ever break any?"

"Yeah, a lot of eggs break. We usually get about a twenty-five-gallon bucket a day—just of broken ones."

"What do they do with them?"

"They dump them when they spread manure. It goes in with that."

"OK." Then, Dr. Dotterer hands him his completed form.

"Two thumbs up?"

"Yep. Have a great time at camp."

"Thanks. See you later."

Having seen her last patient of the day, Dr. Dotterer then goes over to her desk to review her charts and to call back the patients who have called in the past two hours. Then, she gets a call from another doctor, trying to coordinate a patient's medicines between hospital discharge, the family doctor, and the cardiologist. There's often miscommunication when patients go from the hospital, to specialists, and back to their family doctor. Then, there's a phone call to the pharmacy to call in a prescription. And finally, a call back to the daughter of a 94-year-old man who had phoned earlier to get the results of some tests that the neurologist had ordered, and the results are not good. Dr. Dotterer tells her that it looks like her father has a large inoperable brain tumor. She suggests that the daughter call the neurologist tomorrow to discuss this further, but that someone in the family should sleep over his house to be with him. The daughter had suspected as much, and was clearly choking back tears, realizing there isn't going to be much to do but try and keep him comfortable. Dr. Dotterer then asks the woman to call back tomorrow after she speaks to the neurologist, and "let me know how I can be of help."

• • • • •

Chris's husband, Dick, is a sub-sub-specialist—he's an echocardiologist, a nuclear cardiologist, and a lipidologist. He grew up in suburban Philadelphia, did his residency at Geisinger Medical Center, and then spent two years working for the NHSC (National Health Service Corps) in the small town of Orbisonia, Pennsylvania before completing his cardiology fellowship. Then he joined the full-time staff at Geisinger, where he's been ever since. Their five children are now all between 20 and 30 years of age—two from Chris's prior marriage, and three from Dick's prior marriage (his first wife died of cancer). Chris relates, "I was on service with him when I was a med student and he was a senior resident, so I knew him back then. Later on, he had heard from somebody at Susquehanna that I had gotten a divorce, and I knew that his wife had died. And we had been friendly referring physicians. Then, a patient of mine had a heart attack while on vacation and needed bypass surgery when he came back. So I called Dick up and asked him to see the man, and we talked a little bit about the patient, and then he said, 'You want to go out to dinner?' And that was that. It was great."

Today, Chris and Dick live out in the country, about ten miles from her office. Two of the kids are living home with them. "I appreciate living out here every day," Chris says, as she looks around her property. "My house is an important part of who I am. We have 40 acres. Our property goes farther than you can see. We rent some of the land to a Mennonite farmer, and he has organic dairy cows, and grows organic alfalfa and clover hay for his cows, so he can sell organic milk.

"My other desire besides being a doctor," Chris says smiling, "was to be a farmer, so I sort of handle it by doing odd little things. I planted an orchard this spring. I have baby pheasant chicks that I hatch in the spring—I have an incubator. I get the eggs at the wild game hatchery south of Sunbury in the Herndon area. They set 50,000 eggs one day a week, every week in the spring. [Setting means putting them into an incubator.] That's a lot. I bought two dozen, but I didn't have a very good hatch. Only ten of them hatched, and two of those died, which is not unusual, so I have eight, which is plenty actually. And then I keep them over the summer, and let them go in the fall. We're in a pheasant protected area. I figure OK, I'll add to the population. And my orchard has seven apple trees, five peach trees, five pears, and four plums. I had an apricot tree before—I need another one. And I have an asparagus bed, and a vegetable garden."

Walking around the house, one hears the constant sound of birds chirping. Chris points out, "That's my purple martin houses. I grew the gourds, then hollowed them out and painted them and made the holes and stuff. You can see a purple martin sitting on one. I've got more gourds started in the garden, and more drying in the basement from last year yet. I'll probably stop with a dozen or so. That green thing out there is my pheasant pen. Once they're big enough I'll put them out there. I built that by hand. Dick helped some, but most of it I did myself. This is my little kitchen garden with basil, and lettuce, and nasturtium. And here are the baby pheasants. They're about two and a half weeks old now. They can be vicious—they can peck each other to death."

Then, walking out toward the barn—an old barn with a stone foundation, red painted boards for walls, and a kayak laying upside down on the side—we pass two of Chris's dogs. Past the barn is a fenced in garden in the midst of a large field, and to the left is a small pond with a dock, bordered in back by a thick grove of trees. "We have three dogs," she says, "Bernese mountain dogs. We have a pond, and they like to swim in the pond. And we swim in it. We stock it with trout sometimes, but no one really fishes in it anymore.

And we have cats. Here's my garden. Those are the gourds, the asparagus, tomatoes, some rhubarb, some honeydew over there. And Brussels sprouts and green peppers. It is fun! There's the barn—we have two riding mowers. And we get deer come around. My daughter has a horse, but she boards it on a farm a few miles away."

Then, heading over to an area of the deck behind the house, she says, "Here's my other hobby—bonsai. This is a hawthorne, an oak, a maple, a crape myrtle, a Japanese elm. I really like the deciduous trees. This is a kumquat. This is a flowering cherry, which is really pretty. These are sycamores. Here's a gardenia. It's fun. I have a greenhouse over there—it's for my bonsai stuff. It's an overwintering cold greenhouse. So it's just to keep things above freezing, 'cause they have to have some dormant time. I don't know how I have the time to do all this. They do require a lot of care, but a lot of this is like, 'whenever you feel like doing it' care. I don't sit down a lot. I have a hard time sitting down, honestly. I like to be on the move."

As to what Chris doesn't like about living rural, she says, "Oh, there's not all the entertainment possibilities. You don't get first-run movies, you can't go to a show. But being near a university helps with that. Both Bucknell and Susquehanna have artist series, and they bring in international orchestras. So you don't get to choose which things to go to, you just go to everything they've chosen for you. But that works out just fine. When I first lived here, the mall wasn't here, so we had to drive to Harrisburg to buy clothes—that was a problem. Now, we hardly ever leave town to go shopping. We don't have a big bookstore here. Recently, we drove out to Elk County to see the elk, and we made a point of stopping by State College to go to the bookstore, and went to an Indian restaurant there. We have some good restaurants here, but certainly not the variety. And we don't have big sports events. We usually go to see the Phillies once a year. It would be nice for Dick if we were closer, he'd go to more games. We leave town every couple of months, and a lot of that is kid related. We'll go and visit them. Or my parents—they still live in Pittsburgh."

As for other activities, Chris says, "We kayak on the river, and take the kayaks when we go on vacation. We used to ski before I tore the ligament in my knee. And, my husband started playing golf a year or two ago. He bought me a set of golf clubs for my birthday recently. He said 'I want you to play golf with me.' It's a bit of fun. I'm not very strong, and I can't hit it very far. But there's a par 3 around, and I'm getting better."

The past two years, Chris has also gone on mission trips to the Dominican Republic. "There's an organization that has a clinic there," she explains. They've developed a hospital, and a school, and they're working pretty hard, but it's a pretty small organization. One of my husband's colleagues is on the board of this organization, and they've been going every year, and they take medical students every year. Actually we don't work in the clinic there, we go out—speaking of access. We take a bus or a truck or whatever an hour and a half out in the countryside and set up shop in a church, which is about the size of my waiting room, and see people. We bring everything we need. All their medicines—we hit up the drug companies here for samples. Each person takes a seventy-pound bag of supplies in addition to one suitcase. Everybody saves plastic peanut butter jars—you can get a whole year's worth of blood pressure medicines in a peanut butter jar!"

• • • • •

The town of Selinsgrove was founded in 1787 by Anthony Selin, who fought in the Revolutionary War with George Washington. It sits on the shore of the Susquehanna River, one of the largest rivers flowing into the Atlantic Ocean. The population of Selinsgrove is 5,383, and the major employer is Susquehanna University. There's also a lot of lot of farming, family-owned businesses, and small manufacturing in the area. Driving along the river, Chris points out the town's "famous fabric inflatable dam over the River. It raises the water level six feet—so the area on the left becomes Lake Augusta in the summer. It's used for recreation."

• • • • •

Although she is aware that most recently trained family physicians enter group practice—in fact fewer than 15 percent enter solo practice or partnerships—Chris clearly believes that "the future of rural practice would be better if there are more people in solo practice or partnerships than if there are big groups. New graduates aren't even told there's an option. I worked for a couple of years for somebody else before I opened up. Going directly from the end of your residency to opening up your own office would be really, really hard. But I think a lot of people ought to keep open the possibility of working for someone for a while, get a couple of years under your belt until you feel comfortable with all these things, and then think about opening up on your own." Then, Chris says something that captures what most of the doctors in this book seemed to express, either verbally or nonverbally, but that one rarely still hears nowadays from today's physicians in metropolitan areas: "I think that medicine is the best way you can have fun, be intellectually challenged, feel like you're really making a difference in people's lives, and feel autonomous. I don't think there's any other job like it!"

It does appear that what Chris Dotterer has carved out for her professional and personal life would be very difficult to do in a city. "So," she says, "somebody who thinks like me needs to come to the country. And this is the kind of care that I think everybody ought to have. So I feel pretty good about what I do. And I enjoy what I do. I'm not immune to all the problems of medicine today. They come and they drive you crazy, but I can set them aside. I probably am more satisfied than most physicians. If I was working for somebody else, I wouldn't be anywhere as satisfied as I am. 'Cause I'd be fighting all these battles that don't make sense. And I can play classical music if I want during my office hours. I have a patient who sings in the Susquehanna Valley Chorale, which is a classical chorale. It's really very good. And she also does solos at weddings and some other events. She came in and told me that the first time she ever heard any classical music was here in my office as a patient. And it got her interested in classical music. That's so neat!"

BLOOMSBURG, PENNSYLVANIA

> The secret of the care of the patient is in caring for the patient.
> —Frances W. Peabody, MD, 1925

> Our product is healing relationships.
> —Donald Berwick, MD, 2002

For Catherine O'Neil, all roads definitely did not lead to Rome. In fact, Rome, Pennsylvania, where she grew up, was only "one street basically—a very, very small town. There are a couple of trailer parks that make up most of the town's population," Catherine explains, "but I doubt that there's more than 500 people in the town. There are mostly farmers outside the town. And kids from my town had to be bused in with kids from five other small towns so that we could actually get enough people to have a decent sized class.

"My mom was a teacher," she continues, "but had to quit when she got pregnant with me because she wasn't allowed to be a teacher and be pregnant in those times. After that, she ran a day care out of our house with about six to eight kids, and I was part of that until I went to kindergarten. And then when I was twelve, she went back for her master's degree and went back into teaching. And she did that until a few years ago—she just recently retired. My dad also was a teacher initially, but then he worked on computers for a while, and ended up working for a rural electric company. He also ran a pizza shop in our small town—it was the only place to get any kind of food without driving fifteen minutes away. I helped with that—I even had to make pizza when I was five, because the help didn't show up."

On the weekends, Catherine would go to her grandparents' fishing cabin, about 15 to 20 minutes from her house. It was on the Susquehanna River near the town of French Asylum (the area where a number of the French nobility went into exile after fleeing the French Revolution, and where Marie Antoinette was planning to come, if she had made it before she was beheaded).

"I spent tons of time at my grandparents' camp," Catherine recalls. "It was neat. It was on a farm. They built this cabin—it had two rooms with bunk beds, and it had a refrigerator and a sink with running water. But there was no toilet, there was an outhouse. And it had a long picnic table that we would all sit at. And in our family, actually half of us are left handed, half of us aren't, so one side would be the lefties, and one side would be the righties. And we would go down every weekend; I mean it would be a regular thing. Friday night my brother and I would go down and normally stay overnight with our grandparents. I would sleep with my grandmother, he with our grandfather, and we would play Yahtzee and pinochle, and go fishing. And I also hunted for about three years—I actually shot two doe." Then smiling, she continues, "But then I realized that you could go shopping, and not have to get up quite as early in the morning and not be cold. So that's when I kind of decided that hunting was a bad idea. But, I still have my shotguns. And I still go fishing out in our little pond, though there's not much to catch there, just little sunfish. Yeah, I fished from when I was probably two—I have pictures of myself with my other grandfather (he was a big fisherman)—all the way up until I was in medical school, when I came up on weekends. Until my grandparents passed away. That was pretty much how we grew up."

Initially, when she was in high school, Catherine wanted to be a special education teacher. But as she headed into her senior year, "my mom kind of discouraged me from that. She thought that since I was good at science and math, I should pick something in that field." So, she decided to become a pharmacist and attend Lock Haven University, which had a joint program with the pharmacy school at Temple University. Although Catherine's parents both went to college at Bloomsburg University—at "Bloom"—as did her brother, "I decided not to."

Catherine did very well at Lock Haven, and in her second year she was accepted at two pharmacy schools. Then, her advisor called her in to his office and asked her why she wanted to be a pharmacist. "And I said, 'I want to help people, and I like science, so it seems like the perfect combination.' I don't know what I thought pharmacy was at that point, but that was my perspective. And he said, 'Well, if you really want to help people, don't you think you might help them more if you were a family doctor? You seem more like the family doctor type than a pharmacist.' Before then, I had never thought about medicine. But I thought, maybe he's right. And I wasn't anxious to leave Lock Haven—I liked it. After visiting pharmacy schools in Philadelphia, the city seemed a little overwhelming. And to be honest, I had a boyfriend at the time too. And I thought, well, a little closer to home might not be so bad."

So over the next few months, she started to think seriously about medicine. "I met with a doctor—she was an internist—and I just remember being so naïve, not having any clue—I didn't even know what an internist was. I thought that all doctors did the same thing. I didn't realize that there were specialties. But actually she was a good person to interview, because she had just had her second baby and was managing to do the full-time doctor, full-

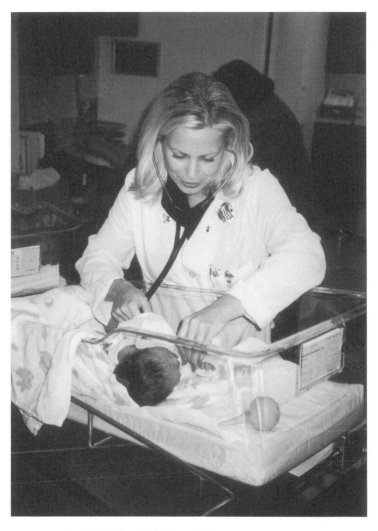

Dr. Catherine O'Neil examining a newborn baby.

time mom scenario, and that seemed to be working OK. I also worked in the skilled nursing unit at the local hospital. I was really interested in geriatrics, and I wanted to see what it was like working with the elderly. And I really enjoyed that. And I also worked at a camp for the severely handicapped, as a sort of a nurse's aide—caring for adults with tubes and things—to see if I could handle that.

"And I talked to my own family doctor," she continues. "He was definitely a big influence. He actually had been a plumber for many years, and then went back to medical school, because they needed a family doctor in the town. And that's what he did. He was in the next town over, since we didn't have a doctor in Rome. He took care of everyone, he really did. He delivered me, and he stayed there for at least twenty years afterward. He farmed too. So he was a farmer, he was the plumber, and our family doctor. And he had the classic typical doctor's office: one little door, one little waiting room, in the back two little exam rooms. He was a great, great man. I talked to him quite a bit when I was making my decision about medicine. I made an appointment for an exam, and asked him a lot of questions about what he liked, if he thought it would be a good idea for me. He said it was the best decision he ever made in his life, and he highly recommended it. He was really very positive about it. And also, my advisor at Lock Haven was very supportive."

Catherine completed her last two years at Lock Haven, and applied to medical school. Her mom was actually the one who first read about the PSAP, and said, "This sounds like you—we're in a small town, and this is a special program for people who want to come back to a small town." "That was my plan," recalls Catherine. "I really didn't have much interest in specialties. I watched my grandparents as they were aging. They did fine when they were with their family doctor. But if they got sicker, and went to the hospital or to the specialist, they felt lost. They weren't quite sure what had happened, the doctors didn't really talk to them, or if they did, it didn't make much sense. And I saw how little confidence and security they felt with these doctors. Well I wanted to be that link, I wanted to be that person to figure out what was going on with them, and be able to explain things, and make them feel comfortable with what was going on. So I really thought I could take care of people like my grandparents all day long. I could just help them, and make them feel better." Catherine's medical school application echoed those aspirations, stating "The desire to help people has always been my goal. I hope to return to a rural area to practice family medicine."

· · · · ·

"To be honest," Catherine says, "I really did not like the first two years of medical school. I had done really well in college, where I worked hard, but not terribly hard. But in medical school, I felt overwhelmed. In med school, there is so much information that you can't even take notes to keep up, so I lost my whole method of studying that I used in college. So I thought the first two years were rough. And, my parents ended up getting divorced my first year of medical school—that wasn't easy, definitely not. But I did fine. You know I didn't get A's all the time, and that was a big adjustment, and I think that happens to a lot of people in medical school. Once I got over that, I was OK. Also, I worked in the Department of Family Medicine in the research assistantship program between the first two years. I worked on a project in a low-income section of Philadelphia, and basically tried to find out why most of the young people there don't use the health care resources that they have. We wrote up our results, and presented them at the Pennsylvania Academy of Family Physicians research meeting.

"And then the clinical rotations were wonderful," she continues. "I loved the second two years. Third year was good—that's when it started being more manageable for me. It wasn't based just on how much I could memorize, but how I could apply it. And that seemed to be something easier for me to do. And there was more people interaction, which is much more my mode than just sitting and studying. Third year family medicine at Latrobe was fantastic—it was good old family medicine. I was thrilled. It was exactly what I was hoping it would be. Sit down, talk to a person, get comfortable, start an interaction, try and get them feeling better, and see them back in a couple weeks, and see that most of the time they actually got better. And I liked getting out to the different hospitals, and seeing what the different specialties were like. I definitely didn't want to do any of them, but I got something out of all of them."

During medical school, Catherine began dating one of her classmates, a young man who planned to become an emergency room physician. They participated in the "couples match" for their residency program, and matched together at Geisinger Medical Center in Danville, Pennsylvania (where Chris Dotterer had also taken her residency training). They got married right before they graduated medical school, but then divorced during her residency. Although this caused some difficult personal times, Catherine felt that her residency training at Geisinger was "a great experience for small town family medicine."

As she was finishing her training and deciding where she wanted to practice, she was concerned about repaying the more than $100,000 in loans that she had taken out during medical school. She had also started to become serious with one of her fellow family practice residents, Chris O'Neil, who was a year behind her. Because Chris had grown up in Bloomsburg and was planning to return to his hometown, and since Catherine also had a cousin and two friends from college in the area, she decided to look for a practice there. So in 1999 she joined Family Care Associates in Bloomsburg, as did Chris the following year. And Catherine and Chris were married in October 2000.

· · · · ·

Family Care Associates—ten minutes from Catherine's home—is a red brick building connected to the back of Bloomsburg Hospital. In small towns, one can almost always find the hospital by looking for the biggest building in town, often near the center of town or up on a hill overlooking the area. Hospitals also serve as a major employer in many small towns.

The first thing in the morning, Catherine goes into the hospital and heads to the newborn nursery, where she washes, gowns, and enters to do a discharge exam on a two-day-old newborn. After learning from the nurse that the baby is doing fine and that her mom is doing really well with nursing the baby, Catherine goes over to the bassinet, unwraps the baby, and examines her. As she begins, the baby starts to cry, and Catherine calms the baby, talking to her. "Hi sweetheart. Hi pumpkin." As the baby settles, she continues, "I bet mommy will be ready to take you. You're going home today—you can check that place out. Yeah, you can."

Then she asks if the nurse's work with the baby has been completed, so that she can take the baby out to her mother. In the mother's room with the baby, Catherine discusses the fact that the baby has a "normal" amount of jaundice (a yellowish color to her skin due to the temporary increase in bilirubin that all newborn babies develop during the first few days of life). She continues, asking the mother, "Is your breast milk coming in yet?"

"I certainly feel like something is coming in."

Dr. O'Neil explains that the baby is perfectly healthy and discusses a number of issues in preparation of taking the baby home, including using a thermometer, when to call the doctor, fever, stools, sleep, feeding, baths, umbilical cord, visitors, air conditioning, and sun protection. "You'll be able to judge," she says reassuringly. "So don't be afraid to give us a call. If something isn't quite right, parents usually know. We'd much rather take a look at her. And try and sleep when she sleeps, it's the most important thing. Things that are dirty will still be dirty when you wake up—you'll get them done. Get friends to help. And don't feel guilty. Do you have any other questions?"

"Not now."

"We'll want you to come into the office with her in two weeks. And congratulations! She's sooo cute. She's great, enjoy her."

"Thank you."

• • • • •

Seeing Catherine as she cares for her patients, it is obvious that she works hard to address their needs—both the ones they express verbally, and those that she senses nonverbally. When patients comment on issues or concerns that some doctors might just let pass, or if they seem anxious about something, Catherine addresses it, tries to find out what's really going on, and reassures them when appropriate. She has a wonderful way of talking with people that seems to almost take away some part of their anxiety. Her calming and reassuring manner and caring attitude actually appears to make patients feel good, so that people visibly feel better when they leave her office.

"I think that's part of the art of being a family doctor," she says. "For specialists, they have the lab, they have the X-ray, they have everything there. They don't have to figure out if this is something that's going to affect this person's life when they walk out the door or not, because they have the information right there to tell you whether to take out the gallbladder, or not." But family doctors have to decide how serious a patient's problem is, and whether or not they need specific treatment, additional tests, consultations with a specialist, hospitalization, or surgery. And at the same time, they also need to address the patient's worries and anxieties about their health and their life. Obviously they have to diagnose and treat patients' medical problems. "But if I don't address their concerns also," Catherine continues, "and I know they're going to worry about it when they go home, I haven't done them any good."

The first patient Dr. O'Neil sees in the office this morning is a 47-year-old woman who recently had a hysterectomy for a large uterine fibroid.

"So how are you doing since your hysterectomy?"

"I'm doing wonderful."

"Are you?"

"I am. I just didn't realize."

"That's great. And did you have your ovaries taken also?"

"I did. I wanted to share with you what I'm taking for hormone replacement. Is this a very mild kind?"

Looking at the pills, Dr. O'Neil says, "Yep. It's a very good one."

"And the only side effect is in the early morning I get very warm, flushed."

"And how's your sleep been?"

"Beautiful."

"Good, that's the most important thing. If any of that gets worse, and I don't think it will, we can always go up on the dose to better control it. Any mood swings at all?"

Laughing, the patient says, "Not that I admit to. Maybe a few, but nothing that I can't tolerate."

"OK. We got your blood work back. Are you still on iron?"

"No, and I didn't know if I needed to be or not."

"Your blood count is great. Before your surgery it was 8. Now its 13.8. So you really don't need to take the iron."

"I had started to take a multiple vitamin right after the surgery, and I thought maybe now I'll keep on taking it."

"There's actually no harm with taking just one."

"And calcium?"

"You definitely should be taking 600 milligrams of calcium twice a day. I can write that down."

"I got those chewable . . ."

"Yeah, they're good. And they come with the vitamin D in them, which you need to absorb it." Then, looking at the woman's chart, Dr. O'Neil says, "And you're due for your mammogram in two months. Did the gynecologist do a breast exam when she saw you for your hysterectomy?"

"No. She said to come back to you for my routine care."

Getting up from her desk and walking up to the exam table to begin her examination, Dr. O'Neil glances at the woman's feet and says, "Nice shoes. Are they comfy?"

"Oh, my God, yes."

Examining her eyes, and then mouth, Dr. O'Neil asks, "Have you had a regular eye and dental exam?"

"I have them both scheduled. I work for the university, so I schedule everything over the summer, when I'm off."

"Very good. Any problems with chest pain, breathing, your bowels? I don't have to ask you about your periods anymore." After getting negative responses to all these, and upon completing her examination, Dr. O'Neil continues, "OK, let's have you come back in a few months for a breast exam, pelvic and rectal exam, and then we'll have everything all tied up. OK?"

"Sounds good to me. I have another question that I wanted to ask while I was here. I had gone to a dermatologist years ago, and he had prescribed this topical cream for my face. It keeps me from breaking out, and I wanted to know if I could get a prescription."

Looking at the tube of cream, Dr. O'Neil says, "Absolutely. You're just using it at bedtime?"

"Yes, once a day, or even every other day."

"Good. And we'll get you set up for the mammogram. Just keep up with the things you're doing."

"OK. Thank you very much. Have a great summer."

· · · · ·

Although many women physicians think about how they are going to balance motherhood and practicing medicine, Catherine seems exceedingly comfortable in doing both. Seeing her today, there is little question as to how much she enjoys Riley, her six-month-old son. She beams when she talks about him and when she looks at him. And she has pictures of Riley all over her office—blond, blue eyed, a big smile, and really cute. "Being a mother is great! It really is," Catherine says, smiling. "It's the one thing that's better than promised. I worked until the day before Riley was born—I was blessed with a good pregnancy. Recovery went almost as well, and I returned to work full-time six weeks to the day after my delivery. While it's hard to leave my son in the morning—because he is simply the most beautiful thing I've ever seen!—I have worked out my schedule so Tuesdays and Thursdays are half days. It's a part-time feel with full-time hours." And her husband Chris has been helping out with their patients in the hospital, "which has been a huge help."

"The time demands actually haven't been bad. We have a college student, who was actually a friend of ours, come to the house and babysit. That's been a big help. And the office staff are very sensitive about my schedule and not booking too many people close to lunchtime, so I have time to use the breast pump, and not booking extra people close to the end of the day. So if they're going to double-book me they do it earlier in the morning or the afternoon, knowing that I will have time to get caught up. That's been a big help. Our office is very good, very sensitive to that."

Dr. O'Neil asks her next patient—an 18-year-old young woman here for a college physical—"So how's school this year?"

"Oh, good."

"And you're going to go to the university now?"

"I'm on my way."

"Good for you. What are you going to take there?"

"I want to be a lawyer. And I have a busy summer."

"What are you going to do?"

"I'm going to France. It's a three and a half week program, we're going to be traveling around. It's a French language trip, and we're going to see everything. I've never been to France before, so I'm really excited. And I love French, so it's the perfect trip to take."

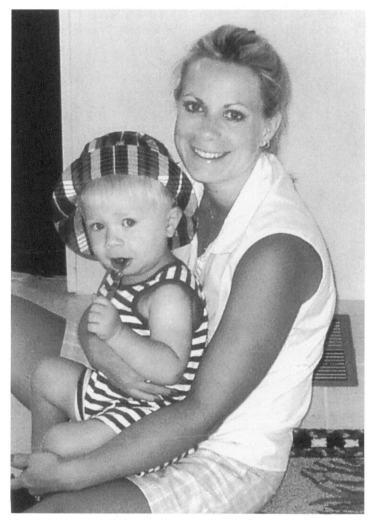

Dr. Catherine O'Neil with her son Riley. (Courtesy of Dr. Catherine O'Neil)

"Yeah, how did you get involved with that?"

"I took four years of French in school. And this group advertises this travel program, and it looked awesome to me. So my friend and I signed up for it."

"Wow!"

"Yeah, very cool."

"Don't forget to wear your—"

"Sunscreen."

"See, you knew before I even said it. Good, good, good. Anything else exciting?"

"I just got back from California last night. My grandparents live there."

"Gee, I want you're life," Dr. O'Neil says, kidding. "Can I have your life?"

"Oh, it's busier than you think. But, I'm sure it's not half as busy as yours. When did you have your baby?"

"In December."

"Oh, that's so cool. Congratulations. What's his name?"

"Riley."

"How's he doing?"

"He's doing really well."

Looking at the pictures on the wall and on the desk, the patient says, "He's a cutey."

"He's good. And of course he's already mastered 'Dada,' but not 'Mama.' "

"I'm sure any day now."

"OK, hop on up the table." Then, almost as if she were a big sister, Dr. O'Neil asks, "So, any boyfriends at school?"

"No."

As she examines the young woman's abdomen, she asks, "Does it hurt where I'm pushing? Then, looking at the woman's wrist, she adds, "Let's see your watch . . . that's pretty."

"Thank you."

"How's your eating?"

"Good."

"Good. Well, you look wonderful."

"Thanks."

"You're doing fantastic." Then Dr. O'Neil says jokingly, "Well, I guess I'll let you go to college, if that's what you want to do."

"All right," the patient responds, smiling.

"OK, you're all set. Wear your sunscreen. Wear your seatbelt. Good luck with everything."

"Thank you very much. And I hope your baby says 'Mama' soon."

"I do too. I'm going to be working on it."

"Great. Thanks very much."

The next patient is a 32-year-old woman with a rash on her arm. She has four children, and brought her three-year-old daughter with her to the office today.

"Hi," Dr. O'Neil says as she walks into the room. Then, looking at the woman's rash, she asks, "When did that start?"

"Last month, it was just a little dot. Then it spread down here. I tried some cortisone cream, and it's not working. I wash it, but it's just not going away. It's itchy, but if you touch it, it hurts."

"Exposure to anything?"

"No. There was another time, and I went to a dermatologist and he gave me some pills."

"Yeah, I wonder if you weren't on an antibiotic. I think you have some impetigo, a minor skin infection. I'm going to treat you for a week with an antibiotic, and if it doesn't get better, call me, and we'll get you to see the dermatologist."

"You don't think this could be skin cancer? My dad has something on his nose, and he says that's what it is."

"No. Definitely not."

"Good. So how old is your baby now?"

"Six months."

Dr. O'Neil then turns to the woman's three-year-old child, and asks, "Are you doing anything fun today?"

The child shakes her head yes.

"What are you doing?"

"We're gonna go to the movies."

"You are?"

Dr. O'Neil writes out a prescription for the antibiotic and gives it to the woman, saying, "Hopefully this will take care of it." And then she says to the child, "OK, have fun at the movies."

"Thank you."

"You're welcome. Take care."

• • • • •

"The best thing about practicing family medicine in a small town," says Catherine, "is getting to know all the families, and really understanding how different families function. And the support that you get from the families. I mean even having the baby was such an easy experience here. It was so much easier for me being here than it would have been if I were in a city. I don't think folks there would have even known if I had a child. Whereas here, my gosh, you feel like you're part of a family, which is excellent. There's not two patients that go by, when somebody doesn't remind me of my son, tell me how beautiful he is, congratulate me, ask me how he's doing. On the other hand, that's also the toughest part sometimes. You're always part of these people's families, and like any relatives," she says, smiling, "you need a little break sometimes. And there's not anywhere to really break around here.

"And I like the school districts," she continues. "We know most of the teachers and the principal. Actually Chris grew up and went to school with most all of them. So, I like that. And the fair—the Bloomsburg Fair! It's the largest fair on the east coast. You've never seen anything like it. I've come down to the fair since I was two years old—Rome is about two hours north of here. The schools shut down for a whole week. They have concerts every night, they have a demolition derby, comedians, horse and tractor pulls, an animal section, a big farm equipment section, buildings with agriculture, horticulture, arts and crafts—it's huge. And rides, and the best food. It's the last week of September each year. It is really quite impressive. The Bloomsburg Fair. People come from a long way away."

Catherine says that she could never see herself living in a city, primarily because she "could never picture myself raising children in a city. Because that isn't how I grew up. I grew up going fishing, going hunting, hanging out on weekends. I grew up with the nearest mall being an hour away." Which brings her to the hardest thing about living in a small town—shopping. "Yeah, the one thing we don't have around here is shopping—especially clothes." Then laughing, she says, "But it's good. It saves money. We go to Wilkes Barre or Scranton about once every other month—they're about forty-five minutes to an hour away. We get our fill, and then we go home. When we go to a city like New York or Philly, the biggest thing is the restaurants. We go out to eat, especially since we don't have a lot of different ethnic restaurants here. I used to miss that. But now that I've become a mother, I don't miss it anymore. I don't even think about it anymore. Before the baby was born, we also liked to travel quite a bit—visit friends, go to the beach, go skiing a few times a year. But we also like to just stay around here, mow lawns, have friends over, barbecue, sit around the patio in the back of the house and look over the pond,"—referring to the small pond in the backyard that Chris built and landscaped.

· · · · ·

Today, Family Care Associates is a true family practice—the family of Drs. Catherine and Chris O'Neil (and their partners) taking care of the families in Bloomsburg. Living and practicing with Chris, Catherine has a unique ability to see some of the differences between being a male and female physician. Catherine says that it's not that different in a small town than in the city, but "there definitely is a difference. I can see that with Chris and me. There definitely are things that people think I can and can't do, and there are things that they seem to think he can do better. And it's not because of our experience, but because that's what people think. For example, if it's a female problem, I must know what it is. Or if a pregnant woman calls here at night and gets Chris, she'll say 'Well, really I see your wife—I kind of thought I'd be talking to her.' So, absolutely, there is a bias."

There are also differences in style. Catherine describes herself as "more of a nurturer. I'm not a 'This is how it is, this is what you need to do, boom' kind of person. I may do that sometimes, but then I back it up with, 'Yes, I understand it's hard to lose weight, or I understand it's hard to quit smoking.' Some people want to be told what to do, and that's it, and not be given all the other options. I do have primarily women and kids as patients—that's self-selection. Chris has a lot more men patients. Women in general come to the doctor more often, but if you look at my schedule most are women, while his schedule is more men. Even some women that normally see Chris will come to me for their gynecologic exams."

· · · · ·

Catherine thinks that it's easier to maintain a higher standard of living in a small town. "Part of it is expectations," she says, "in a larger city, keeping up with the Joneses. You don't have that as much in a small town. Anything you have is good. Doctors—even family doctors—are at the high end of income in town. But Chris and I both have loans, and the repayments are larger than I thought. I am paying mine off over ten years, and I pay $1,600 a month. And, if reimbursements continue to decrease, and medical school tuition is as high as it is, I'm concerned that communities like this are going to have a harder time getting physicians. And I think that's bad. I think that's going to be an issue. It may have to get to a crisis first. But really, now we have it pretty good here."

Perhaps because Dr. O'Neil is the most recent graduate of the ten doctors in this book (having graduated medical school in 1996), she seems to express less intense resentment toward "managed care" than other physicians. She admits that it results in "a lot of paperwork, arguing, and still not always getting people to get the care that you'd like to. But I think that we're so used to it. And I think that coming out of residency—being trained at a hospital that had their own health plan—it was kind of ingrained in you what paperwork was needed, and what you needed a referral for. I think that if we hadn't been brought up in that environment, I might feel a little bit differently about it. But I know to look at the front of the chart before I start writing out a referral. I know I need to fill out a certain form, and that there are certain specialists that some patients can go to. Actually, a much bigger problem is that one of the local health plans dropped their prescription coverage for their patients, so that's been our biggest stressor, to be honest. We have a bunch of elderly patients who have no prescription drug coverage whatever, but are on tons of medications. Luckily we do get a good sample supply, but that's been our biggest problem. Of course, I think care could be better if we didn't have managed care."

• • • • •

Wearing her white lab coat, her stethoscope folded into a front pocket, Dr. O'Neil enters one of the exam rooms in her office. On the wall is a bulletin board covered with pictures of the children she takes care of—and of course all around the room are pictures of Riley. Sitting in a chair is her next patient, a 34-year-old woman who has been having irregular menstrual periods.

"How often do they come?" Dr. O'Neil asks.

"About every other week."

"Are they particularly heavy?"

"No, but I always get a really bad headache."

"How long has that been going on?"

"About a year."

"What do you use for birth control?"

"I had my tubes tied—six years ago."

"How old are your children?"

"14, 13, 11, 10, and 6."

"Boy, let the fun begin."

"Uh-huh."

"We did a bunch of blood tests last week, and everything was normal. Have you ever had an ultrasound?"

"No."

"And would you consider any kind of birth control, just to control your periods?"

"I had used the pills before, but it made my blood pressure really high."

"Oh, did it? OK. Are you still teaching? Is that going all right?"

"Uh-huh."

"Are you drinking coffee or caffeine?"

"No, and I'm on the Weight Watchers again."

"Oh, are you? How are you doing?"

"I went from 193 to 180 on my scale at home."

"Yay! That's excellent."

"And I'm walking and exercising, a lot."

Looking at her chart, Dr. O'Neil confirms "You've lost fourteen and a quarter pounds in the past four months. That's excellent. Do you walk every day?"

"Yes."

"Great. OK, I'll step outside for a minute, and you can put on a gown."

As soon as Dr. O'Neil steps outside, one of the nurses pulls her aside and takes her into an adjoining procedure room, where a 19-year-old young man has a tick on his back, which Dr. O'Neil removes. Then, she goes back in and performs a pelvic exam on her patient, which is normal. When she returns again after the patient has dressed, the woman asks, "Is there anything you can give me for cramps?"

"Well, have you tried ibuprofen?"

"Yeah, lots of it. Can you overdose on it?" she asks, laughing.

"Yes, you can hurt your kidneys," Dr. O'Neil says seriously. "That's not a good thing at all. You don't want to do that. Who's your prescription plan through?"

"Through my health insurance. I don't know."

"There's a new medicine out, which a lot of women have said works pretty well. I can write you a prescription for a few pills and some refills, and see if it works."

"OK."

"Then I want to get you set up for the ultrasound."

"Well, I quit smoking so I could live longer, and now I'm so fat."

"You're doing wonderful. Just keep walking. That's the best thing for it."

"OK. See you. Have a good day."

The next patient is a 26-year-old young man with a sinus headache. He's a teacher in town, and his mother works as a nurse at the hospital.

"You've been having some pain?"

"Friday afternoon it started. I just thought I'd started with a mild headache, and it just progressively got worse. Right across . . . all through here," he says, pointing from one side of his forehead to the other. "Then it started going up in my temple and into my ear. I've been trying to take Sudafed and Tylenol. Over the weekend, I was taking 30 milligrams of Sudafed, but when I went to work Monday I took 60 milligrams, and I liked that better. It gave me six hours of relief. But, I wanted to come in and have you check it out, because I'm miserable at night."

"Any colored discharge from your nose?"

"It started to turn yellow-ish yesterday."

Then Dr. O'Neil asks a number of questions, one at a time: "Have you had fevers, chills, coughing, sore throat, sneezing?"

"No (to all). I just started sneezing yesterday."

"You haven't picked up any bad habits, like smoking?"

"No!" the man says emphatically. "I usually take an antihistamine when I go over to my brother's house because of the dog, but I haven't been there lately. We're really busy, we're moving into Grammy's house—we originally were going in to help take care of her."

Examining his throat, Dr. O'Neil says, "Say 'ahh.' How's she doing?"

"She died . . ."

Shocked, Dr. O'Neil abruptly stops her exam. "She did? I didn't know that? Nobody told me."

"Oh, we called and left a message. I just figured they'd tell the whole office."

"No, I didn't know that. Ohhhh! Poor Grammy, I took care of her for a long time. Oh, I'm so sorry to hear of that."

"She's in a better place."

"Oh, absolutely."

"She passed away eating a dish of ice cream," the patient says, and both he and Dr. O'Neil laugh at this. "The next thing you know . . . at least she didn't suffer. It was quick for her. She was home."

"Yeah."

"She was happy till the end, so we were happy. And she didn't suffer, so we were happy about that."

Continuing with her examination, Dr. O'Neil asks, "When you move your head forward like this, do you feel pressure?"

"Oh, yeah."

"I really think you have sinusitis."

"That's what I was wondering."

"You've had this before. You do well on azithromycin, don't you?"

"Yeah."

"Well, here's a prescription. Take them one a day for five days. And try plain old Robitussin, and salt water nasal spray—they're both good things too."

"OK, we have that at home."

"And call me if you're not getting better."

"OK. Thank you. How's the baby doing? He's gorgeous."

"Great. Thank you."

The next patient is a 56-year-old man with high cholesterol and high blood pressure. Dr. O'Neil asks him, "So, we increased your blood pressure medicine last time, and you haven't had any side effects from that?"

"No."

"Well, it didn't make your blood pressure much better. Have you checked it yourself?"

"No, I don't know what it should be."

"Well, less than 140 over 80 is ideal. You have your bottom number down, but your top number is still up. Has anything changed in your diet?"

"No. You asked me last time I was here if I had been going to my eye doctor, and I had been there, and she says my eyes are healthy. I was also to the orthopedist for my knee."

"What's going on with your knee?"

"I had terrible pain there, and he sent me for blood and X-rays. I had everything done at once. I called him, and he said everything was fine, and the only thing he could do would be to give me a shot."

"Did you do that?"

"No, because he said it would only work for four days."

"Did he give you a diagnosis?"

"No, he couldn't find anything?"

"How's it been?"

"It isn't any better. It's my right one."

"I'll check it out. And the main reason you came in was to check on your cholesterol. Have you been exercising?"

"You know me."

"Well I have to ask—you never know. Comparing your cholesterol with the one six months ago, there is no difference. Your fasting cholesterol is 280—it was 277. Your triglycerides are also a little elevated, and your bad cholesterol, your LDL, is now 190—it was 188. What do all these numbers mean? The most important number is the LDL of 190. With you having high blood pressure, you're already at risk for having a heart attack or stroke, and cholesterol is another risk factor. And when you put those together, it really increases your risk, so we really need to try and get aggressive and treat both of them. Our goal is to get the bad cholesterol down to 100. And even if you dieted and exercised your heart out, I don't know that you could get it all the way down to 100. This is more the kind of cholesterol that comes along with family genes. Your mom and dad gave you this, and there's not a lot that you can do about it. Not that I would ever discourage you from good diet and exercise, because that's always good. But I really don't think that if we only did that, we could get it down. And the more aggressive we are earlier, the better off people do. The quicker we can get that down to less than 100, the less cholesterol that's floating around your arteries, and the less that's forming plaque, so the less chance . . ."

"What does the pill do?"

"Well, what the pill does is help your body eliminate cholesterol. And the downside is that it goes through the liver, so we always check your liver enzymes first, before we start you on something. And yours are fine. If you develop any symptoms, especially muscle aches, let me know, because that's another side effect of the medication. We'll start out with a low dose of the medication, and then we'll titrate you up until we get you to a good dose, and make sure your liver is tolerating it OK, and make sure your cholesterol is doing OK. So we'll check you every six to eight weeks till you're stable.

The medications do work very well. There are occasional side effects, as we discussed."

"OK."

"Let me see your knee."

"It was a little warm, less so now. And it hurts all over."

After examining his knee, Dr. O'Neil says, "Well, it sounds like the joint is irritated. I think that ice will be good. And anti-inflammatory medication. But the injection may work a little longer, especially if he puts steroid in it. We could also send you to physical therapy if you would rather. I would try the shot first, to be honest with you."

"Can I call and let you know?"

"Sure. I also want to start you on a weak water pill for your blood pressure, and see how it does. Just one pill a day so you don't urinate all night."

"Do you know anything about glucosamine and chondrointin?"

"The glucosamine does work for your joints. And I have some samples of the cholesterol medicine for you. I'll see you in a month to check your blood pressure."

"OK. Thank you."

Next, Dr. O'Neil sees a 46-year-old woman who presents with foot pain. Then, she sees a 13-year-old boy who comes in for a baseball physical examination. Dr. O'Neil tells him, "It's always embarrassing when you guys are twelve to thirteen and are already taller than me, but you've been for a while." Then she discusses his health concerns, how things are going at school, what he's going to do for the summer, and about his parents. His examination is perfectly normal, so she discusses sunblock and safety and fills out his physical exam form.

In between patients, Dr. O'Neil reviews lab tests and asks her nurse to call patients with the results—both normal and abnormal. She also writes notes in her charts and discusses any questions she might have with her partners that happen to be in the hall between the patient rooms. She also answers questions from nurses regarding phone calls. There's a patient with an abnormal lab test who needs to be seen but says he can't come in, so she arranges for a visiting nurse to check on him tomorrow. A child with a ruptured eardrum who was seen yesterday—his mom called to check in and say that he is doing OK. And a two-year-old girl who put a bean in her ear—Dr. O'Neil tells the nurse to have her come into the office today.

• • • • •

Family Care Associates is owned by Bloomsburg Hospital, and Catherine is an employee of the hospital. Her own practice is currently closed to new patients, even though she's only been here three years. She sees about 25 to 30 patients a day in the office, and takes care of multiple family members. "That young man that we had in today, the one whose grandmother had passed away, I take care of his sisters' children, so that's four generations. And we get involved in dying and counseling—we have a great hospice program in town. That's why I was so devastated that I didn't know that his grand-mother had died. I had taken care of that woman for quite a while, and when I went off for my delivery she went to hospice. Yeah, I was really upset that no one told me she had died. It's very personal. Absolutely."

The practice doesn't deliver babies, but they do many office procedures, including gynecological procedures such as endometrial biopsies and cryo-therapy. And "we're going to start working on campus in the University Health Service—we'll all take turns doing that two to three hours a day. That's going to be fun. We also work at the high school and elementary school—we do the sports physicals, school physicals, attend at the sports games. We don't do many actual home visits, but we do make an occasional social visit to make sure a patient is doing OK, bake some cookies or something. Just a few times a year, not that often." As for call, Catherine is on call only every seventh night and weekend, but sometimes it feels as if it's more often, since with both she and Chris, one of them is on call almost every third night. "With both of us having call beepers, it's a little stressful. But, when we're off, we're totally off.

"Some of my women patients work at the local factories around here—the ribbon factory, the carpet factory, there are a lot of blue collar workers. Many work at home taking care of their children. We have quite a few professors from the university. Magee Carpets, the newspaper, and the university are the biggest employers. The majority of my patients—about sixty to seventy per-cent—are from Bloomsburg, and the rest are from outlying areas. There are a lot of small towns in the areas, but it's quite a drive for some of them—about a half hour."

There are six physicians in Catherine's group, which is the largest group practice I visited. Advantages of being in a larger group include having less professional isolation and less frequent night call. Disadvantages include a larger practice to cover at night when you are on call, and the difficulties inherent in working with multiple partners—although the doctors in Family Care Associates seem to get along exceptionally well. "There are about twelve to fifteen other family doctors in town," Catherine says, "and we're getting two more in our practice soon—that will be good. We're probably the biggest practice in town—we have about 20,000 patients in the practice. Our office probably takes care of thirty percent of the population in town. The hospital also owns some other practices in other towns in addition to ours. We haven't really had trouble recruiting. If some of the older docs in town start retiring, then we'll need more doctors, 'cause we're pretty busy." Sometimes, the avail-ability of specialists is a problem, and this is getting worse since the malprac-tice insurance crisis has forced some doctors to leave the state. "We don't have cardiology here—we can consult them, but it could be a day or two till they come down. We do have internists, and they are very good, and serve as our consultants for cardiac patients when we need it. That's what I did recently when I had a 52-year-old man who was having a heart attack.

"I think the prestige of family doctors is higher here than in the city," Catherine says. "The family doctors here are really well respected. And people come to us for pretty much anything—things that if you were in the city, you wouldn't even think of going to your family doctor for. I think the prestige is just as high as for the surgeons and the specialists in the area. And I think the specialists have a good relationship with family doctors in town. They respect us and trust us."

• • • • •

While all of the small communities in Pennsylvania are commonly referred to as "towns," they are technically defined as boroughs. Bloomsburg is actually Pennsylvania's only official "town," due to a special Act of Incorporation passed in 1870. It sits along the north branch of the Susquehanna River, and serves as the county seat of Columbia County. The population, 12,375, is the largest of the communities in this book. Walking through the center of town today, one sees banners hung from each light post announcing the "Bloomsburg Bicentennial: 1802–2002."

The Susquehannock Indians were the first occupants of the Susquehanna River valley, at a time when the river was a major route to central New York State. Later, when squatters and land speculators moved in, a small fort was built to protect the settlers from Indian attacks. Iron ore was discovered nearby, and was a major industry here for 75 years. Around 1900, the iron ore was depleted, as was the agricultural base, and textile mills and small manufacturers began to locate in the area. Today, the permanent population increases for much of the year with the additional 8,000 college students from Bloomsburg University, whose campus is adjacent to downtown. Since Wal-Mart arrived, some of the downtown shops are struggling to survive, but "Wal-Mart is doing well because it's convenient, and they have parking," says Catherine. "But, this is definitely a college town."

• • • • •

Driving from the office to Catherine's home, one passes along a long ridge that parallels other strips of low mountain ridges in the distance. Small valleys are tucked between the ridges, filled with large farms alternating with wooded areas. Walking around Catherine's home, one passes the small pond behind the house, the enormous red wood barn with its adjoining fenced in area for the dogs, and a large farmed field extending up the gently sloping land, bordered in the back by a forest. "Our house is a farmette," Catherine says, "and we have approximately thirty acres and a little barn—and two golden retrievers. Of course, Chris has to have his two tractors, a bulldozer, and a souped-up lawnmower, and keeps them in the barn. His parents own the land that's adjacent to ours—they own about 130 acres altogether. Their house is actually across the road from ours. They love to baby sit. We're going to buy about sixty acres adjacent to our land from them. And then we're going to build a new home on that land next year—we already have plans and a builder. Once they get started, it will take six to seven months. We're going to keep our present house and barn and rent them out.

"We rent out the land behind us to farmers who raise mostly soybeans and corn," she continues. "They're very nice. We had our first anniversary party in the barn last year, and the farmers came up and set it all up for us. They soundproofed the barn, piling up bales of hay against the walls since we had a band, and didn't want it to be too loud for the neighbors. It was great—definitely country living."

• • • • •

The next patient in the office is a 42-year-old woman who is here for a routine pap test. As Dr. O'Neil gets ready to go into the room to see her, her nurse tells her that the patient also wants a mammogram—she's never had one before—because she has a friend with breast cancer. As she enters the room, Dr. O'Neil says "I heard you had some bad news . . ."

"Yaaah."

"When did you find out about your friend?"

"Just recently, but it turns out that she found a lump a year ago, and just let it go."

"Oh my goodness!"

"She didn't want to have chemo or radiation before her son's wedding, and so she just let it go."

"Oh my. And now she's . . ."

"Not doing well."

"Is she from around here?"

"No, but we've been friends since college. I mean I know when my aunt died from cancer, it took her a long time. But for her, it got really bad very quickly. It's in her bones and everything."

"That's got to be sad."

Wiping away tears, the patient says, "Yeah, it is like sooo sad. . . . She's only forty-two. Oh, God!"

"Well, for you mammograms are definitely a good screening test. Do you have any breast cancer in your family?"

"No."

"And are you doing self-breast exams?"

"Uh-huh."

"Have you found anything that concerns you?"

"No."

"And are your periods regular?"

"Yes."

"OK. Well, let's do a pap test and pelvic examination, and schedule you for a mammogram. I'll call you as soon as I hear the results."

"OK. Thank you."

The following patient is a 50-year-old woman concerned about her toenails. Dr. O'Neil tells her that she has a fungus, and gives her some sample medications. Then Dr. O'Neil instructs her to have some blood tests taken first, and says that she will call tomorrow with the results. If they are normal, the woman can start taking the medicine.

Next, is a 91-year-old man, who comes in with his daughter. He has a lot of chronic medical problems, including a history of depression, and takes a number of medications. His daughter brought him in a week ago, because he was complaining of muscle aches, and he had a little anemia, so Dr. O'Neil did some additional blood tests. The repeat test for anemia was now reported as normal, but another test of his urine was abnormal. Dr. O'Neil was ambivalent as to how much further to pursue this, and whether or not to put this elderly man through a lot of additional testing, when it may not be very likely to benefit him. But she was also not yet sure exactly what the medical significance of these results were. So she asked him and his daughter to come back today to discuss this together, and to see what they would like to do next.

Daughter: "He's also getting more of those spots on his hands and arms."

Dr. O'Neil looks at these and says, "They are getting a bit darker, more waxy. See how I can almost peel that off. They're not harmful at all."

Daughter: "Oh, that's good."

"They're very benign things. They are just extra growths of skin."

Daughter: "They don't bother you, Dad? Do they?"

"If they bother him," Dr. O'Neil adds, "we can always take them off." Then, turning toward the patient, she asks, "How's your arthritis?"

The patient, who doesn't say much throughout the visit, replies, "Pretty good."

Daughter: "He says it's better, but his knees hurt every day, he says."

"What is he taking for pain?"

Daughter: "Tylenol, twice a day."

"And that's helped a little bit?"

Daughter: "It seems to help some."

"Good. We did all these blood tests. Did you do the home tests on his stool?"

Daughter: "Yes, I brought them in, and your nurse said they were normal."

"Yes, I see. Good. And the good thing is that his blood count went up when we repeated it, and was normal. Are you taking any extra vitamins or iron?"

Daughter: "Another doctor had given him vitamin C and E, but that's been years ago."

"The only other thing that we had gotten—and I know that my nurse had called you—was the urine test. We were looking to see if there was any blood there, and that came back OK. But the one thing that came back a little unusual was that there was some bilirubin in it . . ."

Daughter: "What's that?"

Dr. O'Neil asks the man, "Do you still have your gallbladder?"

The patient shakes his head no.

"Well, bilirubin is related to the gallbladder and also the liver. So the next step would be to repeat the urine test, but also take a closer look at the liver, which we can do with further blood tests. And the next step after that would be to look at the liver with an ultrasound. Now this is a lot of stuff to do for some bilirubin in the urine, and I wanted to talk to you and see what you thought about that. This isn't a common thing, so I can't say this is definitely normal or that definitely there's nothing wrong. And that's why I would want to start small with a urine test and blood test, and see what came out. If the blood tests were completely normal and the urine went back to normal, then we would be done with it. But if it weren't, then we may go ahead with the ultrasound to see if there's something wrong with the liver, see if there were a tumor or anything else to cause that to be abnormal. To me, you don't look like somebody that's having problems with your liver right now, so it's kind of up to you. Can I take a look at you up on the table?" After the patient gets up on the exam table, Dr. O'Neil begins to examine him. "What did you have for breakfast?"

"Cheerios."

"Oh, good. Well, how do you feel about pursuing this bilirubin business? Does that sound OK? It also may be that some of your medications are affecting the liver."

The daughter then asks her father, "We need to check it out, right, Dad?" Then, to Dr. O'Neil, she says, "I was thinking it might be one of his medicines too." She turns again to her father and continues, "You want to have your blood and urine checked again, just to see? Right? Right?"

Patient: (In a barely audible voice) "OK."

Daughter: "How high was it? A little high, alarmingly high?"

"Well, it was actually quite a bit. It was three-plus. How's he eating?"

"He gets meals on wheels for dinner time. And we buy lunch meat for supper."

"Well, that's good." Then, Dr. O'Neil asks the patient a number of questions regarding problems with his eating, his bowels, his stomach, his urine— all of which the patient answers with a very weak "No." Then, hearing that the daughter—with her father's OK—agrees with this step-by-step plan, she continues, "Well, let's start with these tests, and if any are abnormal, then we'll get an ultrasound. Sometimes I think all I do is keep sending you to the hospital for tests. Well, it keeps you busy, out of trouble."

Daughter: "Thank you so much. You're an excellent person and doctor. We're lucky to have you around."

"Thank you."

In the next room is a 62-year-old man who is here to follow up on a rash on his face. Dr. O'Neil had seen him last week and thought it looked like poison ivy, although he repeatedly denied any contact with anything, including poison ivy. Nevertheless she treated him with steroid pills.

"Oh, you are looking better."

"Yeah, this started going down into the lip there, and it scared me yesterday, so I called. But now it dried up a bit. It's all done on the nose, it's all done up here. I just have a few spots left."

"Yeah, you look much better. Does your jaw feel better?"

"Yeah, I only have four pills left."

"I definitely think it was a reaction to something—like poison ivy."

"Well, I was working at my son's one day, burning brush, and it could have been. So maybe I might have got a little smoke, and my face was the only part that wasn't covered."

"Yeah, I think you're on the mend."

Then the patient asks, "Are these pills any good for poison ivy?"

A bit surprised at this question, Dr. O'Neil says, "Yes."

"Oh, I'll give it to my son, he's suffering from it."

More surprised, Dr. O'Neil says, "Where'd he get it from?"

"Poison ivy? Oh, he was weeding with shorts on. Just across the street from where he lives."

Then, a bit incredulous as to where this story was going, considering that the patient had denied being exposed to poison ivy last week, Dr. O'Neil asked, "The same area you were in?"

"Yeah. I was burning brush, and he was weeding. So I'm suspecting that was what it was. I generally don't get it, but I had a bad sunburn, and it was peeling, and maybe I was susceptible." Then laughing, he says, "Why do I come to the doctor if I know all these things?"

"Yep. You take care."

Then, Dr. O'Neil is interrupted by her nurse. The parents of a 17-year-old with anorexia are on the phone. They are having problems getting her admitted to an inpatient treatment facility. The next patient is a 72-year-old man with a history of heart disease and prostate cancer, who is here for a check up, and is doing well. Then, she sees a 76-year-old man, a patient of one of her partners, who had been seen in the emergency room recently with chest pain, which turned out to be gastritis.

"So you're feeling a lot better than you were on Sunday?"

"Yeah."

"Were you nauseated?"

"No, I just had that awful pain right up here," the man says, pointing to the center of his chest.

"Have you ever had a lighter version of that before?"

"I think I had another attack about a year or so ago. I was in the emergency room for it, and they couldn't find anything."

"Do you have a family history of heart problems?"

"My father had a slight heart problem, but nothing serious, you know."

"How old did he live to be?"

"Eighty-three or eighty-four."

"Did he die from a heart problem?"

"I think a little bit of everything. Old age."

"But that's young these days, you know."

"Yeah, I know, I'm planning to be 100."

"And you don't smoke or drink alcohol?"

"Nope."

"And who lives home with you?"

"Nobody." Then, the man pauses, looks down at the ground and in a lower, more subdued tone, says, "My wife died six years ago. I'm home alone."

"Do you have pets?"

"No, when I want to go, I don't want to have anybody to take care of."

"Well, come on over to the table here, let me check you out. As she examines the patient, Dr. O'Neil asks, "Were you dizzy or lightheaded or sweaty? Did you feel any palpitations?"

The patient says no to all of these, then points to the top of his abdomen and says, "It hurts inside there."

Examining him, she says, "Does it hurt when I push?"

"Yes. There's a spot there that isn't right." Then, as Dr. O'Neil continues to push gently in the center of his abdomen, he says, "Ow!"

"Are you sore there?"

"Yes."

"That's right where your stomach is. I wonder if you just have too much acid in your stomach. You can get referred pain, 'cause your stomach goes into your esophagus which goes into your chest, and you can get some pain up there."

"I'm tender there."

"Hmm. Well, I think we should get you on something for acid in your tummy—at least for a short period of time, to see if we can get this to settle down and go away."

"I hope."

"Do you have a prescription plan?"

"No."

"OK, let me see what we have for samples. Your other medicines are for your blood pressure and your thyroid, right?"

"Yeah."

Dr. O'Neil goes to the closet where the sample medications are stored, says hi to her husband, who also happens to be there getting medicine for his patient, and is then interrupted by her nurse, who asks about refilling a prescription for a patient on the phone. Then, she re-enters the room. "I'm back," she says. "I got you a 'goody' bag. Do you take any arthritis medications?"

"No."

"How much coffee do you drink?"

"Maybe one or two cups a day."

"Does that seem to make a difference?"

"No."

"We'll get you started on this medicine, which suppresses acid in your stomach. Just take one pill a day. I gave you enough for a month's worth, and hopefully that will be enough time to settle down that acid, and make this better. If this is not getting better, and you're getting pain on the right side, we should consider doing an ultrasound of your gallbladder. Well, try this out, and don't be afraid to call me back if it's not working."

In the next room is a 26-year-old woman with anxiety. After quickly reading what the nurse has written on the chart, Dr. O'Neil walks in and says, "I hear you're doing a little bit better."

"Yeah, I seem to be better. I'm not as emotional."

"Good."

"But I'm eating like crazy."

"Have you gained any weight?"

"Yeah. But I'm trying to exercise every day. I don't want to gain any weight. You know how I am about that."

"Well this new formulation of your anxiety medicine should have less of a side effect of that. Now that your appetite has returned, of course, you'll gain the weight back that you lost. But you'll have control over that, especially if you're exercising and watching your diet."

"It seems like I'm eating a lot of cereal. And bad stuff, like ice cream."

"Is ice cream bad?" Dr. O'Neil asks, smiling.

"Comfort food, you know."

"Are you sleeping OK?"

"Better. That's OK. I'm feeling a lot better."

"How's your energy level?"

"Never that good. I'm tired. But I can get through the day."

"If you feel like the medicine is making you sleepy, you can take it at night."

"OK. I think I'll do that."

"Well, let me listen to your heart and lungs." Then, after examining the woman, Dr. O'Neil says, "I'm going to have you come back at the end of the summer to make sure everything's going OK. If you have *any* problem before then, give me a call."

"OK. Thank you."

"I'm glad you're feeling better."

The next patient is an 18-year-old young woman with obsessive compulsive disorder. She is phobic about thunderstorms, and crawls under her twin sister's bed when they occur. Dr. O'Neil opens the door to the room and says warmly, "Hello, Linda."

Startled, the patient jumps up and says, "Oh!"

"Did I scare you?"

"Yeah, Yeah."

"How are you doing?"

"All right."

"Give me the low down."

"Well, I've been sleeping in my room more often, when there's thunderstorms. And, um, I have a job now."

"What's that?"

"I work for a woman, Mrs. Phillips, and help her around her farm."

"Well that's good. So how are you doing with all that?"

"Doing all right. I just got back from work today. And yesterday I worked. Tomorrow's my free day."

"When you work for her, are you able to keep doing stuff, or do you have to go back and check?"

"Usually I keep working until she says it's time for a break, or if I finish one job, and she gives me another job. Or I go down to her house for a glass of juice or a soda or something."

"Your grandmother sent me a note—I guess you probably brought it along, right?"

"Uh-huh."

"And she says she's worried that you're having a little more trouble with storms."

"I haven't been having trouble with storms."

"She said that if it starts to cloud over and gets a little dark, that you're worried it's going to thunder and lightning."

"All I do is unplug my stuff. That's all I do."

"OK. Why do you suppose she's worried about it?"

"Because, right away, as soon as it starts to get dark, I assume there's gonna be something happening. I just take precautions and unplug my stuff, because two years in a row we had bad cases of lightning. So I figured, well, I'm not going to take a chance with my stuff."

"So, it still worries you pretty much?"

"Uh-huh."

"You know," Dr. O'Neil says, "I have a couple thoughts. One of them is, the dose of the medicine that you're on—you've grown, and the dose hasn't grown quite as much as you have, or quite as quickly. And I'd like to have you be a little bit more comfortable with things."

"Uh-huh."

"It must kind of get in the way sometimes."

"Right."

"I mean, what if you want to listen to your CDs, and you have to go unplug it because it's getting dark?"

"Right. I have a battery-operated stereo."

Smiling warmly, Dr. O'Neil says, "You always have an answer."

"Whenever I have to unplug my good stuff, I still have cards I can rearrange."

"OK, but what I'm thinking, it would be nice to . . ."

"Right. Not worry about it."

"To not worry about it so much. Yep. The other thing, I know that you were working with that counselor a couple years ago."

"Right."

"Do you think it would make sense to see if we could get that started up again?"

"I don't know. Possibly. I don't know if I'll have time this summer, 'cause I have lots of things to do."

"OK. Think about it, all right?"

"I will."

"Or maybe after the summer. If you start having trouble again. You can think about that."

"Right now, it's like a low-level thing, it's not like real high up there—like elevated."

"Does it stop you from doing things you might want to do?"

"Nah."

"What do you do if it thunders when you're at work?"

"Well, I don't know what I would do. If I was like inside a building, not outside, I would still work."

"OK, so you sort have planned out how you might cope with it?"

"Uh-huh. But if I was outside, with all those trees. Huh, I might try to think that a tree can't come down on me."

"Well that's good. I was just trying to think what the other things were that you worried about. The storms were the biggest, and the dark, weren't they?" Then, reviewing her chart, Dr. O'Neil continues. "OK. Yeah, you went up to this dose of medicine quite a few years ago, when you weighed almost thirty-five pounds less."

"It was a long time ago. I've gone from 88 to 121."

"Well, that's good. I like to see that."

"I've been eating more."

"You've grown nicely. So I'm going to increase your dose of medicine a little. You may even need a bigger dose than this, but we'll go up one step at a time. Anything else I should know about?"

"Nope, just my foot." The patient has a small A-V malformation—what looks like a dime-sized vascular bubble—on the back of her left foot, between her big toe and second toe. It was operated on twice already, but still swells up, like a large varicose vein.

"Does it hurt you?"

"Not really."

"Do you wear your stocking?"

"Not really."

"You don't have to if it doesn't bother you."

"No, it doesn't bother me."

Then, knowing that Linda's grandmother has high cholesterol, Dr. O'Neil continues, "You know, the last time I checked your cholesterol was two years ago. We need to check yours again. Are you watching your diet?"

"My grandma is."

"OK, Linda, did we cover everything?"

"So far, yes."

"Do you need to talk any more now?"

"No, I'm fine. OK. Thank you." Then, walking out, the patient asks, "Do you want this door shut?"

"No, thank you. Bye." Early on, when the patient originally started talking, she denied that she was having any problems with the storms. Rather than confront her directly, however, Dr. O'Neil comfortably found a way to convince her that it would be better to increase her dose of medicine—which she clearly needed.

• • • • •

As for balancing her personal and professional life, Catherine says, "It gets a little tricky sometimes, especially with us both being at work all the time. It's great, because I get to see Chris all day. But sometimes it's bad because you need an 'off' switch too. Sometimes we have to just say, 'No, we're not going to talk about work at home anymore,' and that's it. I think you have to work at it every day. I don't think it comes easily.

"And I see my patients out of the office all the time—pretty much anywhere you walk into—Giant, Wal-Mart, restaurants, church, anywhere. We were with Chris's parents and their friends, and I saw patients that I didn't even know were friends of theirs." She and Chris remember talking as residents about why they never saw any of the attending doctors out at dinner. Now they understand. When Catherine first came to town, she hated to go to the grocery store or Wal-Mart, "because you can't go down an aisle without running into four to five people. There's no quick trip to anything. Once—the night we had just come back from our honeymoon in Hawaii—I stopped in the store to get some milk for the morning, and a patient came up to me and said, 'Hi. How did my cholesterol test come out?' In my mind, I was still sitting on a beach in Hawaii. It's hard. Sometimes you're tired, and people don't realize." Catherine and Chris are planning to build their new house farther up the hill, away from the road, so they can have some more privacy. "Now, people all know where we live, which is both good and bad. We walk out with the garbage, and people driving buy honk their horn to say hi. And people were coming up to the back door with baby gifts when I was barely able to walk around. But overall, it's very nice. And I definitely think it's very rewarding to be in a small town. As much as we complain about not being able to go to Wal-Mart—still you get to know people's whole families, and you get to see them at church, or the football games, or wherever.

"And, it's been better when I go shopping, now that I have the baby, because now people stop and make a fuss over the baby. It used to be as soon as you talk about one medical problem, they would be asking about another. Now they realize that you're also a person, you have chores, you have to buy diapers and things. I think that's also happened even in the office. Before, when I first got here, some folks said 'I thought you were going to be older,' or 'I thought you were going to be taller.' But now that I've become a mom, it really has made a difference. So overall, it's been really nice. Oh my gosh, you can't believe the gifts from patients. And they always ask—more picture, more pictures. But you can see there are already a lot of pictures in the office."

Today, Catherine O'Neil appears to have it all. She balances being a family doctor and a new mother with equanimity and poise. She herself thinks that her present life is pretty close to her original image. "We've had a few students who have come through the office and shadow me. I say, 'Make sure that you really, really know what you're getting into, and know how much it's going to cost, and be prepared for that, because it can be a shock. Just make sure you're going to love it.' For me, it actually has worked out to be what I expected. And I love it. I really do enjoy it. I have a very good life now. I am very lucky. So it worked out perfect!"

CHAPTER $\qquad$ | **8**

LOCK HAVEN,
PENNSYLVANIA

It is not quite true that you can't go home again.
—Wallace Stegner, *Angle of Repose*

It was days like this that made Thane Turner want to practice family medicine for the rest of his life. Late at night, he had one of those perfect deliveries. A happy couple, their first child, a beautiful baby girl. Dr. Turner knew the family, having gone to high school with the father's older brother. As he left the delivery room on the way home, he walked by the waiting area where the extended family had gathered. Everyone rushed up to him and said, "Thank you, Doctor!"

Earlier in the day, Dr. Turner had seen an 80-year-old woman in his office. It was the first time he had seen her since her husband had died three weeks ago. Dr. Turner had known the couple ever since he had moved into town as a child. Now, he took care of three generations of this family, including their son—who had been Thane's high school gym teacher—his wife, and their two children. The woman's husband had been diagnosed with pancreatic cancer a year earlier, and when it spread extensively, Dr. Turner sat down with both of them to discuss the options, including a living will. The man said that he didn't want to die at home, that he wanted to be in the hospital. So when he became terminally ill soon thereafter, Dr. Turner admitted him to the hospital and kept him comfortable. Shortly before he died, he decided that he didn't want any further medical support, and when his IV stopped working, he asked that it not be restarted. With his wife at his side, he said, "We've already discussed this, and we've decided." He died shortly thereafter. After his death, his wife and family sent Dr. Turner a kind note, thanking him for his compassionate and personal care. Now, the wife was in the office for a checkup.

She had a past history of a heart attack and had a high cholesterol level. When Dr. Turner came into the room, her eyes welled up and she thanked him again for caring for her husband and for helping him to die in the way that he had wanted—and she hugged him. Then Dr. Turner, sensing that she may have put her own health issues on hold for the past few months because of her husband's illness, asked her, "How much chest pain have you been having?"

"More," she responded quietly.

"How long has this been going on?" he asked.

"For the past year," she said, even quieter, as she lowered her gaze.

"You know, you need to start paying attention to your own health," Dr. Turner said gently. And he arranged for her to have a stress test to evaluate her heart.

Later, the last of the 30 patients that Dr. Turner saw in the office that day was a 48-year-old man who came in because his knees were hurting. By the end of the visit it was apparent that he wasn't there just for his knees, but because he was depressed and needed to talk to someone. Because Dr. Turner had been well trained in the biopsychosocial model of medical care and in counseling, he was able to deal with these problems and ready to spend the extra time that was needed. And by the time the man left the office, he felt better. It had been a long and difficult day, but one in which Dr. Thane Turner had dealt with birth, death, and everything in between.

· · · · ·

Type "Dr. Thane Turner" into Google, the Internet search engine, and a CNN news story appears about Dr. Turner's return to his hometown of Lock Haven, Pennsylvania, to practice rural family medicine. Today's most modern technology—computers, the Internet, cable TV broadcast around the world—telling the story of rural family practice that most people believe is a relic from the past. But Thane Turner isn't an old-fashioned horse-and-buggy country doctor from the early 1900s, he's a young, modern, rural family physician of the new twenty-first century.

Having lived in Lock Haven since he was in the eighth grade, Thane Turner knew and appreciated the town and its people, and he wanted to return home to care for the friends and family he had known most of his life. When you meet him, his wide grin openly expresses his delight at being a family doctor in his hometown. "It's very satisfying, and so I'm not looking to say I could have done this somewhere else. It's all here!" Dr. Turner provides comprehensive family medicine common to rural areas, everything from treating patients for their colds and heart attacks to delivering babies. "Practicing medicine in the country," he says, "allows me to provide a wide range of care to all family members in an area where the availability of general and specialty medical care is low. My practice gives me the opportunity to learn not only my patients' medical history, but also the history of their family and their life experiences." Today, Dr. Turner is firmly established as one of Lock Haven's

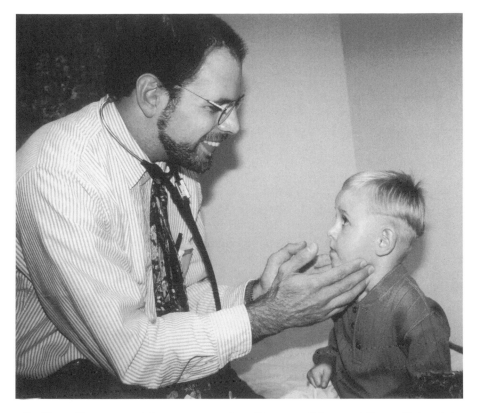

Dr. Thane Turner examining a young patient. (Courtesy of Thomas Jefferson University)

most respected family doctors. He and his wife Rachel have three children and enjoy living in Lock Haven.

• • • • •

With his stethoscope draped around his neck, Dr. Turner walks into an examination room to start seeing his patients on this typical morning. His first patient is an 11-year-old boy with a possible infection in his thumb, and whose mother has concerns regarding the family's contact with a farmhand who was found to have tuberculosis. Next, a call from the hospital that one of his patients, an 84-year-old retired coal miner with severe chronic lung disease, was being admitted to the hospital with increasing difficulty breathing. Dr. Turner discusses his care with the doctors in the emergency room and makes plans to see him in the hospital later in the day. Then, an adorable one-and-a-half-year-old girl that Dr. Turner had delivered comes in for her well child checkup and three immunizations.

Next, there is an older couple who have known Dr. Turner and his parents since the Turners arrived in Lock Haven. The husband, in his mid-80s, wants to discuss the results of his "slightly high" prostate cancer test that was performed during a recent community screening. His wife, who is in her mid-70s, has mild lung disease and had a high cholesterol level at the screening. But like her husband, she doesn't like taking medicines unless she "absolutely needs them," a fact she mentions multiple times during the visit. Dr. Turner had diagnosed a skin cancer on her cheek six months ago and had referred her to the dermatologist, who had removed it. The dermatologist asked her to return for a follow-up appointment, but as with many people who live in small rural towns, she doesn't want to travel 30 miles to "have him spend five minutes to check it and charge me sixty dollars." So, she asks if Dr. Turner could check it instead. After a brief discussion, she agrees to see the dermatologist for one more visit, after which Dr. Turner will provide further follow-up care. She also asks Dr. Turner to check a number of other lesions on her skin—she is "getting more all the time"—and Dr. Turner reassures her that none are cancer. Finally, her husband complains of some pain in the side of his neck, and is worried that he might develop a stroke, as his father had. Dr. Turner examines him and finds no evidence of any serious problems. But because his blood pressure is minimally elevated for the first time today—Dr. Turner suspects it is due to anxiety—he arranges for his nurse to recheck his blood pressure in a few weeks.

The next patient is an active seven-month-old little boy who was brought in by his mother to check on his bronchiolitis and ear infection, diagnosed two days ago, both of which are getting much better. Then comes a young man with chronic anxiety and depression—common problems in family practice—and fibromyalgia, a chronic pain syndrome. Although still affected by a number of symptoms, he has been doing a bit better lately, and Dr. Turner adjusts some of his medications, and spends time counseling him about his problems. The next patient is a teacher with pain in his left knee. Then there is a healthy 16-year-old boy, accompanied by his mother, who comes in for a high school physical to play basketball. Dr. Turner asks, "What are the two most important health problems for people your age?" Looking somewhat embarrassed, the teen replies, "I don't know." But when Dr. Turner says they are alcohol and its related problems with car accidents, and sexually transmitted diseases, the boy doesn't seem surprised. Dr. Turner then discusses "never getting in a car with anyone who has had anything to drink," and how sexually transmitted diseases are "entirely preventable."

· · · · ·

For Thane Turner, being a doctor had always meant being a family doctor—and living in a small town was what he had known and liked. So when he heard about the PSAP, it felt like a perfect fit. In fact, what he wrote in his application to medical school in 1988—"Having been raised in a small community setting, I can see both the need and value of a family physician. Therefore I wish to practice in a field where I can develop a more personal relationship with my patients"—is uncannily similar to his current description of life as a rural family doctor.

Thane was born in Lancaster County, Pennsylvania, and his family had moved to a number of small towns early in his life before settling in Lock Haven when his father became the head wrestling coach at Lock Haven University. Wrestling was also Thane's major extracurricular activity as he was growing up, and during high school he finished as one of the top five high school wrestlers in the Junior National Championship competition. He was also on the varsity wrestling team at Lock Haven University, which during his last two years of college was ranked in the top ten of Division I college wrestling teams in the country. While wrestling was and continues to be an important part of his life, Thane also entered college committed to pursuing a career in medicine, in part motivated by the medical problems in his own family. His oldest brother, Terry, died of leukemia as a small child, shortly before Thane was born. Then, tragically, when Thane was 19, a second older brother, Troy, also developed a rare form of cancer and died at the age of 24.

Thane excelled at Lock Haven University, and was elected to Phi Beta Kappa. He also knew Catherine O'Neil, who was a few years behind him. During the summer between his first and second years of medical school he worked in the Department of Family Medicine, where he did research on medical student career choices, and was coauthor of two resultant publications in the journals *Academic Medicine* and *Family Medicine*. Then in the last two years of medical school, his rural rotations confirmed his decision to become a rural family doctor. During his third year, he took his required family practice clerkship at the Geisinger Family Practice Center. Then, in his fourth and final year of medical school, he took a six-week rural family practice preceptorship at the private office of a Jefferson alumnus, Dr. Randy Westgate, in Mountville, a small town a few miles from Lancaster, Pennsylvania. Thane found this experience "extremely helpful to reaffirm my vision of rural family practice. I also needed to see Randy Westgate eat dinner with his kids. I needed to know that he could coach his kid's soccer team." Thane also spent a one-month elective at a hospital on the Navajo Indian Reservation in Shiprock, New Mexico.

After graduation from medical school, Dr. Turner decided to move to a smaller community, and "matched" for his family medicine residency at Lancaster General Hospital. During his third and final year, he was selected as chief resident, an honor afforded the best resident of the class. When it came time for Dr. Turner to decide where to practice, the fact that he and Rachel were both from Lock Haven made the decision to return easier. At this time, they had already had their first child, Ellen, and the pull of being near family was strong. Balancing his personal and professional goals was extremely important to him. "It was important to find a community where high quality care was provided, though with a smaller town feel, where I could know people, and have an impact."

"When I was in Lancaster," recounts Thane, "my own family doctor sent out some feelers about our interest in coming back." So Thane and Rachel went back to Lock Haven to take a look. On the drive up, "Rachel was ready to say 'we're coming' but she didn't want to put pressure on me. But as I went through the things that I wanted to do, it matched. It worked. I can remember being in the car driving home and Rachel asking that amazing question: 'When you started this whole thing, what did you want to do?' When I had applied to the PSAP, I had to write this essay about what I wanted to do, so we pulled it out and read it. And I realized that I have to be out in a small town doing this. I have to be where I know people. As much as it bothers me sometimes when I run into people at the donut shop asking me about their medicines, that's who I am. I'm that kind of guy, and I love to talk to people. And that wasn't going to happen in Lancaster, and it wasn't going to happen in Philly either. That's part of what rural family medicine is.

"You know, our progression was: We loved Center City Philly, we loved the experience, the relationships," Thane says. "But at the end of four years, we definitely knew we didn't want to stay in the city. That was always a little hard for me professionally. I struggled with the vision of staying at the university and joining the faculty. So we thought Lancaster was the answer— Amish country, where you could have the best of both worlds: a large hospital where you get to do everything, but also living rural. But in reality, Lancaster was becoming a bigger city every day. I lived in Lancaster for three years, and I don't think I ever ran into one of my patients. Whereas when you live in Lock Haven, almost everybody knows who you are. It's just that type of town. So what we liked about Lancaster was all the shopping and the restaurants. But the thing that we didn't like—we just didn't know anyone in town. And it still took a long time to get from your house to the hospital."

So in 1996, Thane joined his former family doctor, Dr. Frank Parker at Lock Haven Family Practice. Their office, a one-story tan building with a parking lot in front, is located on the main road just outside the center of town. The view from the front of the office is a wide vista of the nearby ridge of mountains. "Frank built this office about twenty years ago," Thane explains, "and when I came, we expanded the space and redid all the examining rooms. We've been blessed. The practice is really, really busy. The model works—just deliver good quality primary care and people will find a way through your front door. Frank's done a great job. He's the old-time family doctor. When he did obstetrics, he delivered 300 babies a year. We laugh now—I'm delivering kids of kids he delivered. He knew me growing up. He actually did my marriage physical in this same office—Rachel and I were here in this office. Sure there were lots of problems we didn't know about coming in. There were a lot of things that Frank was naïve about too. Some of his patients who he had been seeing for twenty years weren't real anxious to see a new young doctor. Now we laugh that some days I'm so busy, he's seeing some of my patients."

Like many rural physicians today, Thane and his partner do not own their own practice. Lock Haven Family Practice is part of a larger health system: the Susquehanna Health System in Williamsport that also owns two hospitals. There are four family physicians in Lock Haven who work for Susquehanna Physician Services. "I like working for a health system," Thane says. "For me, it offered me loan repayment, some guaranteed contracts for three years, and saw me through the lean days. I couldn't be in Lock Haven without that. And I was fortunate; in one and a half years my practice was already making money, which is faster than the three years I was given. I'm also glad that I work for a health system, because I don't want to worry about things like billing and office safety compliance.

"In this town," according to Thane, "family practice is very strong. It is a town where family practice is respected. There are still problems between specialists and primary care doctors here—the same as everywhere. And managed care made that worse for a time, but it's better now. I know our patients respect us, and I have patients who won't take medicine that a specialist gives them unless I say it's OK. And family practice will always have that role."

· · · · ·

"Our scope of practice is cradle to grave," Thane says proudly. "We do a lot more than family docs do in the city. The OB part of practice is a blast. It's just a constant influx of patients and new families. Doing OB leads to some of your most loyal patients and some of the strongest relationships that you create. I see that even today with Frank, when there's a college student in the office, and their mom says 'that's the doctor who delivered you.' Already for me, some of the first kids I delivered are getting ready for school, and are starting to come in for their kindergarten physicals.

"One of the other things I like about family practice is seeing lots of kids," says Thane. "I had to see kids. It's probably the thing our practice loves the most. And another advantage of doing OB is that you also get to take care of a lot of kids. But on the other hand, I had to decide at the end of the day, are kids *all* I want to see. You know, I really enjoyed that visit today with Mrs. Jones too." About half of Dr. Turner's practice consists of caring for entire families—multiple family members, and multiple generations. "A grandmother, a mother, her daughter, and then I deliver the baby. I wanted all those levels."

Geriatrics is probably five to ten percent of their practice, although Thane's partner does more of the nursing home work. They also have a number of patients in the extended care facility connected to the hospital. Dr. Turner sees about 28 to 30 patients in the office most days, from 8:30 AM to about 5:00 PM, with patients scheduled every 15 minutes. "During the flu season," he says, "we go right through the lunch hour. We also remove 'lumps and bumps,' suture cuts, put on casts for broken bones, and do cast removals. Of course, all the same life problems you see in urban areas—counseling issues, divorces, the destructiveness of alcoholism—are all here."

Today, Thane doesn't have any patients in the hospital, but usually the practice has about two patients, and on some weekends they can have as many as four to five admissions. "It's a small rural hospital," he says. "Some weekends you can admit somebody to the Intensive Care Unit [ICU], and then admit someone to the medical-surgical floor, and have somebody in pediatrics, and for me I can have somebody in OB. And that's exciting. For me, that's what it was all about. That was part of my vision of rural family practice.

Lock Haven has a small eight-bed ICU. We admit patients with chest pain who we suspect might be having a heart attack, or patients with heart failure. There's a cardiologist from Williamsport who comes up on Wednesdays. Although I was extremely well trained in cardiology, the reality is that if I had stayed in Lancaster, I wouldn't have gotten privileges in their ICU. They trained me so well that I'm doing it here, but the irony is that I wouldn't be able to do it there.

"We often transfer patients who are more seriously ill, or who need a specialist we don't have in town. We just opened up a dialysis center. We also admit kids to the hospital, but don't have a pediatric intensive care unit, so we transfer children who require those services. We do have a high-risk newborn nursery, and use oxygen tents, and insert umbilical artery catheters. But if newborns need a neonatal ICU, we transfer them."

Having been a competitive wrestler in high school and college, Thane often gets called by the university to serve as the doctor for local sports events, especially for wrestling. He and another doctor in town do all of the high school sports physicals in town, and he also provides care to people who are in a local missionary training institute in town.

· · · · ·

Lock Haven is a town of 9,149 in central Pennsylvania, located between the west branch of the Susquehanna River and Bald Eagle Creek. Originally called Old Town in pre-Revolutionary War days, the name was changed to Lock Haven: "Lock" because of the canal with locks connecting the river with the creek, and "Haven" since the area was a safe place for milling lumber and was a defense fort for protection from the Indians.

From the highway, the town of Lock Haven stretches out lengthwise nestled beneath the long low mountain ridge that forms the backdrop for the area. The cluster of orange brick buildings of Lock Haven University, where both Thane and Rachel attended college, dominates one side of town. As with other small towns, maintaining a stable economic base has been a constant problem. "The university is the largest employer in town," Thane says, "and the hospital is number two." This is similar to many small rural towns, where health care plays a major part in its economy. In fact, health care represents up to 20 percent of the employment and income in a rural community, with estimates that each family doctor in a town contributes more than $1 million per year and 50 jobs in the local economy. Continuing his description of the economy in Lock Haven, Thane says, "Woolrich woolen mill is three miles down the road and is a big employer, as is the school district. There is also a little bit of farming in the area and a few other small industries. Lock Haven was the home of Piper Aircraft, but it left in the 1970s. And the International Paper mill is about to close, and 400 jobs will be lost. It was the longest functioning paper mill on the same site in the United States. Rachel's granddad worked at the paper mill."

· · · · ·

Without having to think, Dr. Turner quickly says, "the best part of being a rural family doctor is the relationships, and the ability to make an impact on a community. When folks heard that I was coming back, the community was really excited. People in town knew me. In Lock Haven, wrestling is big—it's spelled with all capital letters. We moved here before I started high school, and I went to the university, and wrestled, and academically did extremely well. My wife was the valedictorian, and I was number two in our graduating class. So we're well known on a wide range of fields—by the sports people, the academic people, former teachers, etc. For me, it is a bit unique here, since I went back to my hometown, and my dad was the sports coach here. But I think the doctor always holds a special place in just about every small town.

"Primary care is the appreciation of the relationships with patients, combined with continuity of care," Thane explains. "I didn't want to be a subspecialist that was primarily hospital based. I come in and round on my patients at 7AM, and am out of the hospital at 7:45, and some days we don't go back until one of us stops by the hospital on the way home. We live our life over here in the office. I'm glad that is what I do. Like my kid says, 'My Dad's a doctor!' That's what I am. That's what I do. And it's exciting."

• • • • •

Thane says that his wife Rachel "is the epitome of a rural kid. She lived in the same house all her life. Her older sister's here. When we moved to Philly, I was taking her parents 'baby' away. We started dating late in high school—we were in the same class, we're six months apart in age. We both graduated from Lock Haven University in 1989, got married in June, Rachel started physical therapy [PT] school at Hahnemann University (in Philadelphia) in July, and I started at Jefferson in September. She went to PT school for 2 years, and then worked at Magee Rehabilitation Hospital during my last two years of medical school. Then she worked as a physical therapist in Lancaster. We had Ellen during my last year of residency, and that's when she started staying home. Now she does occasional work at two local hospitals."

As with the other five doctors in this book whose spouses also grew up in a rural area, Thane and Rachel illustrate the important role that a spouse has on the location decisions of physicians—as with most people. Having a rural-raised spouse is a very important factor in ending up rural. In fact, looking at all Jefferson graduates who were practicing in rural Pennsylvania (in any specialty) during a 20-year period, 79 percent either grew up rural or had a spouse who did.

Today, the Turner's are "doing really, really well." They have three children; two girls and a boy. Ellen, the oldest, is now six and in kindergarten. Avery is four, and the youngest—Caleb—just turned two. For Thane, the kids are definitely the greatest part of life. "And Lock Haven is a good place for kids," he says. "Every now and then I've taken one of the kids with me into the hospital when I make rounds, or do some quick things, but they're not quite to the age where I can do that very often yet. One of the things I did this morning was take Caleb for his two-year-old checkup. I told Rachel I'd take care of that, and I also did a few charts, while he ran around in here in the office."

· · · · ·

One of the biggest challenges facing Dr. Turner in rural family practice, as with almost all physicians in all locations, was carving out time for his family—what he refers to as "the time thing. I had some struggles early on about just how overwhelming rural medicine really is. It's everywhere. It's in the donut shop, it's in the church. And I knew that, I guess, coming in. But then I came to realize that you do have to step back and ask, 'What are all the positives? Why am I doing this?' One thing we did early on, when I first came here, my partner and I each took a half day off. It's a small town thing—people joke about it—everything shuts down Wednesday afternoon. Now, we are committed to taking a whole day off with the other person just working harder that day to do whatever is necessary. And that's helped.

"Since there are four of us in town who cover for each other, we are each on call one night a week," Thane says. "I take Wednesday nights. Then we each take call every fourth weekend. It's variable, it can be easy, or it may not be. I have nights when I sleep the whole night. Or I can have nights when I get phone calls every hour. You have this vision when you're in residency—you picture you have five or six admissions and have to run around all night when you're on call. But a lot of nights, no. Today, for example, we don't have anyone in the hospital, and there are days like that." Because Dr. Turner is the only doctor in his practice, and one of the few in town who deliver babies, he's also on call for his own pregnant patients all the time. There are two obstetricians in town, two other family doctors who do obstetrics, and a midwife. Overall, there are about 400 deliveries in town each year, and Thane does about 40 of these. He and his partner are planning to hire a new family doctor soon, one that will be able to share OB call, which will make a big difference in Dr. Turner's night call schedule. But, "rural medicine, at least in this town, isn't as bad as I think I pictured it," he says, "even considering that I'm the only one in our practice taking OB call. For example, I've delivered all my babies that are due for the next six weeks. So Rachel and I will probably sign out a couple of these upcoming weekends. No one is likely to deliver, and I have backup—just in case. Patients really understand that you can't be available all the time."

As for spending time with his kids, Thane considers this a constant challenge, although "I work pretty consistently to try and be home for dinner with the kids, spend time with them after dinner for homework, and be able to put them to bed. I do try to be pretty involved in those types of things, going to school functions, and picking them up at soccer practice. I want to be a big part of their lives, and I think I actually have more control over those decisions in a rural community than if I were in a bigger community. For my wife and I, our family, our marriage, our faith—those are the most important things. So you need to make time for them."

• • • • •

Economic factors are frequently raised as one of the reasons that rural areas have a shortage of physicians. Compared with physicians in metropolitan areas, rural doctors nationally do have lower average incomes. But it turns out that a lot of that difference is due to the larger proportion of family physicians and other generalists in rural areas who also have lower incomes than specialists. In fact, for family physicians, net income is very similar for those practicing in rural and urban areas. On the other hand, as mentioned by all of the doctors I visited, the cost of living in rural areas, especially for housing, is much lower than in other areas—with the result being that the standard of living for many rural family physicians is quite high, in many instances higher than for urban family physicians. "You really can make a good living as a rural family physician," says Thane. "When I came out here, I bought thirteen acres of land for less than what one acre costs in the city. And then we built what for many people would be a very big house. It's two miles from the office, and almost half of that is the access road to the house! I drive up a three-quarter mile lane and you'd think I was up in the middle of the mountain—in the middle of nowhere. That's the best part. We knew we wanted to have four or five kids. So when the opportunity came, we worked with a guy I went to high school with, to build it half finished, and over time we're gradually finishing bedrooms as we go. And we finished the basement. But if you just look at the size of our house—five bedrooms, 4,000 square feet—and took that to Lancaster or Philly, I don't think a family doctor could afford it. But I can in rural America. And we live very comfortably and still pay off my school loans. Of course when I first came here, I made less income starting out, but that's increased significantly over time.

"For Rachel and me, we say 'Thank you for the advantages of living in a small town.' Yes, we have to drive thirty minutes to get to the mall, but for us, having the land, and the space, and the bigger house is important. Do we have so much money we don't have to think about what we buy? No, of course not. And sure, family doctors everywhere make less than specialists. But those aren't going to be the things that are going to satisfy you anyway. That's not what's going to make you happy. It's 'Are you doing what you really want to do?' "

• • • • •

Because of the important role his medical school rural preceptorship played in solidifying his own career goals, Dr. Turner—like Bill Thompson—now serves as a preceptor for current PSAP and other Jefferson medical students. "The preceptorship has been great," he says. "Serving as a preceptor has allowed me to experience the benefits and impact of the PSAP from the other side. I was able to keep my teaching skills sharp and bond with my students in much the same way as I did with my advisor. As a whole, the PSAP gives both students and teachers the opportunity to learn the dramatic and interesting differences between the practice of family medicine in Center City Philadelphia, and rural Pennsylvania.

"We also teach in the rural physician assistant program at Lock Haven University, and have freshman medical students from Penn State College of Medicine. There's a lot of different ways to have an impact. Actually, what I have to offer is much more helpful in this setting than it would ever be standing in front of 200 students."

• • • • •

As for life outside of his family and medicine, Thane says simply, "My church is one of the most important things in my life." A major outside activity is sports. "We have season tickets to the Penn State football games, and usually go to two to three games each year. Also, I run my Dad's Web page for the Messiah College Wrestling Team, where he is the coach now. I also go to the national wrestling finals, and have covered it for the Harrisburg newspaper—I had my press pass. I go to the wrestling matches here at Lock Haven University. And we're active in the university's alumni association—we want to help others to be successful.

"The thing that we miss the most that we did before we had kids is the hiking and the biking. Our kids are just not old enough yet. But we talk about doing more of that, as the kids get older. The dike that they built in town here has a walking trail on top of it, and they light it at night, and lots of people walk on it. So Rachel will often walk up there—put some of the kids in a stroller—it's about three to four miles long. It's beautiful along the river."

Friends are also important to the Turners. "My best friend growing up," says Thane, "is now the veterinarian in town, and was somewhat instrumental in setting up my first interview to come back here. And since we came back we really reestablished that friendship again. Actually, he had forty acres of land, and we bought thirteen of it, and we're neighbors, but live acres apart from each other."

For the Turner's, another big advantage of living in Lock Haven is having family around. "There's sixteen years between my wife and her sister," Thane says. "Her sister was actually our ninth grade teacher. Neat stuff like that happens in small towns like this. Now, her kids are basically grown. Her youngest is sixteen years old—I just did her driver's license physical exam yesterday. And she's excited that she has nieces and nephews, and likes to babysit for us. Rachel's mom and dad are also here, and my folks are only about two hours away. Rachel and I do more together than some other couples. We go out to dinner together or go to the movies. And so it's not uncommon that we quickly get a babysitter and go do something—just not on Wednesdays or my weekend on call."

• • • • •

While most of Dr. Turner's time is taken up with the day-to-day role of caring for his friends and neighbors in Lock Haven, he also thinks about the impact of national health policy issues on his patients—as do many of his PSAP colleagues that I visited. "The number one thing where I hurt the most for my patients," he says, "is the cost of prescription drugs. Day to day it is. You know, you're sitting with a 70-year-old woman with diabetes, and her hemoglobin A1C blood test [measuring long term diabetic control] is starting to go up a little bit. She has no other medical problems, and she's making a decision not to take any more medicines because she really can't afford it. And I know the research says she's probably going to live longer if she takes it. She's in a mind-set of 'I'm seventy, I'm not going to live that much longer'— but I'm thinking that plenty of 90-year-olds come in here, and I don't know that we're not going to have twenty more years together. And so I shut the door at the end of the day, just saying 'How do I deal with that?' You can only find so many samples of medicines. So, if I was going to say the one big thing that was hurting our patients the most, it's the prescription drug cost. And that's the thing that breaks your heart the most—those people that take $600 to $700 per month of drugs."

• • • • •

For Thane, "the reward in the long run has been the satisfaction that I'm doing what Jefferson and the PSAP wanted to create for a certain portion of their graduates—awesome primary care doctors. Sure, they also produce lots of great teachers and researchers. But part of what they want to do is what I'm doing, so I'm proud of that. You do have to be well trained, but if you are, you can have such an impact, and have such a great time. I'm convinced that good quality primary care is going to win the day. I don't care who the president is, or what insurance plans we take, I am convinced that it's all going to start with primary care. I don't know how managed care will change. But I still believe the ball gets rolling when the patient comes through the front door, and that will still be true years and years from now.

"In medical education," Thane is convinced, "we need to encourage those interested in rural family practice, and provide them with opportunities, and give them role models. And we need to make sure they understand that it's a tough job to be on the front lines of medicine, so you'd better be well trained. It's really rewarding, though it's also hard in ways I didn't think would be hard."

• • • • •

So, can you go home again? Thane Turner says, "You can't go home the same way. You can't go home and be who you were. So much happened to us in the process. We got married, had lived in Philadelphia, decided what we were going to be, lived through residency, had a six-figure debt, our faith was challenged in so many ways, and we grew in such a different way. And our view of the world was so different. So you can't go back and be who you were. But you can go back! And you can fit in. And it's fun. When I have a student in my office and they walk in the room, patients often get a kick out of telling them about all their connections and relationships to me. That's neat for me, and I like that."

So, for Dr. Thane Turner, the best thing about being a family doctor in a small town is "knowing the people, and having the relationships. And having the chance—when somebody's in trouble, or needs something—to use the skills and training that you were provided, and help them through it."

MOREHEAD CITY, NORTH CAROLINA

> I still hope that someday there could be a wedding between scientific proficiency and the sort of earnest solicitude and untiring sympathy of the old country doctor.
>
> —E. B. White

Sitting at the desk in his office, Joe Nutz looks at the two computer monitors sitting side by side on his desk. Both are connected to one computer, one mouse, and one keyboard, and his screen saver—a panoramic picture of his favorite place, Cape Lookout on the North Carolina coast—crosses the two screens, half suspended on each one. As Joe moves the mouse, the different windows he has open—his patient schedule, his e-mail—jump from one monitor to the other, just as if you were alternating between the two windows on a single monitor, except that Joe can see both full windows at the same time. "Actually, I have a new system coming," he says. "It has four flat-panel LCD monitors that you can put next to each other, because once you have two, all of a sudden the two monitors aren't good enough, and you want to go to four. I can keep my patient schedule up here on one monitor, my electronic medical records up here on another, I can keep my Web browser open over here, and I have one for doing whatever else I want over here, like my e-mail. Once you get into that, you'll never want to go back. You just won't. When you're on the fly, the fewer clicks the better. It's all about information."

Also sitting on Joe's desk is a tablet computer that works off of a radio frequency. He plans to use this in the new office he is building, which will be a twenty-first-century state-of-the-art computerized medical office. When he moves into his new office in a few months, he plans to implement his computerized medical record system, and to carry the tablet computer from room to room instead of a paper chart. As he enters each patient's rooms, he will download their medical chart onto the tablet computer, and write his note

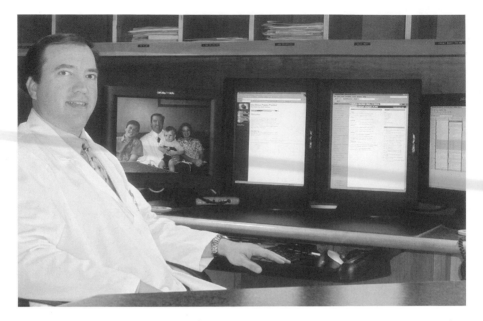

Dr. Joe Nutz sitting in front of his four computer monitors. (Courtesy of Dr. Joe Nutz)

directly on the tablet and thus directly onto the computerized medical record. "Once I get my computerized medical record," he explains, "if I'm going to send a patient off to a specialist, before they leave the room my note can get faxed off to the specialist with a picture of the patient attached. For refilling patient's medicines, I can just hit the fax button and fax it to the pharmacy. It takes up so much time now for the nurses to call it in."

Compared to most other professions and industries, medicine is far behind in using computers to assist doctors in improving quality health care and in increasing efficiency. Hospitals have only recently begun to develop computerized order entry, including medication ordering, which can almost totally eliminate the errors inherent in poor handwriting and verbal orders given from doctor to nurse. However most doctors offices still keep all patient information in a paper format, and doctors continue to collect reams of medical information about their patients, including notes from their prior visits, in paper charts—recording information in a way that is rarely looked at again or used in subsequent visits, and hard to find if it is needed.

Computers are a big part of Joe's practice. "I always wanted to computerize the practice," he says. "I do not want these paper charts. I hate paper and charts! When I first started the practice, it got so busy so quickly that I couldn't get it up and running in time. But now I'm taking another go at it. I already have it so that everything that's in the office—the billing stuff, my faxes—I can also get at from home, except for the actual clinical records. I have my whole house networked, so I have four computers at home, and I have a fifty-four-inch big screen TV that's a computer, and I can sit there from my couch and bring up all this stuff. And the electronic medical record system I am getting is Web based, and I can get hold of it from any computer too. Even with a palm pilot, if it's wireless. I'm working on it now, and my goal is to get it up and running before my new partner gets here, and before we move into the new office in a few months. I've been thinking about this for a long time. My EKG machine is all digital, my lung function testing machine is all digital—so you can download the results. All my faxes come in through the computers, so they can be tagged right onto the medical records. So we are moving towards a paperless office. But this is the hardest thing I have tried so far.

"Even now," he continues, "I print out patient information off the computer and give it to people, or sometimes forward it to patients via e-mail. When patients come in, I try to collect their e-mail address, and eventually I want to have the whole thing set up so I can send out reminders when it's time for flu shots, or this or that. And they can send me e-mail. Now, only a few people contact me by e-mail about their health—I haven't really pushed that yet.

"We're also putting digital TVs in the new office. Debbie [his nurse practitioner] and I are going to make our own videos with messages we want people to hear—like about getting flu shots during influenza season—and flash them up every twenty minutes or so. And I'm putting a patient computer in the waiting room so people can start to put some patient information in, and we will link it to the computerized record. And I'm going to walk around the office from room to room with my computerized pen tablet. It's an all wireless network system. I've been working on this new office for a year."

· · · · ·

Joe Nutz grew up in Raceland, Kentucky. As he says in his southern Kentucky accent (a smooth, almost musical, and soothing voice), "All I remember is Kentucky. Most of my life was spent in Raceland—I remember that from the first grade on." Raceland is in eastern Kentucky with a population of 1,200, and "my dad was chief of police. I was known as 'Joe's boy.' And I could not get away with anything. He knew everything in that town. I was scrutinized from first grade all the way up to my senior year. I guess, looking back on it, it was good, but it was tough sometimes. Yeah, I remember when I got my driver's license, I was in the next town, and I'd squeal my wheels a little bit, and the police would see me, and he knew about it right off the bat. But if my baseball games were in town, he'd drive up in his police cruiser and watch me play ball. All the kids would love him, because he'd take his radar gun and shoot the baseballs, so they knew how fast they were throwing them. And he'd help us out in practices. My mom owned a restaurant. She owned a couple different restaurants, but the one I remember was called the Dairy Cheer. That was a hit, cause after baseball games, if we won, everybody'd go down there for a free milkshake. And it was right next to our house. I peeled potatoes for the french fries. I peeled a lot of potatoes.

"I always felt like I wanted to be a physician," Joe recalls. "My mom tells me that Dr. Jones, our own family doctor, used to give me shots all the time. And she says I used to tell him 'You know I'm going to be a doctor some day, and I'm gonna get you back!' Yeah, I always thought about medicine, and I always worked toward it." His first real experience with illness was when his family "took care of my aunt. She had breast cancer and she lived in our house. She actually took over my room. I remember seeing my parents care for her."

After high school, Joe went to Ashland Community College. It was close to where he grew up, and he lived home for the first two years of college. "Nobody in my family had actually gone to college except for my sister and me—in my entire family, cousins and everybody. So we were the brains of the group back there in the backwoods of Kentucky. But they also used to say, 'When you going to graduate?' They'd be out working construction or on the assembly line, they'd have their houses and kids, and I'd still be in school." During his first two years of college, Joe was a personal assistant for an elderly lawyer in town. "I'd go over and fix his meals at night and hand out his pills—he took about 20 pills. He used to like to talk and talk, and I'd sit there and listen to him. I shared call with another guy, so one of us would be there every evening, from about 5:00 PM, and we'd sleep through the night there."

Then, after finishing up at community college, Joe transferred to the University of Kentucky in Lexington, where he completed his last two years of college. "I applied to medical school after college, but didn't get in. During my second year of college my parents got divorced and my grades were bad—things took a dip. There were real family problems there for a while. But then everything turned back around. So I went to graduate school after that. I stayed at the University of Kentucky, and that's where I met Petra. I was in Biochemistry 501, and she was trying to find Physiology 502, and I had to show her where to go. We dated for a year, we were engaged for a year, and then we got married. Then she got into veterinary school at the University of Pennsylvania, and she took me up to Philadelphia. So I transferred to the Philadelphia College of Pharmacy and Science and went to graduate school for two more years up there. I was heading toward a PhD degree in pharmacology and toxicology. I worked hard at it—and I did really well—but I didn't enjoy it. I was always a people person. And to be locked in a lab, and doing things with rats and cats, and pain studies—I mean it was all technically challenging, there was a little surgery, and the research—but it just wasn't interacting with people. So I really wasn't happy with that. My heart was always in medicine, so I started to look around again at medical school. It was rough there for a while, but I wasn't going to stop."

So Joe decided to apply to medical school again, this time his application bolstered by a strong academic record from graduate school. When he heard about the PSAP, he remembers thinking that it fit him. "I mean I always wanted to be a general practitioner, you know, somebody that does a little bit of everything." When he applied to Jefferson, Joe wrote that his career plans were: "To have a successful family practice." "And I always saw myself going back to a small town," he continues. "I really didn't care for Philadelphia. It was just too big, too impersonal. I used to argue with my medical school advisor—he was from the New York City area—and he'd say, 'Philadelphia is such a small town.' And I was like, 'No—this is huge!' And I remember thinking, it's all your perspective. I'm coming from little Raceland all the way to Philadelphia, and he's stepping down to Philadelphia from New York City."

• • • • •

For Joe, moving to Philadelphia was a "real shocker. I'm from a small town, and when we first moved into West Philadelphia, there was a guy hanging out the window, two stories up, beating a stick against the wall screaming racial obscenities. And I'm like, 'Where am I? What am I doing?' Later, after I got into medical school, we moved farther out and found a place that was really nice. We actually had a little patio, and there was a park across the street—and we thought we had it made. We'd take the trolley car in to school." Joe remembers first being on a bus in Philadelphia. "I wanted to get off at my stop. I saw other people pull the cord and the bus driver stopped. And I pulled it, and he didn't stop. So next time I pulled it again, and he still didn't stop. I guess you have to step down onto the step first and pull it or something—I guess there was a trick I was missing. And so the next time I pulled it, and I yelled 'Yo! Stop the bus!' like I was Rocky. I thought well, that's how they talk around here—and people looked at me, and started laughing. Yeah, I remember saying in my southern accent, 'Yo, stop the bus!' "

When Joe started medical school, his wife was in her third year of veterinary school. Then, as he was finishing his second year, Petra was graduating, and they had their first child, Steven. "I remember studying for part one of my medical boards holding him in my arms. That was busy—and it was tough." Petra got a job working at a local veterinary hospital for a few years, and their daughter, Jessie was born just before Joe graduated from Jefferson. (Their third child, Eric, was just born shortly before my visit). During his third year, Joe remembers seeing lots of kids during his family practice clerkship. "I was into kids, 'cause we had one at home. The other medical students weren't used to handling babies, and I was flipping them over, changing diapers—and I understood the parents and what they were going through." He also liked anesthesiology. "Because I liked pharmacology and toxicology. But I didn't do that, probably for the same reason I didn't stay in research—I mean you really don't have that people interaction. I liked the science of it, but everybody sleeps on you. They're either waking up or going to sleep, and that's about it. I mean I really and truly enjoy sitting there and talking with the person, and taking care of them, and seein' where they live at, seein' them around town. I enjoy that."

Joe really enjoyed his senior family practice preceptorship with Dr. Rich Pierotti in Harleysville, Pennsylvania, but "I'm not sure there was any one person who turned me on to family practice—no one that I actually said, 'I want to be exactly like this person.' It was just kind of like it fit. I really enjoyed my OB rotations, I enjoyed my internal medicine rotations in the hospital, I really enjoyed my family practice rotations. I couldn't see myself just being a surgeon, and as for internal medicine, they didn't see kids, and I felt like 'that's not medicine, if you can't take care of children.' So family practice just seemed to have all the components. And of course the family practice department was very supportive. You know, you looked at the Family Medicine Department, and you just felt comfortable there. I remember my interview for medical school was there when I was just a little 'wanna-be' doctor. And my medical school advisor was there. And I did a research project there after my first year, on alcoholism. And we saw babies and adults in the office, and made home visits. I enjoyed that."

For residency, Joe decided to go to Hamot Hospital in Erie, Pennsylvania. It was close to Petra's home. "That was one of the drawing factors," Joe explains. "It was hard, with the kids, and Petra was practicing veterinary medicine. She was practicing seventy-some hours a week, and I was working 100 hours a week. So in Erie, her mom was there, and she watched Jessie for several months. I think it was hard on them, but they would do anything they could for us. I enjoyed the residency program at Hamot—I really did. They had good faculty, and it was a good program—a lot of hands on experience. I remember they were teaching us about practice management and coding and I'm thinking 'What's this coding? I don't want to learn this stuff.' And now, Oh my gosh!" Joe's exclamation about "coding" reflects the huge effort that all doctors now put into learning about coding, the structured and legal format by which physicians bill and get reimbursed from the government and insurance companies. In general, doctors have to code each office visit on a 1–5 scale, from a brief visit to a comprehensive examination. While this appears simple enough, the requirements for selecting each level are actually extraordinarily complex. For example, in order to bill for a "level 4" or "detailed" visit, there must be written documentation in the chart for that specific patient visit that the doctor did two of the following three: (1) asked questions related to at least four areas of the history of the present illness, reviewed the history related to two to nine body systems, and updated either: the past history, family history, or social history; (2) performed an examination that included at least five body systems, or two elements from six organ systems or body parts, or at least 12 elements from two or more organ systems or body parts; and (3) included a level of "medical decision making complexity" that included two of the following three: there were multiple diagnoses or a new problem, there were multiple data items to be reviewed or diagnostic studies ordered, and there was a moderate risk of complications. Without written documentation in the chart for two of these three areas for each patient visit billed for a "detailed" visit—irrespective of whether or not it was actually performed—doctors are now liable for committing fraud!

"After Petra went through her first winter in Erie," Joe continues, "and we had snow up to her chin for six to seven months, she said, 'Now I know why I used to say I'd never come back here when I was growing up.' So after all that snow, we decided we're not going to stay here. Then, after I finished my residency we started looking for small towns, all the way from as far up as Norfolk all the way down to Savannah. 'Cause we knew we liked the water and we didn't like the snow. And we didn't like large towns. So I just started calling some hospitals. One headhunter got my name and kept trying to get me to go to a town that was sixty miles inland, saying 'You can get to the ocean in just an hour.' And I told him, 'If I can't hit the water with a rock, it's too far away.' Growing up, I did a lot of boating in lakes, fresh water, rivers, and so forth, and we always vacationed on the coast. And I didn't want to wait till I retired to come to a place like this. I was looking for a small town, good hospital, good practice, and good schools, so I chose Morehead because it had everything we really wanted, and we've been happy.

"I moved down here in 1995, so I've been here seven years. Compared to Raceland, this here's a metropolis. My first day in the office was cancelled because of Hurricane Allison. They said it had been thirty years since they had a hurricane, and we've had six of them since then—so I've seen more hurricanes than most of the locals around here. Some were Category 3 hurricanes, but we haven't had to evacuate yet. You can get 100-mile-an-hour wind and horizontal rain. So you learn where the cracks in your house are, and how to board up windows, and get through a hurricane."

· · · · ·

When Joe first came to Morehead City, North Carolina, he joined the practice of the physician who helped recruit him to town. But after a few years, he became aware of serious accounting errors associated with his partner, and because of this he decided to leave the practice and open his own office. "When I walked in here," he recalls, "all I had was a stethoscope and an otoscope—I had no furniture. But basically, the entire staff went with me, so I had a complete staff. The head of the hospital helped me out and got me some computer tables and a couple other things, and I had this place up and running in a couple of weeks. And my neighbor owned the building, so he helped get me in here. As soon as I walked in here, patients were following me. It's a small town, and people were asking, 'Where'd Joe go?' 'Where'd Dr. Nutz go?' So I started four years ago with no charts, and I've built the practice to over 5,000 patients. I closed the practice down for new patients for a while, but now I'm trying to build it up so that my new partner can walk in. So it all worked out pretty good.

"And my staff here, some of them have been running an office for twenty years," he continues. "So they teach me things. I've learned so much. I have a billing manager, an office manager, and my head nurse has been a nurse for twenty years, and she knows just about everybody in town—no matter if they're bankers, or fisherman, or whatever they do. And our receptionist has been doing this for twenty years too, and everybody looks to her. When I left, patients left the other practice and followed her—the receptionist. They wanted to be with her.

"I have a wonderful nurse practitioner, Debbie, who helps me out," Joe explains. "She's great, and everybody loves her. I do inpatient medicine and pediatrics, and normally have about four patients in the hospital. Right now, I'm chief of the medicine department in the hospital. Then I see about twenty to twenty-five patients a day in the office, and Debbie sees about the same number. And another twenty people come in for labs, nurse visits. That kind of keeps me busy. Right now, I have maybe five babies in my practice. I had two recent newborns—right about the time our son Eric was born two months ago, so they're growing up together. And I'll get to watch them the rest of their lives, as long as they stay here. I do a number of outpatient surgical procedures—mostly lumps and bumps, skin cancers—you know down here on the coast you see a lot of suspicious lesions. There's not a week goes by, I don't do some sort of office surgery.

"I keep a medical box in the back of the truck here," Joe continues, "and occasionally I'll do home visits. I just do home visits for people that can't get out to see me—it's just too much a burden for them, or they're terminally ill, and in hospice care. And rather than have the ambulance bring them in to see me—it's so uncomfortable for them—I'll just go see them. I learned that at Jefferson—we did home visits when I was in medical school. So, I packed me a box—it's actually a fishing box—and I keep all my medical gear in it. I can draw blood, and I have an EKG machine—I can just about run a medical "code" [resuscitation] from it. And I've sutured up many a person in the middle of the night. Home visits are really a kind of quality medicine too. I mean you're actually going to that person's home, seeing them, taking care of them, and they really appreciate that."

As for being on call, Joe says, "I was on call every other weekend for the last three years. The practice has really grown a lot recently, and I do get paged a lot. But now there are two other doctors in our call group, and I'm on every third weekend, which is heaven. And when my new partner comes, I'll be on once a month. And that's gonna be fine. I was in a call group that had seven people, and that's just too busy. You'd be on every six weeks or so, but when you were on, you were on. You just basically lived in the hospital and had constant phone calls. Every other weekend was nice—you could sit home and do things, but you were tied down. But once a month is going to be perfect. Also, my nurse practitioner takes first call. So if somebody has a cold, runny nose, fever, I don't hear about that. If it's the emergency room, the hospital, or the nursing home, I tell them to call me. And I try to teach my patients what is and what is not an emergency, so—" Then, just as he's talking about being on call, Joe's pager beeps. It's a call from the hospital about a sick patient of one of the other doctors he covers for. But he quickly answers the question and continues, "It's really rare when I have to pick up and go into the hospital. The ER docs are really good."

Concerning the number of physicians in the area, Joe says, "There are about nine to ten family doctors in the community now, and about seven internists, a few older general practitioners, and three pediatricians. We use nurse practitioners, and that helps a lot. I couldn't make it without mine, I just couldn't do it. We need two to three more family docs, and one more internist. I'll be bringing one of them in. Also, there's definitely a shortage of mental health professionals in small towns."

· · · · ·

Dr. Nutz has three patients in the hospital today. The first patient is a 71-year-old man with a history of multiple sclerosis, and his legs are getting weaker. He had been discharged from the nursing home a few days ago, and called Dr. Nutz at 3:00 in the morning—he had another fall. He went to the ER, where he was found to have multiple bruises. Then, he developed a bad reaction to the shot of pain medicine that he was given, got very confused, and was admitted for the night. He has a son in town, but both the son and his wife work, and are unable to watch him during the day.

The next patient is a 54-year-old woman with recurrent diverticulitis (inflammation of her intestines) over the past year. Dr. Nutz has known her for about three years, and treated her with antibiotics a number of times for this problem, but whenever he stops the medicine, the inflammation flares up again. She had developed a very thickened part of her colon, so the surgeons decided to remove that part. "She's feeling better already," he reports. Then, reviewing her chart, he continues, "I just follow her along with the surgeons. They took the tube out of her nose—that's always a good sign. Her blood pressure is good, and she's afebrile. So if she starts eating, she should go home tomorrow." In the room, Dr. Nutz tells her half jokingly, "If you can eat hospital food—that's called the 'food test'—you're ready to go home."

The last patient is a 36-year-old fisherman who Dr. Nutz has taken care of for the past five years. "I've seen him through a couple different things. And I see him all the time at the Golden Corral restaurant. He's not supposed to be there—it's a steak house buffet, all you can eat. He has high cholesterol, and he always kind of looks the other way when I see him there." The man came in with appendicitis the day before yesterday, and the surgeon removed his appendix. Dr. Nutz says, "He seems to be doing pretty well now. He's on a clear liquid diet, no fever. His blood pressure is up a little. His electrolytes are pretty good." Once in the room, the patient tells Dr. Nutz, "I tried to convince the surgeon that beer was a clear liquid."

· · · · ·

Joe says that even though his wife, Petra, "grew up in a big city, she's pretty comfortable not living in a city. She likes it down here. You know, we lived around so many malls and everything, so I think she misses the malls. There's not a mall here. We go over to the new mall in Raleigh every few months. It's about three to four hours away, so we don't go that often. We'll spend a day there, and we'll get our fill of it, and that's about it. And then we walk out of there thinking, 'I'm glad we don't live around a big city, we'd spend all of our money in the malls.' I mean they're all the same, there's just the same shoe stores, and clothing stores, and places to eat. We get everything we need here from Wal-Mart, Lowe's, Sears, or we buy it on line.

"My wife's a veterinarian," Joe points out. "Her practice is in town too, although she hasn't gone back to practice since Eric was born. But if I put someone in the hospital who has a dog, for example, she'll send someone out to get the puppy and they'll put that puppy in her hospital. Then when I go round on the patient, she'll ask me 'How's my puppy doing?,' and I'll say, 'she's doing fine. She's eating and they're taking care of her.' So we take care of the entire family."

Joe and Petra's son Steven is now 12, their daughter Jessie is ten, and their newest son Eric is two months. "I think the schools are academically challenging here," Joe says. "That's one of the reasons we chose this place, because the public schools are so good." Compared to growing up as the son of the chief of police, as Joe did, he thinks that growing up as "Dr. Nutz's kids" is probably nicer. "My dad went around and he wrote tickets, he disciplined people, he ran kids off the street, he ran a tight ship. So I had to put up with that side of it. I'm out there basically helping people out—spending my nights with people when their grandma's dying, or when their babies are born, and taking care of them. So the kids see a whole different world than I did. They see people coming up saying that they know you, and that you helped them out, and they take pride in that. Jessie is very talented in art, and she loves the arts. Steven has a real interest in medicine. I think he sees how much I enjoy it. All the people kind of gather around me all the time in a small town. I have him tagging along with me sometimes. He's already told me he's going to join me in practice. He's already picked out a place in my new office."

Joe lives in the adjacent town of Newport. "That's the mailing address," he says. "We live on the water—the Bogue Sound. We live a couple streets back from the sound, but we have community boat docks and boat ramps and community pools and tennis courts and all this stuff. So you can park your boat there and leave it. I used to be able to sit on my back deck and see the water, but since I've moved there, there's probably about twenty-five to thirty houses that have been built, and I can't see the water as easily now—I have to look between driveways. My lot is about three-quarters of an acre— it's a nice house. And it's less than ten minutes from the office or hospital— it's about ten miles. And I can be at the hospital from my office in two and a half minutes."

• • • • •

Morehead City, one of North Carolina's deepwater ports, is located at the very southern end of the Cape Hatteras and Cape Lookout National Seashores. It sits on the mainland, with the Bogue Sound separating it from the small ocean side resort town of Atlantic Beach. It is home to a number of marine research facilities, including the Institute of Marine Sciences, the Duke University Marine Laboratory, and the North Carolina Division of Marine Fisheries. It is also home to the Ferry Division of the North Carolina Department of Transportation, and serves as a port for the US Marine Corps at Camp Lejeune. In recent years the town has developed a large charter-fishing fleet, and continues to serve as a modern port terminal.

"Morehead City is a small town," Joe says, "but it's the big city in Carteret County." Most of Joe's patients come from Morehead City and the adjacent towns of Newport, Beaufort, and Atlantic Beach. The population of Morehead City is a little over 7,500. The entire county, which only has 12 family doctors, has about 50,000 people. "In the summer, it grows to 150,000, when 100,000 tourists come in here—half for boating, half for the beaches. A lot of 'weekenders' come down here—you can see them trailering their boats from towns an hour away, like New Bern or Kinston. Morehead has a number of boat docks and boat ramps. It's also the state port, and they do a lot of import/ export through here. I'm the family doc for a couple of the companies that work down at the port. There's also a small waterfront area in Morehead, which is kind of the hub of everything." Driving past the waterfront, Joe points out the charter boats that he's been out on fishing for bluefin, marlin, and tuna. "There's the Bill Collector, the Wave Runner, the Magnitude." Then, passing Jack's Fishing Store, Joe says, "This guy right here, Jack, he's taught me a lot of things about fishing. He got me all hooked up, gives me lessons on how to rig bait, what to look for. I get a couple other old guys out there who've been fishing off these waters for twenty-some years—I don't take boating courses—I take guys out who've been out there forever. They tell you how to sniff the wind, how to look at the water—you know, you smell certain things. You look for birds—where the birds are diving there's fish, where the water changes there arc currents. You learn to read the depth finder—the bottom where the fish are—so I got a kind of informal training that way.

"My boat is twenty-five feet," Joe says. "I keep it dry stacked in town. When I want to go out, I just call them and they put ice and bait in it, and oil, and put it out in the water. When I come back, they clean it off and flush it out. They have a fork lift and pick your boat up and keep it out of the water. It's like keeping your car in the garage." Then Joe continues, "It can be pretty scary out in the ocean. About two weeks ago I got stranded twenty-six miles off shore! I hadn't had my boat out in a while because first Petra was pregnant, and then Eric was born, and it got hectic afterwards. So it had been a few months. And I got stranded—they had to jump start my boat, because the batteries were dead. I got out there, turned the boat off to bottom fish a little bit, and it wouldn't start back up. So luckily I had my anchor dropped, and there was one other boat out there. My short wave radio—nothing was working. So I started blowing my whistle, and waving my orange flag, and finally guys came over after about a half hour. Another boat was circling us, but they were catching fish and they weren't going to stop. I had my cousin from Kentucky out there with me, and I'm thinking 'We're twenty-six miles out and can't see land!' So anyway, one of the guys called Sea Tow—that's like AAA—they come out and gave us a jump. I learned my lesson on that one, as far as getting a backup handheld radio, and a backup battery jumper. We weren't even late coming back—we just didn't catch many fish that day.

"The biggest fish I've caught so far is probably about fifty pounds—a tuna," Joe says. "It was actually the very first fish I pulled in. It was about this big," he continues, putting his hands about eighteen inches apart, "and I fought that thing and fought it. And I thought, 'This must be the 400-pound marlin they're talking about.' And I bring it in—and it's like this big—a 50-pound tuna. I started my nurse practitioner Debbie off on fishing, so she's been fishing with me a number of times, and now she absolutely loves it. She's caught a 400-pound blue marlin—that's a big fish! But I haven't caught the 400-pound blue marlin yet.

"Yeah, I've fallen in love with the water," Joe says. "I get out on my boat a couple times a month. I even get out in the winter sometimes—we have some beautiful days in January. I love to fish, and Stevie and Jessie like to fish. Petra hasn't quite been bitten by the fishing bug yet. But she likes to go out. Our favorite place to go is Cape Lookout. We'll drop anchor, and we'll walk along the beach, and she's happy just sitting on the beach, or just picking up shells. You can walk up the lighthouse, and on the other side of the island is the ocean. You can see dolphins in the water around here—sometimes so many you can't count them. It's really amazing. And there are wild ponies on the islands around here. It's like going back in time. There are deserted beaches everywhere, and the water's crystal clear—that's why they call this area the Crystal Coast. It's just so peaceful and quiet. You don't have any large rivers coming out into the sound, stirring up the water by dumping sediment. Kids swim in the sound in the summer."

Leaving Morehead City on the only road heading inland, there is one small town after another—Havelock, New Bern—it's just one straight road. It goes right through the large Croatan National Forest—an Indian name—that consists of 160,000 acres of forests, swamps, and salt marshes, much of which is roadless. As a result of being at the end of this large tract of wilderness forest, and the lack of a major highway, this area of the North Carolina coast is much more isolated than the more popular resorts of the Outer Banks to the north, or the area around Wilmington to the south. As Joe says, "People around here are so laid back sometimes. If the fish are biting, you know you're not going to be getting any work done on your house, or your lawn cut, because they will run out there and fish. They've been doing it all their lives. So if the fish are biting, sometimes things go kinda slow around here. They call it 'the Carteret way.' You get used to it."

• • • • •

After making hospital rounds, Joe goes over to his office, a one-story brick building in a small office complex—the sign "Sea Breeze Family Practice" next to the front door. Once inside, he sits down at his L-shaped desk. On the left side of the desk sit his two computer monitors; angled at the intersection where the two arms of the desk meet are his keyboard and mouse. On the right side is an open area to work, his phone, and pictures of his kids. When he turns on his computer, a reminder list of things to do pops up on the right monitor—buy a Christmas candle for his kids, take his kids to Tae Kwan Do tonight at 6:45, and pick out countertops for his new office. Then he looks at the second monitor screen on the left and reviews today's patient schedule.

"My youngest patient right now is probably about four weeks old," he says. "My oldest is 106. I went to her 104th birthday party over at the museum—and she was older than some of the stuff in the museum. And I said, 'Mrs. G., what's your secret?' And her mind is very clear, and she said, 'Well, I have no enemies.' And this was in front of everybody, and I'm like, 'You don't?' And she's like, "Yeah, they've all died.' So everybody was laughing, 'cause she's so sharp and witty."

His first patient in the office today is an 86-year-old man with arthritis and atrial fibrillation (an irregular heart beat). Dr. Nutz has known him for a long time. "He's really nice." Walking into the exam room, he is wearing his knee-length white doctor's coat, carries his dictating machine in his pocket, and has his stethoscope draped around his neck. Dr. Nutz asks the man, "Well, how are you doing today?"

"I think I'm doing great."

"Are you? Good."

"I was a little tired yesterday, but I'm doing good today."

"Good. And how's the arthritis doin' for you?"

"That was bad yesterday."

"Was it? Was it the weather changes?"

"I think maybe that's what it was."

"OK. Are you still taking the arthritis medicine, and does that seem to help OK?"

"I take one tablet. I know you said I should take two, but I take one."

"Why don't you take two, if it's a bad day?"

"I've got a lot of medicine."

"Yeah, you do have a lot here, don't you? Are you having any headaches or indigestion?"

"No."

"Are you sleeping OK?"

"Yes, I fall asleep maybe about 11:00 or 12:00, and I get up at 6:00 in the morning."

"Do you stay active?"

"I try to."

"What kind of things do you like doing?"

"Well, I mostly just walk around the neighborhood."

"So you keep an eye on all the neighbors," Dr. Nutz says, smiling.

"Yep, I go around and talk with them."

"Where do you live at?"

"I live at High Manor Court."

"OK, so you have a lot of close neighbors there. And you're taking your Coumadin like you're supposed to? Because your blood level is just perfect."

"I take it just like I was told."

"You've been doing really good with that for the last two years."

"I'll be eighty-seven next week. I'm taking care of my own house."

"Are you living with your son?"

"No, I live by myself. I live in Morehead, and he lives in Newport."

"Does he help you out, though?"

"Oh yes, he takes me grocery shopping. He's busy himself."

"Yeah. Are you happy?" Dr. Nutz occasionally likes to ask this question of his patients. It gives him a sense of how they are doing in their life overall, and forces people to think about what they have to be happy about in life. "They usually pick out something that they're happy about, and if they're not, then I know what's going on," he explains. "And if they're not doing the things they used to do, like getting out and walk, or they can't make it to church for a prolonged period of time, I know something's wrong too. So it's kind of a gauge for me." He frequently asks this question either in between other routine medical questions, or while he is in the middle of examining a patient—whenever there is a lull in the conversation. And since he's been asking this question of patients for a number of years, it has become routine and he oftentimes asks it without even thinking, which leads him to tell a story. He recounts that a year ago, when he was doing a complete physical examination of a middle-aged man, he had just begun to perform a rectal examination when he asked—without being aware of the timing—"Are you happy?" He remembers the patient being a bit taken aback—and speechless for a few seconds—before Dr. Nutz realized what had happened, quickly explained that the question was in no way related to the exam, and both had a good laugh.

So he asks, "Are you happy?"

"Yes, I'm happy."

"What are you happy about?"

"I have good friends, I have good church members. Like yesterday I wasn't feeling too good, I didn't make it to church yesterday. My friends brought me some good things to eat. I have good friends."

Then, taking out his stethoscope and placing it on the patient's back, Dr. Nutz says, "Let me take a listen to you."

Laughing, the patient says, "Do you think I'm still breathing? I got my first flu shot when you first came."

"Well, you take good care of yourself."

"I live by myself. You got to take good care of yourself."

"That's right."

"I'm getting old," the man says, laughing.

"No, I told you, you're in your prime. You keep enjoying yourself. Nice deep breath. Well you're doing absolutely wonderful. Why don't we recheck that Coumadin level for you in about a month? OK? I'll set that up for you. If everything's doing OK, I'll see you in four months. But if you're having any problems, let me know. Tell your son I said hi. Bye-bye."

The next patient is a 72-year-old woman who arrives for a three-month follow-up visit for high cholesterol, diabetes, and arthritis. "She's really sweet," Joe says. "Her husband is in the Rotary Club with me, and her brother goes to my church." After quickly reviewing her chart, he enters the room, greets her, and says, "We're here today to kind of follow up on your laboratory tests. Are you still walking with Linda?"

"We haven't walked for six weeks. She's had a knee problem, so she hasn't . . . But we started something exciting last week—water aerobics. And I'm hoping that it will help me too. I just want to hear all my good or bad reports. Is it getting there?"

"Yeah, you're getting there. Are you still taking your cholesterol medicine every day?"

"Yeah."

Then, showing her the lab reports, Dr. Nutz says, "This is kind of where you've been the last couple of years. You've started on forty milligrams of your medicine, and it used to be up there—pretty high—but now you're on 80 mg and you got your total cholesterol down to 183."

"That's awful."

"No—that's much better than last time. Better than the last two times. And you continue to get it lower on the same dose of medicine, so you're continuing to make some headway."

"It's supposed to be under 100, though, isn't it?"

"No, your total cholesterol should be under 200, and it is. Your bad cholesterol, your LDL—that's what clogs up your arteries—that's what should be down under 100, and you've got that down to 108. So that's pretty good, that's pretty close."

"You're going to show me the range on here, and I can take a copy home to put in my folder?"

"Yes you can. And you can see that your good cholesterol dropped down from 55 to 50, and your triglycerides pretty much stayed the same."

"Is that bad?"

"That's normal. And this is a copy of everything in detail. Remember, this is your result listed here, and that result should fall within the reference range over here, and it gets starred if it falls outside of that range. And also, all your liver function tests are normal. So here, your total cholesterol is 183, so that's within the normal range. And your good cholesterol is 50, and you want that above 40, so you're doing good with that. And your LDL is 108, so you're not too far off your mark, just a couple points."

"So maybe I can go to Dunkin' Donuts and get a maple frosted on the way home, and a cup of coffee?"

"Sure—as long as you don't eat it. You can go there and buy all you want—just don't eat them."

"I just crave that."

"After church yesterday, my wife and kids split up from me—I was going to go do some work, and I saw them going to Dunkin' Donuts."

"I used to get a wheat bagel."

"Yeah, that's not bad for you."

"Oh, they're awful!"

"And your thyroid tests are normal, so you're doing OK with your thyroid. Actually, things are looking OK here today."

"Pretty good for an old lady?"

"Pretty good for any lady."

"OK." Then, pulling out a newspaper clipping, she says, "Well, here she comes—I'm the one that comes with all my things that I need. It's the health thing in the paper. I just want to ask you about this. What's this 'CRP check for virtually everybody getting a cholesterol check'?"

Taking a quick look at the article, Dr. Nutz responds, "Well, they're trying to gather more risk factors for heart disease. But we're already trying to be real aggressive in preventing any of that. That test there isn't used regularly yet."

"OK. I just wondered. I just wanted to ask your opinion of it. You know, here comes Judy with all the clippings."

"That's fine, that keeps me on my toes. But that's a C-reactive protein test— I'd hold off on that for the time being."

"Oh no, I just wanted to know what it was. And I thought well, maybe Dr. Nutz thinks I should have that."

"What else do you have there?"

"Just my prescriptions that I need."

"OK, let's give you a ninety-day supply, then you won't have to keep running back and forth. That way you can spend your time with Jim walking the beaches."

"OK. I'm glad you have him going to a cardiac man. I'm thankful for you. And you have such a nice family. Your wife put my dog down. And we always read about your children in the paper."

"Thank you. And you got your flu shot—good for you. So you should be all set for a while. Your last bone density test was in 2001, so you should get another maybe in 2003 or 2004. You need to keep up the medicine. Well, we'll let you work on things for four months, and then we'll recheck things. Everything looks wonderful. I'll have them make a photocopy of your results for you."

The following patient is a 61-year-old woman who works at a local grocery store. She has diabetes, hypertension, and recently had a bad rash on her legs. She also has a daughter who has had juvenile-onset diabetes for more than 30 years now. "She loves people," Joe explains. "And she just enjoys herself."

"How are you doing?" he asks.

"I'm much, much better," the woman says, in a *very* southern accent. "But my husband is real bad off—he just had major surgery."

When Joe talks with patients who have a deep southern accent, his own accent intensifies. "He did? What kind of surgery did he have?"

"He had two blockages in his heart. He had excellent surgeons. That's why I had it done here. I trust them, and I can get around in Morehead City. I'm a small city person—I don't like these big cities. I like small towns. He's doing real good now. He just got out of intensive care and he's on the second floor. He's getting good attention there."

"Yeah, the nurses know what they're doing down there. And I'm sure you're looking over things there."

"Oh, yeah, I'm the director in charge."

"Well, your blood pressure looks wonderful, and your rash is doing better?"

"Yeah, much, much better. I hope I never have that again."

"Yeah, how about your sugars? Have they started to drop down some?"

"They fluctuate. But you know what, I've been eating with my sister, and she's an excellent cook, so I've got to curtail that. She's the kind that makes those tiny biscuits, you know, everyone the same size, and you can eat them just like a chicken pickin' up corn. So I got to stay away from there. Little tiny biscuits, and I eat too many. But, I know what I got to do, and I got to do it."

"Did you bring your blood sugars with you?"

"Yes I did. I wasn't going to show 'em unless you asked for them."

"You got to show them."

"I knew you'd want to see these. You're not going to like them."

"Well, I thought you were trying to smooth things over there."

"Yeah, I'm trying to use my very southern charm."

Dr. Nutz looks at the paper where the patient has kept a record of her blood sugars, and exclaims, "315!"

"They're too high. My cousin is here from Georgia—Sandy's daughter. So she's really cooking all the goodies."

"And you got the holidays coming up."

"I know. And my blood sugar's too high. But I'm much, much better otherwise."

Trying to encourage her to watch her diet, Dr. Nutz says, "You can make it look like you're sampling things—a little bit of everything, but split it out on the plate."

"That's what I got to do."

"Yeah, put little bits all over the plate. 'Cause around here, if you don't eat, people think there's something wrong with you."

"You know, that is the truth. And everywhere you go, there's something to eat. I said yesterday, I'm going to church. I don't care what I look like 'cause the Lord won't care. I don't care if my hair's not perfect and everything. And I did, and of course, they had something to eat. But I didn't eat—I didn't need to, not with blood sugars like this."

"Just hold it in your hand and talk."

"You know what I really like—oysters. And they'll really run your blood sugar up. They're so rich. Even if you stew them, it'll run your blood sugar up."

"So—you know what to do?"

"Yeah, I've been a diabetic since 1988, so I know when I'm bad."

Looking at the paper with her blood sugars again, Dr. Nutz says, "Well, why don't you do this. It looks like you've had quite a fluctuation—you get them down to 125 sometimes."

"And I feel so much better when they're down."

"Rather than bumping up the insulin again . . ."

"Yeah, I'm still taking 60 in the morning and 40 at night."

"Why don't you try really hard?"

"You know what, sweets has not done this. Good food has done this. I come from a home where my granddaddy had his own fruit market, my grandmother always had a wonderful garden. And my daddy—his garden was his hobby—and he used to make us go up and down these rows and weed. And the reason he grew this stuff was to give it to his friends. Daddy didn't sell it. You know some people would sell air if they could bottle it up. I didn't come from a home like that. You know, I'm a grandmother now—you haven't lived until you're a grandparent. Billy is in preschool. He's an only child, but I'm not going to worry about what I don't have, I'm going to enjoy what I've got. He's going to be just like his granny, though, a people person."

"Well you are that. Are you still working full time?"

"No, I'm not going to do anything until my husband gets all right. No, I'm taking care of him now. But then I will go back to work, 'cause I like to work. I love people."

"You're why Carteret County has a good name. People come over here and visit and say, 'I met the nicest person over at the grocery store.' No chest pains or breathing problems?"

"No sir, I just have to curtail my appetite."

"Uh-huh. It's a small town—I'll be watching. Well, why don't you keep up with these same medicines."

"I will, and I'll keep track of what I eat. I'll bring you some more sheets of my blood sugars, and I hope they'll be better."

"Yeah, I hope so. Remember, smaller portions, eat slow, and talk while the rest are eating."

"I will. I can do that."

"I'm glad you're doing better."

"Thank you. Thank God for doctors like you being here. We need good doctors down here."

"I'll see you in a couple months unless you need something sooner."

"Thank you, Dr. Nutz."

The next patient in the office is an 87-year-old man who has terminal heart disease. He goes in and out of the hospital. "The heart doctors won't even look at him anymore," Joe says, "because there's nothing they can do. When I put him in the hospital, it's more for support. There's not much I can really do."

Then, Dr. Nutz sees a 48-year-old man with a prior history of alcohol abuse, but who hasn't had a drink in over five years now. He has high cholesterol and high blood pressure, and he's developed narrowing of the arteries in his leg, which causes him to have severe pain when he walks. But he has trouble paying for his medicines. "He couldn't afford them, and there's a couple of plans where the drug companies pay for your medicine for a while. So I have him on some of those. So I always ask people if they can afford their medicines or not, and I try and get them hooked up with one of these programs if I can."

"Well, you look good. Are you feeling good?"

"I'm feeling really good, except you know, I went to the doctor about the pain down my legs. I had some blockage, but not enough for surgery. And he gave me this prescription that took my breath away—$104! I can't take that. It's more than I can take."

"Let me check and see what I can do. I'll have to look and see who makes it. Did you check with the Rx Program to see if it's covered under that?"

"No, I haven't."

"Well, I'll get you some samples, and we'll look at a couple of these programs, and see if we can help you out."

"$104—and I don't know if it's even going to be good for me!"

"Well, let me get you some samples, and if it works, then we'll work hard to get you some. And if it doesn't work, then . . ."

"That's one thing I like about you, Dr. Nutz—you're so nice. They finally decided this was from hardening of the arteries. And he wants me to walk and walk and walk and walk. Now every step I walk my legs are killing me. If I stop, they don't hurt a bit. If I sat on my butt the rest of my life, I'd never have any pains so far as the legs."

"No, that's one of those diseases that if you sit around and do nothing, it gets worse and worse. But if you walk, you build up these collaterals—little arteries that go around the blockages—and that helps open things up for you. Maybe just try walking half the way. But at least do something. But each day if you walk half way, the next couple weeks you try three-fourths, eventually you'll make it. And it really will help."

"OK."

"And you had some laboratory tests done as well. The last time you were here we put you on a new cholesterol drug. Now are you getting those samples?"

"Yes."

" 'Cause I don't want you to run out. It helps keeping that plaque from building up any further. We checked your thyroid test, and that looks really good for you. And your blood count's fine. You can look right here—this is your result. You can take this page home with you. So your white count's doing just fine for you. And your hemoglobin and hematocrit are fine, so you're not anemic at all. And the characteristics of your red blood cells—how big they are, and how much hemoglobin there is—are all normal; the platelets that clot the blood are normal. The different kinds of blood cells—looked at two different ways—are all perfect. You're a perfect specimen of health."

"I'm in good shape. How was the cholesterol?"

"It's too early to check that, you just had the last one done last month. It was 345, which is pretty high, but you're taking the new medicine, so you should be checking that in another two months. You've got to stick to that diet over the holidays. You've got to!"

"I cheat a lot."

"You can't do that. Are you having any chest pains or blurred vision or headaches?"

"No."

"And are you happy?"

"Am I happy? Sure."

"What about?"

Laughing, the patient says, "Well, I'm happy to be alive, for one thing. That's the most important thing."

"How about those sugars. Are you checking them?"

"They're doing good."

"What kind of sugars are you getting?"

"Well, I haven't had any for two to three mornings. The last time I did it was about 110 to 120. My sugar really does good."

"OK. So in two months we'll get together again. And I'll get you some samples. And it is important that you walk. It helps with everything."

"I know it is."

"And it's nice weather to do it."

"Yeah, it's beautiful out there today."

"Let me have you get up on the table. Take your time. Normally I'd let you sit in the chair, but I want to make you exercise. $104?"

"Yeah, $104!"

"I'll try and get you some samples."

"I'd appreciate that."

Then, in the next room, is an 85-year-old woman, the wife of a retired fisherman. She used to bake a lot and would always bring an apple pie in for Dr. Nutz when she had an appointment. But, she's been getting frailer, and a few weeks ago, she had a fall and cracked a few ribs and hurt her back. Her husband is taking care of her now. Also, her blood pressure has been very low recently, and Dr. Nutz stopped her blood pressure medicine last week and is following up on that today.

Looking first at her husband, Dr. Nutz asks, "Well, how's she doing?" Then, turning to the patient, he asks, "How you doing Mrs. N.?"

"I'm probably doing all right," she responds.

"Probably OK?"

"Well, it's hard to sit. I'm hurting a little bit, but that's normal, I guess."

"No, we don't like to have pain. But your blood pressure's come up there a lot."

Her husband reports that "She sleeps a lot. She hasn't been getting up, and sometimes she sits in the den, and she doesn't even watch television like she used to. I go in there and she sleeps. I don't know . . ."

"How much pain medicine is she taking?"

"I cut it back to one in the morning, one at night," her husband responds.

"OK. Does that seem to be holding your pain OK?"

"The way I sit, laying back in the chair—most times I put a pillow right back here for pain—and that helps."

"A little pillow helps back there. Do you try putting a heating pad back there as well?"

"Yeah. It helps a little bit."

"So overall you kinda think you're holding your own?"

Then her husband adds, "And she staggers a lot when she walks."

"Does she? Does she have a cane?"

"No," he says.

Dr. Nutz says, "Well, I guess she doesn't need one since she has you." Everyone laughs, and he continues, "But we need to give her a cane."

"A cane for what?" the woman asks, not very happy about hearing this.

"Just an extra leg so that if you're kind of off balance, that could help keep you from falling."

"Oh."

"Just keep it around—just in case."

"It'll help you when you pull up," her husband explains to her.

Dr. Nutz adds, "Yeah, you have quite a bit of arthritis there, and sometimes it's not as easy to get around. And if you get a sudden pain, we don't want to have you falling down or having another problem. Let me write a prescription for the cane."

"Where do I get it filled?" her husband asks.

"Well, do you know John C.? He works for the Aging Center."

Husband: "Yes, I do."

"Well, call him up, and ask him what to do, and he'll probably take care of it. He's absolutely wonderful."

Husband: "He's almost as good as you are."

"Yeah, he's a good guy," Dr. Nutz says, laughing shyly. "We have a lot of older people down here, and he kind of organizes things down here. So we'll try and get this, 'cause we absolutely don't want you to fall down."

The woman's husband then asks, "And she doesn't need to drive either, am I correct to say that?"

Shocked at the possibility, Dr. Nutz asks, "Are you still driving?"

Husband: "No, no, no. But she says she'd like to."

"Yeah, OK. Probably it would be better, with the aches and pains, I'd hold off on that for right now." Then, pointing at her husband, Dr. Nutz adds, "And you have a chauffeur! You're moving up in the world. Anywhere you want to go, you just say 'I have my own chauffeur.' You have just the person."

Then, after talking a bit with the couple about their grandchild, Dr. Nutz adds, "How's your energy level? Are you eating good?"

"I reckon I am," the patient answers, smiling. "I'm eating three meals a day."

"Well that's pretty good. Your weight is holding its own for the most part. Your blood pressure is looking better. So that's going to help some too. So I would just keep that up. I would just stay off the blood pressure medicine for now. Your lungs sound really clear, and your heart sounds good. You're still having pain from that fall—and your arthritis—but you're taking less pain medication, so it sounds like you're making some progress. Do you think we could get you up and have you start to walk a little more, get you a little bit more active?"

"Yeah, I can walk."

"OK."

"OK, let's see if we can do that, because everything else seems all right."

Husband: "I think the main thing is that she needs to not just sit, 'cause you don't get stronger when you just sit."

"Exactly. I think that fall just set you back a little bit. Sometime after a fall it takes you three days to get back for every day you just sit. You've been sitting for a while, so it's going to take you a few weeks to get you back up to your normal routines there. I'm glad you're off the blood pressure medicine. That's good. And your blood pressure is definitely coming up. Let me help you down there. And you really should try to use the cane. The last thing you want is another fall."

Husband: "So you want me to call John?"

"Yeah, tell him I wrote a scrip for the cane. If there's a form I need to fill out, he can give it to me at the Rotary Club—whatever he wants to do. I'll just follow up with him. You keep up the good work."

• • • • •

"I think the one thing that stands out," Joe says, "is that I feel really comfortable in a small town. I've always been in a small town, and just walking around, you know, I know everyone. I would guess I know at least half of the people in Morehead City—I've had some interaction with them somehow. Whether I've taken care of their grandmother, or my wife sees their dog, or our kids have played soccer together, or something like that. I know my kids' teachers, and I take care of them and see them here in the office, and I'm the county school doctor, so I know the people that are around my children. And I guess I get a sense of satisfaction when I sit there and I help someone out. Or I'll take care of someone's grandmother in the hospital, and then I'll see them in town, and they go out of their way to go across the street just to say hi.

"Then through church I meet a lot of people," he continues. "I'm chairman of the board of directors of the bank—RCB Centura Bank—and president of the Homeowner's Association in my community—so I get to meet a lot of people that way. I know a lot of the business owners around here through the Rotary Club. And I'm real active with all the kids' school functions—soccer, basketball, baseball, whatever it is. And I'm always the team doc—you know whenever somebody gets hurt, the whole crowd in the stands looks at you, and you know you just have to go out. I have my three-minute rule. I've learned that if the kid doesn't get up after three minutes, then I know I need to go out there. I always let mom and dad go first. If they're still laying there, I'll get up and go out there, because I don't want to jump up every time someone falls down. And I know the kids out there. Some of them I've known for years.

"I was program chairman of the Rotary Club, and was responsible for bringing programs every week. We try to get topics about the community. We've had someone talk from the Duke Marine Labs and from the local community college. And 'Queen Anne's Revenge'—that's the mother ship of Blackbeard's fleet—it sunk just two miles off our shore, and they're excavating it. So we had the guy involved in that come and talk to us about what he's doing. You can actually visit that on the Web, it's really interesting. He actually helped me recruit my new partner down here 'cause he likes to dive. So this guy was telling my new partner about the diving spots—all these wrecks we have out here off shore—and how good it was here."

For Joe, the biggest challenge is "when you're tired and you want private time. You want quality time. I always try and put my family first, wherever I go. I always tell people if you're not happy at home, you're not going to be happy at the office. And so I try my hardest to make events and games, and be there when I can. And I do. Almost every night of the week I do something with the kids. Even if I just sit there in my truck and watch them, they know I'm there. And I take them and drop them off at school. I get ten to fifteen minutes of quality time with them in the morning because I drop them off at school. That's why I don't carpool. Everybody says 'Let's carpool,' and I'm like 'No!' I mean I can spend ten to fifteen minutes with them every morning.

"On the other hand," he continues, "the kids sometimes accuse me that everybody else tries to steal that time from them. I can't walk out and just hang out at the dock, just sit with my son to fish or do something 'cause if somebody else comes down there, it always leads to a medical question. I can't walk down the street without people pulling me aside, and talking and asking me questions. If I'm with Steven and Jessie, they start to tug on me. Its not that they're rude children, but they just know we have to get going, and they try to jump in there politely and say 'Dad, we gotta go.' You know, I was in the grocery store line once, and I had a woman raise her blouse and show me this mole and say, 'What do you think about this?' And I was at the car wash the other day getting my truck washed, and there were four people in there that I take care of. One guy was showing me something on his neck, and I said 'Well, you come to the office, and we'll get this taken care of.' And then I walked outside, and another lady was out there, and she was telling me about her problem, and I said, 'I'm glad you're doing better with all this.' Then I went back in and someone else started to ask me a question, and another guy was walking down the hall—he saw me too. And the one guy didn't even know the other guy, but he said 'Listen, don't even ask him a question, 'cause he's already been hit up twice already.' And so we talked about something else.

"So even when I'm off," Joe says, "it's a small town. I still can't walk into Wal-Mart, I can't go outside somewhere, without someone saying 'Hey, how you doing? How about this . . .?' And sometimes they don't really realize that you're supposed to be off. And I mean that's fine—I've gone and helped many people when I wasn't supposed to be on call. That's just the way it is. And, like, when I started this place up, I had people crawling out of the woodwork to help me out. The guy that owned the furniture store came over and said 'Here, Joe, take this.' And he sent his guys over to move stuff for me. Neighbors said, 'Here, you can take this building,' and they come by and help me out when I need it. So, I don't mind that part of it. That's just part of being a small town family practitioner.

"Another thing in a small town, I know what goes on around here. I hear about everything, but I'm always careful about never repeating anything to anyone else. If someone asks me something, I flat out tell them, 'If you want to find out about Mrs. Smith, you gotta ask Mrs. Smith.' And you learn not to say anything abrasive to anybody, 'cause there's always somebody who knows somebody. I mean if you yell, or raise your voice to someone, or something, you have to turn around and be on the same side of the soccer field as the person. You can't do that. Everybody knows you, or they've had some link to you, or heard about you—or my wife, or something."

Driving through town, Joe knows the owner and many of the employees in just about every store and building that he passes. "I have this little link to this building and that building. I learn people by where they work. I drive by and say, 'Oh, I know such and such because they work at the Barnacle Bagel, or this person works at Wal-Mart. And sometimes I'll drive by and see a store and start thinking about the owner—if he didn't come back to see me, whatever happened to him. Or I'll see him at some function, and if he's losing weight . . . you know, you just want to take care of him. And sometimes that's hard." Driving by the hospital, two women come out the front door and wave as Dr. Nutz drives by. He waves back. Their mother, a patient of his, is in the hospital now, in hospice, dying after a recent massive stroke. They recognize his truck—a big, bright red, pick-up with a second row of seats inside the cab. "Yeah, they had a real hard time with it."

"So yeah, I enjoy being out there," he says. "But the best thing about living in a small town is the same thing I don't like about it. It's a double-edged sword. I absolutely love knowing everybody, and I love having that connection with them—but that's why you kind of grin and bear it." And when Joe really wants to separate his personal life from his professional life, "I go out in the boat. You're twenty-six miles off shore, and not many people are going to pull up to you. So that's always good. And the Cape. I mean you'll see a boat out there sometime, but you sit there and you talk. We get quality time fishing. Or, we'll sit on the beach and build a sand castle, something like that."

• • • • •

The next patient in the office is a 38-year-old woman in the early stage of a degenerative neurological disease. Her daughter plays ball with Dr. Nutz's daughter. She's been seeing a neurologist and a chiropractor.

"Well, how are things going?"

"The same. The lumbar spine there is a constant ache."

"Did the chiropractor help you out some?"

"Not much. He just hurt me—cracking my bones, snapping my neck. I've never been to a chiropractor before. My husband swears by them—I swear at 'em."

"Well, if it doesn't help, you're not still going?"

"One more visit tomorrow. We'll see if he does anything for me."

"And the neurologist? Did you meet up with him?"

"Oh, yeah, he changed my medicine. I haven't started it yet."

"He was doing some cognitive testing also. How's that going? Are you doing OK with it?"

"Yes."

"So things are going OK at home? Why don't you have a seat up here on the table. The back's still bothering you? What else are you taking for pain?"

"I was taking that new pain medicine the neurologist gave me."

"Did it help you?"

"I don't know. I suppose it did."

"Are you exercising?"

"Just walking to my mailbox—it's about fifty to seventy-five yards."

"No problems breathing, coughing?"

"No."

"What are you doing for fun?"

"TV. That's about it."

"Well, you gotta exercise—more than walking out to the mailbox. Maybe if you pick up a stone every five feet on the way out, and toss it behind you, then maybe you'll get your exercise. I had a guy one time at a conference, he had a pill bottle, and he put on the label: 'Drop on floor three times daily and pick up.' And he put ten marbles in it. And he had the guy drop out ten marbles and bend over and pick them up. People just don't bend over. When's the last time you just bent over and touched your toes and got back up?"

"That's right."

"But you're doing pretty well with everything else. I'm going to give you some back exercises, and let me know how you're doing over the next three to four weeks or so. Or let me know when I see you out on the ball field. Otherwise, I'll try and touch base with you in a few months or so. Have you had a flu shot?"

"No."

"Do you want to get one today?"

"No, I don't get sick. I take enough medicine that I don't get sick."

"Well, if you get the flu, let me know. There's some medicine that can help you with it. And then I can tell you 'I told you so,' and next year you can get a flu shot. I think we've got you all set for a while. Next time we'll do a complete physical."

The final patient of the morning is a 43-year-old lawyer. He's here for his yearly physical. Dr. Nutz also takes care of his three kids, his wife, and her parents. Dr. Nutz begins, saying, "Well, we get to go head to toe today. If you're a little bit cool, I'll turn the air conditioning off, if you want. 'Cause one of us has got to get undressed. You're really good about coming in for physicals and keeping up. Are you still traveling a lot?"

"Yeah, I just got back late last night, and I'm leaving for Dallas tomorrow. It's never ending."

"How's work?"

"It's actually doing OK."

"Are you still watching your diet on the road?"

"Oh, yeah, I watch it."

"OK, let's run through the numbers first, then I'll run through your concerns, and then I have a list of questions for you."

"Remember, I'm having that surgeon you sent me to take out my gallbladder next month. They need a copy of my EKG and a copy of my labs from last week."

"OK. I'll dictate everything, and I'll send copies of everything to him. Here are your lab tests. The first thing is your sugar is one point high. Does anyone in your family have diabetes?"

"My father has old person diabetes. I don't think he takes medicine for that."

"It's only one point high, and last time we checked it last year it was OK. So I'd just keep up with your diet and exercise. All your kidney tests are normal, your liver function tests are normal. Only one liver test is off a little—a few points off—and it's been like this before. It's one of the liver enzymes that can go up if the liver gets irritated with something or other. In fact this is a bit better than in the past. How about alcohol, are you still drinking a couple drinks a day?"

"Yeah."

"Are you still drinking what—two drinks a day?"

"Yeah, but I hardly had any drinks for two weeks out there."

"You're taking your cholesterol medicine every day?"

"Yeah."

"Well, that's getting better. So I'd just stay on the medication. It dropped from 263 to 188—that's a big drop. That's wonderful!"

"Well, I was hiking the past two weeks in western North Carolina. And I had been exercising a bit before I went, to prepare. When I'm back home, I'm a lazy guy, a couch potato."

"Well, you look good on paper. And your bad cholesterol dropped all the way down from 156 to 106, so that's good. Your good cholesterol, your HDL, stayed about the same. So everything looks much better this time. We'll kind of leave your medicine the way it is right now, knowing that you can do it. And your thyroid tests look normal, your white count is fine, your hemoglobin and hematocrit are all normal. And your PSA test for your prostate is normal. You're doing well—better than last time. You're like a fine wine, doing better with age."

"Yeah, I was having too much damn stress last year."

"Are you learning how to handle it better?"

"Yeah, now I don't give a damn!" he says, laughing. "That's the Carteret County way."

"Anything new turn up in the family—any prostate cancer, diabetes, high blood pressure, colon cancer, thyroid disease, asthma?"

"No."

"And you've had your flu shot. Good for you. And you've had your colonoscopy. You've had everything checked." Then, looking in the man's ear during the examination, Dr. Nutz asks, "Are you hearing OK?"

"Not so good on that side."

"There's some wax in there—try some over-the-counter Debrox. If that doesn't work, I'll wash them out for you. Have you had an eye exam in the last year?"

"I have one scheduled in three months. I get one yearly."

Then over the next few minutes, Dr. Nutz slowly goes through a series of questions and physical maneuvers: "Any heart palpitations? Any moles? Squeeze my fingers. Push my arm down. Any weakness in your arms? Push down. Pull up. Any pain in your knees?"

"Only when I stand all day," the patient says, responding to the only question that applies.

"What do you take for it?"

"Motrin."

"Does that work for you?"

"Usually."

Then Dr. Nutz continues in his slow southern drawl, "Arms up. Close your eyes. Touch your finger to my finger, then touch your nose. Follow my finger with your eyes. Good, you've been practicing. Does this feel the same on both sides? Take a deep breath. Let me see you walk, your regular old Miss America walk. Now with your feet together." Then, shifting gears as he get ready to examine the man's rectum and prostate, Dr. Nutz says, "OK, turn around, drop your drawers. Any trouble urinating? Any problems with erections or ejaculation? Cough. Lean forward, I'll get behind you and check your prostate, and you'll be all set."

"Not my favorite thing. Everything was good till now," the man says, laughing somewhat awkwardly.

After completing the exam, Dr. Nutz concludes, "Well, everything's normal. Your exam is normal. All your lab tests look normal. You did well with everything. I'll see you back in six months to check your cholesterol. Work hard on that diet and exercise. We'll get an EKG for your surgery, and I'll dictate all this and send it to your surgeon."

"Thank you."

· · · · ·

The new office that Joe is currently building in town is not far from his current one. He and two dentists and a developer are building a small medical park and have already broken ground. "We're preserving the sea oak trees on the property," he points out. "I'm falling in love with them. The trees have these limbs that kind of skirt out, but we're just a little bit too far north to get much moss. My new office will be almost one and a half times bigger than my current office. There will be a drainage pond in the back, and we'll have a bridge across it, and probably stock it with some fish and have some fun there. When it's finished, there will be about nine to ten small buildings, each housing one physician practice. There used to be an old sawmill here—everybody used to come here for their lumber—so we held on to the mill name. And this is called Bridges Street, so we called it Bridge Mill Professional Park. It's exciting—it really is. It's about three acres, and the hospital is right down the street there. My new partner will be joining me in the spring—he's just graduated from his residency—and the office should be ready by then."

When Joe hears that some people say that you can't make a living as a rural family doctor, he quickly responds, "It's a misconception. I think I'm in the top quarter of family doctors nationally. And my standard of living is absolutely adequate. I mean, it's all relative—when you look around this small town, and many of the people are fisherman and their average income isn't high. So within the community we're at a pretty high level. Petra and I are still paying off both of our student loans—we had two kids in school, so we had high loans. But we've got it down—I tell everybody it's pretty much like buying a house. It's making a payment. Sure we sit there and think how much extra money we'd have if we weren't making these loan payments. But no, we pretty much have everything we need."

Joe says that managed care "hasn't made that big of an impact down here. I mean we're a small community, and we don't have a large corporation. The largest groups of employees we have are the school system and the hospital. Otherwise most of the people are small town fisherman or work for individual businesses. Managed care is just not here." But as with most physicians nowadays, serious issues with malpractice insurance premiums seem like they are everywhere. "I just learned that they're not going to be renewing anybody's malpractice insurance contract here in North Carolina!" So like the rest of the doctors in the state, he's going to have to find another company to purchase malpractice insurance from, which is likely to mean even higher premiums.

Yet when you ask Joe if he had it to do over, would he still choose family practice—would he still choose to practice in a small rural town—he immediately says, "Absolutely! Absolutely! We love it here! My professional career is going great. Once we move into our new office, I will have a new partner. I enjoy offshore fishing, island hopping, various activities with my children. And I think that's partly why Stevie wants to follow in my footsteps. I know a lot of doctors don't want their kids to go into medicine, but I wouldn't pay attention to them. I don't know why they wouldn't."

Then, turning back to the two computer screens on his desk, Joe says he really doesn't feel professionally isolated. "Being out here in a rural area," he says, "whenever I want medical information, I just go to the Internet. I can get books and journals online. I have my dermatology book on my computer, and if I want to look at a picture, I can bring it up and magnify it. I don't really have a bookshelf. I don't buy medical books, it has to be on a CD-ROM. Everybody knows I hate paper. Just about any journal you want you can get on the Internet. I have *Scientific American Medicine*, different anatomy books, lots of books—and they're all on my server, so I can get them from any computer and from home. And also on the Internet, I can get—and this is important," he says, smiling as he looks at his screen saver of his favorite boating destination bridging across the two monitors, "I can get the small craft advisory out there at the Cape!"

BEDFORD, PENNSYLVANIA

> For all its smallness, Northampton had great absorptive powers
> —Tracy Kidder, *Hometown*

> [In the city] our physical contacts are close, but our social contacts are distant.
> —Lewis Wirth, *Urbanism as a Way of Life*

Sitting in the den of his house, Dr. David Baer reflects on caring for his friends and neighbors in the small town of Bedford, Pennsylvania. "When you walk through town, it's like making rounds," he says. "My patients are my neighbors." Then, pointing to the houses next door, across the street, and down the road, he says, "Patient, patient, patient, patient, patient, patient, patient. And if they don't know me, they know my brothers, my mother."

Dave Baer grew up in Bedford, on a farm about ten miles northeast of town. "It was a cow farm," he says, "beef cattle—about 800 and some acres. My dad had the farm, a sawmill, and a logging operation. And he also had some steel trucks on the road. It was kind of a family enterprise. I grew up working on the farm, and from age twelve was pretty much doing the kind of work that dad would have had to pay somebody to do. I started working in the sawmill when I was about twelve, then running chain saws when I was about fifteen. At sixteen, I started actually driving a log truck, which I thought was bizarre—you have to have all these licenses now, but then you just loaded up the truck and went. I hauled mine timbers into Johnstown. I also helped get the cows corralled when they got out, which was pretty frequently. Dad didn't believe too much in keeping fences. So my summers were spent working on the farm, cutting timber, working in the woods." Smiling, he continues, "I got to see early on that medicine was a much better alternative. But it was good growing up on a farm. I regret that my sons will not have that experience, because being a doctor's kid, things come to them pretty easy. Mom is still living on the farm—dad died a year and a half ago. He had liver cancer.

It came on pretty quick. The farm's still there, and my brothers are pretty much running it now—although it's not in full production. It's about fifteen minutes from here.

"I had a notion of what I wanted to do from about the ninth grade on," Dave continues, "although I don't know where it came from. It seemed to be something that came to me intuitively. I did have an uncle who was an anesthesiologist, but I never really knew him that much. And I had some people encouraging me at times. I did have a family doc. He was an interesting man—a Jefferson grad—who had been a pharmacist and then went to medical school. Then, after spending some time in the service in Vietnam, he came back here to practice. Unfortunately he died ten years ago. He was a very bright guy—he was well designed to be a family doctor. He was very versatile in terms of what he could do. In some ways, I saw him as a role model.

"I was not a great student," Dave says. "Everyone said you had to be brilliant to be in medicine, but my experience is you don't have to be brilliant, you have to persevere. That's the biggest quality. I was deeply involved in Boy Scouts when I was growing up. I was also in the Bretheren Church—that was a prominent factor growing up. One of the reasons I went to Juniata College was that it was affiliated with the Church of the Bretheren. And it was close enough to be down the road, but wasn't too far that I couldn't drive home and have laundry done on the weekend. So it made sense. It was a great liberal arts education. I was involved in a lot of things in college. I was student government president my junior year, and I enjoyed that. I realized then that I was a good leader, but a terrible manager. I do a lot of patient management today, but that's more natural for me. But I don't see myself ever being in a managerial role—I enjoy leading the charge, but I hate counting the bullets."

Dave worked in a hospital for two summers when he was in college. "I worked as an orderly," he recalls, "what they called 'the boy.' It was a good experience, basically to see whether I could tolerate it. I remember seeing a C-section, and I thought, 'I've never seen so much blood in my life,' and I just about fainted. I had to walk out, 'cause I thought I was a goner. And one time someone came in with appendicitis and they wanted a glass of water, and so I gave them some water. I thought, 'What's the big deal?' Little did I know they had to be NPO [nothing by mouth, including liquids] before they went to the operating room. The anesthesiologist came down and he was steamed because I—'the boy'—had given this patient water. Nothing untoward happened to the patient, but he was steamed.

"I knew that whatever I was going to do, that I wanted to come back to Bedford. Even when I applied to medical school, even in college, I sort of had a notion of coming back. It was something that—having grown up on the farm—I still feel a connection to that place. We buried dad out there—scattered his ashes on the farm—and it was just a perfectly logical thing. I feel that connection—I don't own it, it owns me. There's a feeling like you belong there. So, I grew up with that, and it just seemed like the right thing, the logical thing for me to do. I had a bit of a sense of a calling to that.

"I also knew leaving here, going to college, that I was going into family

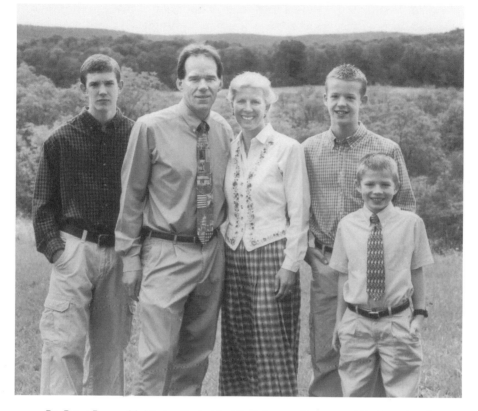

Dr. Dave Baer with his family, behind their house. (Courtesy of Dr. Dave Baer)

practice. My own family doc gave me some insight into what he did. In retrospect, it was an amazing leap, because I don't think there's any profession where there is such a huge distance between what you think you're going to get involved in, and what you ultimately get involved in. But for me family practice was intuitively appealing."

• • • • •

Dave's own family doctor, Dr. Barefoot, was the one who first told him about the PSAP. To Dave, "it made perfect sense. I wanted to be a family doctor in a rural community. And Jefferson just seemed to fit. Dave's application to medical school clearly reflected that, stating "My plans are to return to Bedford or a similar rural district to work as a family practice physician." I did the standard thing—you send off all these applications to all these other schools—which really perplexed my dad. He said, 'Why are you spending money applying to all these other places if you know where you want to go?' I said, 'Dad, you don't understand. People don't get accepted sometimes.' And I got accepted. When I came back from Thanksgiving, I got my matriculation letter. You could tell—it was a thick one as opposed to the thin ones. And I cancelled all my other applications—it was a no-brainer."

So Dave Baer entered Jefferson in 1975, and was in the same class as Chris Dotterer—the second year of the PSAP. "I loved living in Philly," Dave says. "It was a hoot." When Dave was at Jefferson, he lived in the same fraternity house (which is really a boarding house) where his own family doctor, Dr. Barefoot, had lived fifteen years before. And it turns out that both worked as house manager remodeling the house and doing handyman projects in exchange for free rent. But medical school itself was difficult. "It's hard for me to sit still," Dave explains. "I usually don't sit still for more than a short time, so it was really hard to sit through all those lectures. I don't think that's really a great way to do that—try and pound all that stuff into your mind. I read medicine now on my Nordic Track, and found I can do that. But then, for me it was a drudge. It was really painful, but I did it.

"Third year was bewildering," he recalls. "Each rotation resulted in ambivalence. I mean, I could see myself being a psychiatrist for a little while, a surgeon a little while, an internist—I enjoyed all the rotations. I was not a dazzling student, but I learned by doing, not so much by reading. I took family medicine at Latrobe—I had a great time. Then I started connecting with role models, and I started seeing, 'Yeah, I could do that.' And I started to have an identity as a physician, instead of a medical student." Then, in his fourth year, Dave took a preceptorship with Dr. Joel Silverstein in rural Vermont. "What a great time. He was a great teacher. He would actually take time explaining things, and bring you in and introduce you to people, and show you physical findings and stuff. And I'm not sure that I learned so much in content as I did in style and understanding of the notion of what I needed to be doing— more about the practice and the art of medicine. How you practice your craft in the exam room, how you talk to patients, and how you would deal with those issues. He was very influential. You need those role models."

Dave took his residency at St. Margaret's Hospital in suburban Pittsburgh. "It was great," he recalls, "just incredible. St. Maggie's had the fortunate experience of not having any other residencies in-house, and having a treasure trove of experts there. It was a lot of responsibility and a lot of work. I can remember the first day, it was a Sunday. After about two hours of orientation, I ended up admitting about ten patients—doing ten histories and physicals in one day. Wow! But they had some role models that were just very powerful. In the middle of the night, you're struggling with a case saying what in the world am I going to do. And you think, well what would Dr. X do? What would Dr. Y do? And you'd see medicine through the eyes of these people. You'd try and pick their brains and how they went though things, and that role modeling process was just so valuable."

Dave began learning how to do endoscopies (a procedure where doctors look at the stomach through a tube they pass down the patient's throat) when he was a second year resident. "I learned that if I called in the night before and if the doctor who was doing them was on the schedule, I could just go in at 6:00 AM and spend time with him. He was a great teacher." Dave continued doing endoscopies throughout his residency and for one year afterwards, when he was St. Margaret's first "fellow." It was during his fellowship that Dave first met his wife, Lesley, on a blind date. Lesley was working as a dietician in Pittsburgh, having grown up in both rural and urban areas in Canada and the United States. Then, after his fellowship, Dave worked for two years in an emergency room in Indiana, Pennsylvania. "I really didn't want to come back to Bedford until after I was married," he says. "So, we got married, moved back, started practice—all within two months in 1985. It just worked out great."

When he started, Dave opened up a small solo practice, because "well, I had no other option. It was just what you needed to do back then. And I'd been researching it for probably a year or more knowing that I was going to leave the ER. We got back here and realized we hadn't a clue about how to hire staff. So Lesley went to the library and got books on how to hire and fire staff, how to keep books, insurance numbers, exam tables—all the stuff I had no idea about. She was pretty much the office manager for the first five years. Then we had our first son, and it was just not possible to do that. Right now, Lesley is a full-time mother. And she's homeschooling the boys. The Lord put it upon her heart. I was uncertain about homeschooling initially. I encouraged Lesley to explore the possibility. But you know what, it's a great thing. She's been doing that for five years. Back then, it wasn't really trendy, but since then it's really grown a lot here and has become much more of a norm. It works great for us. I have days where I can come home and say 'Hey, let's go fishing.' That doesn't happen very often, but I don't have to worry about getting the boys out of school—we just go fishing. So, it's great. Blake is six, Conner is ten, Kyle is thirteen. They love karate, they play soccer, they ski. I go skiing with them about one time in four or five."

· · · · ·

"I got back here in 1985," Dave relates, "and really the practice was up and running and rolling. I was booked six months after I started. And I dealt with a lot of those issues, paying off the office, getting staff, and hiring, all those kinds of things. I built the new office in 1990, and then in about two years I had a partner and I started to think, 'What am I supposed to do next?' I had been pushing, and then I realized that what I'm supposed to do next is just keep doing what I'm doing now. It feels a little funny to get through medical school, residency, fellowship, all those things—you have kind of a climbing mentality—and then you run into the situation where you're finally doing what you're supposed to be doing."

For Dave, practice in a rural area is quite different than if he were in a city. "Obviously I'm doing endoscopy here, and I wouldn't be doing that in the city. And I'm reading EKGs for the hospital. The responsibility is greater in some ways. I don't have a covey of consultants to see the patient. In some ways I can get the patient in and out of the hospital sooner, because you don't have so many doctors involved. So, I think there's more control. The greatest fear I have is hurting somebody. With the endoscope, it's possible to have a perforation. But you can also miss something, misdiagnose it, overtreat it, undertreat it. So you have that challenge. I joined the medical society for physicians who do endoscopy when I came back here. I go to the meetings, keep up with the literature, but I also realize that I'm not a gastroenterologist. So I refer out some patients to the gastroenterologist. I see a technically difficult polyp and say, 'Not that one.' I just won't do it. I send it on to the guy that has more experience. So you learn what your abilities are, what your skill level is, what you should do, and what you shouldn't do. But that's something I would never do in the city. You just wouldn't get privileges. And I like the sense of autonomy—that there's really no one out here telling me 'you have to do this,' or 'do that.' I should say, not as much as other places.

"But, it also gets pretty lonesome out here at times," he continues, "you know, when the only other person you can talk to—or who can see the patient—is another family doctor. We now have full-time cardiologists on staff—for the past two years. It's a blessing. We have a good working relationship with them. We don't have catheterization available here, so we have to be ready to transfer folks to Johnstown. That's where we send most of our referrals. But the neurologist may not come till next week, or the cardiologists may be out of town. So, it can get pretty lonesome. Fortunately the University of Pittsburgh [which recently bought Dave's practice] has created a system, it's called Med Call, and it's great. You call one number and they'll connect you with any consultant you want. It's incredible. Right there while you hang on the phone. You know they talk about telemedicine, with videos and stuff—that's not going to happen easily, not for a while. But with this system, the university has basically accepted the responsibility of having a consultant available for all of their primary care doctors. And when you call, there's usually a transport coordinator on the line if you need to send the patient down. I probably use it once a week. It's really helped a lot."

While half of the physicians in this book—including Jim Devlin, Bill Thompson, Christine Dotterer, and Joe Nutz—are fiercely committed to owning their own practice, the other half work for a larger organization, typically a hospital or hospital system. Dave Baer is one who started out as a solo practitioner in private practice. But with the changes in health care in the area, he decided to sell his practice to the University of Pittsburgh Health System, which also purchased the local hospital. During the 1990s, hospitals around the country became extremely concerned that they needed to ensure a flow of patients and bought a large number of primary care practices, like Dave's. In some instances, the hospitals were unable to break even financially on these practices, and have sold some of them back to the doctors. In most instances, however, as with Dave Baer and some of the other doctors in this book, the arrangement appears to have worked out satisfactorily for both the doctors and the hospitals.

"The University of Pittsburgh Health System bought me out in 1997," Dave explains. "They own the hospital too—one of nineteen hospitals they own. It's been good. This is probably one of the challenges that health care is going to have—determining what the health care in rural communities is going to look like. Because it's not going to look like solo family doctors. The ability of solo family doctors to survive in a rural environment is so poor— stuck here with billing, payroll, accounts receivable, and personnel management, and OSHA, and CLIA, and HCFA, and HIPPA [These are some of the 'alphabet soup' of acronyms for the increasing number of federal programs with increasing requirements for health care providers. OSHA is the Occupational Safety and Health Administration, which issues safety guidelines for employees; CLIA stands for the Clinical Laboratory Improvement Amendments, which regulates office laboratories; HCFA stands for the Health Care Financing Agency, now called the Center for Medicare and Medicaid; and HIPPA is the Health Information Portability and Privacy Act, a new law regulating medical privacy]. We're not going to get people into rural practices to go into a little house or office, and say 'this is my practice.' That's going to be the exception. So around 1994 to 1995, the hospital and the primary care docs got together and basically created a confederation. I serve on the Hospital Board. And Pitt gave us very honorable proposals on the practices. We pretty much remained independent in terms of the practice styles, but the finances became different because everyone became an employee. I had had plenty of being an employer—I could tell that I was a terrible employer. Fortunately my wife was much better at managing the stuff than I was. When it came down to firing someone, as soon as they started crying, I was a goner. I couldn't do it. I said 'That's OK. We'll work this out somehow.' She would say, 'No, it's just not going to work.' So she was much better at doing this than I was.

"Since then, I think it has been a very wise move. The hospital has continued to grow. We continue to find our decisions are made locally, with input from the system. They take care of personnel management, all the OSHA requirements, HCFA, CLIA, HIPPA, which has left me more time to practice."

• • • • •

Dr. Baer's day starts with two endoscopies, or EGDs (esophago-gastro-duodenoscopy). Entering the Short Procedure Unit at the hospital, he finds his patient lying on the table, hooked up to an IV and a cardiac monitor—and you can hear the regular beep-beep-beeps of his heartbeats. The man is 48 years old, and has a history of high blood pressure and an ulcer a few years ago, which has healed. He was admitted to the hospital recently for recurrent upper abdominal pain.

"Where are you living now?" Dr. Baer asks him.

"After my dad died, I moved up to the house. It's nice—I have five acres."

"Do you mow it?"

"Yes, I do."

"Have you ever had Demerol before?"

"Yes."

Putting on his mask and gloves, Dr. Baer asks the man if he is starting to feel the effect of his IV medications, "Are you getting relaxed? Do you want some more juice?"

"It didn't take much. I didn't sleep all night."

"Are you worried about this?"

"Yeah. There's always that possibility . . ."

"I don't think so."

"I'd like to see what's in there."

The nurse informs the patient that Dr. Baer will take some pictures for him. Dr. Baer sprays his throat with an anesthetic in order to numb his gag reflex, before beginning to pass the endoscope. Then he says, "Open real wide . . ." and slowly begins to slide the endoscope down the back of the man's throat. "Are you OK there?"

"Uh-huh."

"OK. Try and relax. I'm going to try and talk you through this. You're doing great. Deep breath. You're doing fine. OK, it's down. It looks good down here so far." Then Dr. Baer spends about 15 minutes, twisting and turning the endoscope, looking all over the stomach, and then looks at his esophagus as he slowly brings the scope out. "Good. OK, you did great." Then, taking his gloves off, he adds, "Nothing bad. It looks good. All right? There's no cancer. You do have a hiatal hernia. I'll come back and draw you pictures."

Dr. Baer then leaves the room and starts to fill out the chart and all the forms related to the procedure. "It takes as long to do the paperwork as it does to do the procedure," he says, frustrated with this. Later, seeing the patient in the recovery area, he explains what he found. "We did four biopsies looking for Helicobacter. That's an infection that can cause ulcers. Your stomach looked OK." Then, he draws a picture of the stomach and esophagus area, and points out, "Up in here there's a small hiatal hernia. This is the diaphragm that separates your stomach from the chest. When you breathe, it allows the acid to slosh back up there—it's called GERD—gastroesophageal reflux disease. And over the years, you've created an irritation in your esophagus. I brushed it just to make sure it wasn't anything. The rest of the esophagus, vocal cords looked fine. The medicine I'll give you gets rid of the acid, but it doesn't get rid of the reflux. It turns off the acid, but you still have stuff sloshing up in there. I'll give you a brochure that talks about reflux—you had a fair amount of medicine to calm you, so I don't suspect you're going to remember any of this. But the important thing with reflux is to lose some weight and stop smoking."

"I already have."

"That's great. Also, avoid overeating—fatty foods, spicy foods, and foods that have caffeine, fat, or alcohol can be a problem, like coffee, tea. The medicine will take care of the acid, we don't really have anything for the reflux. The treatment is changing your lifestyle."

"I've cut way back on my coffee. So nothing was really wrong?"

"No cancer."

"Because I was really worried."

"I know. You had that look about you. No ulcers, no cancer."

"So, it's a hiatal hernia?"

"Yes. One adult in four has one. So it's that common."

The next patient scheduled for endoscopy is a 58-year-old woman who has had difficulty swallowing. She is currently unemployed and has no medical insurance. Dr. Baer tried to call her yesterday to get some preoperative information, but she has no telephone. She has diabetes and had kidney cancer a few years ago. Back in the Short Procedure Unit, Dr. Baer sees her, and asks, "How are you feeling?"

"Pretty good."

"How's your stomach? Any chest pain, heartburn? Do you still get a bitter taste in the back of your throat? Appetite's been OK?"

The patient says that everything is the same in all these areas.

"I had put you on some antacid medicine. Has it helped?"

"I can't see any difference."

"Any trouble swallowing?"

"Sometimes."

"Well, your blood work was fine."

"How's my cholesterol?"

"Great. Your cholesterol was 166, HDL 55, LDL 95. Have you stopped your aspirin?"

"Yeah."

"You're still on your other medicines, right?"

"Yes."

"OK. What I'm going to do is take a look in your stomach. I'm going to take this scope, pass it down through your mouth and look around down there. The advantage of this over the upper GI X-rays is that you can actually see things, so that if there's anything unusual, I can biopsy it. Whenever you do this, you can get rare complications." Dr. Baer then briefly explains the complications, so that the patient understands the risks involved—bleeding, perforations, missing a cancer. "They're all very rare, but always possible."

"We're going to give you some medication—it kind of numbs up the gag reflex. And some medication to make you a little drowsy. Are you allergic to anything?"

"Nothing except sulfa—it gives me hives. But mostly everything I can take."

"OK. Any questions? I need you to sign this consent form that gives me permission to do this."

Dr. Baer then begins to pass the scope. "OK, try and swallow—a big old gulp for me." The patient begins to gag, and Dr. Baer says, "Relax, you're doing fine. Swallow . . . swallow again. Good, the scope's down there now. Are you OK? Take a deep breath, you're doing great." Ten minutes later, after finishing the endoscopy, Dr. Baer takes the scope out, and puts his hand on the patient's shoulder. "Nothing bad, the only thing is that your stomach doesn't have some of the normal features. I'm going ahead and ordering an upper GI X-ray and a CT scan of the area just to make sure. But I don't see anything bad. I'm going to switch you to a medicine that's a little stronger. I'll be back in a little while to explain this to you, after I write this up."

After completing his paperwork and explaining the findings to the patient, Dr. Baer goes down to the doctor's lounge in the hospital, where he reviews and provides official readings for EKGs and Holter 24-hour heart monitor reports. "This was a turf battle when I came here in 1985," he recalls. "They never questioned my ability to do endoscopy, they questioned my reading EKGs! Even though I had been well trained in this by a cardiologist at St. Maggie's. It's amazing. It was a rural community, and we didn't even have a cardiologist here, and there was no one board certified in internal medicine here at the time." But Dr. Baer finally obtained privileges to read EKGs for the hospital, and has done so ever since.

Next, Dr. Baer stops by the pathology office to discuss the biopsy of the second EGD patient with the pathologist. He explains that he took four biopsies, because he saw decreased rugations and atrophic changes (flattening and irritation of the ridges lining the stomach), and asks the pathologist to examine those areas carefully.

· · · · ·

Bedford was originally founded as a Fort in the 1750s during the time of the French and Indian War. It was located on a new road to Pittsburgh, a road that later became the Pennsylvania Turnpike. With the Fort providing safety, and the area rich with timber and fertile land, the region grew. In 1794, President George Washington stayed here, arriving in response to the Whiskey Rebellion, one of the nations first tax crises. During the nineteenth century, the discovery of curative spring waters and the establishment of the nearby Bedford Springs Hotel by Dr. John Anderson attracted the rich and famous to the area. President James Buchanan used the "Springs" as his summer White House, and it was here that he received the first transatlantic telegram sent by Queen Victoria from England. Presidents Hayes, Garfield, and Benjamin Harrison also stayed at the hotel, which is also the only place that the US Supreme Court is known to have met outside of their Washington chambers.

Dave's office, just down the road from the hospital, actually has an Everett address as it sits a few hundred yards outside the Bedford line. But, his practice really draws from about three-fourths of Bedford County with patients coming from about 20 miles in all directions. Bedford, which is a primary care HPSA (Health Professional Shortage Area) has 3,141 people in town, with about 50,000 in the county. "There are some mountains that create very serious barriers for people coming across them," Dave explains, "and the borders of the county drift into adjoining counties, so we really take care of the central part of the county. The school district is probably the biggest employer in town, next is the hospital, and one of the construction companies. But farming and timbering, which are really pretty much unseen, and light manufacturing are the biggest three in terms of total revenue. We've not really been impacted by the recent recession, although there have been people who have been laid off and pushed into service jobs with a pay cut. The population of the community is pretty stable.

• • • • •

Echoing a common theme among rural doctors, Dave says, "I don't go to grocery stores. The aisles are too wide. I'll do Wal-Mart, but I won't do grocery stores. Wal-Mart is a lot more fast-paced, but grocery stores—there's not a chance. Too slow, too casual, and if you have a grocery cart, boy you'll get nailed in a heartbeat. I enjoy the community contact and the connection, and people are understanding—but sometimes it gets to be a bit stifling—and you really just want to get out of town. And in a small town, whenever you have a bad mistake you have to live with it. Friends are patients, as are teachers, ministers, coworkers, and on and on. When you go to soccer games, patients frequently come to you for sideline consults. You sort of live with that. You learn that some things you can take care of right there—'That's a little poison ivy; here I'll give you some of that.' But there are other things that you say, 'No, I think you better come into the office.'

"I don't resent the phone. Some other doctors seem to, but I don't. Usually it's quick and easy, and a phone call now saves a lot of drudge later on. I mean my beeper is on all the time, you have cell phones, so you're really connected. And I don't really resent that connection. My call is about one night a week and about one weekend every fourth to fifth—so that's livable. And I'm pretty much off when I'm not on call, even though people know how to get a hold of me. Thursday afternoon I take off, but if I get home by 3:00 it's a gift. I work one evening a week—Mondays till about 8:30. I don't do Saturdays and Sundays, if I'm not on call. I've never done OB. When I first started, there were only two of us, and it was every other day and weekend. That was intense! When I first came back, there were a bunch of older docs, and I was the new kid on the block. Now, we're the older docs, and the kids are just coming through."

• • • • •

After leaving the hospital, Dave goes a short way down the road to his office—Pennwood Family Practice—and begins to see his patients. First is a six-year-old boy with a terrible red splotchy rash and swelling all over his face. The boy is here with his mother. Peering over his glasses at the boy's face, Dr. Baer asks, "What gives?"

His mother replies, "Oh—well, he's looking better than he did when he got up. He got up yesterday and he was a little swelled up, a little itchy. I didn't know if it was gonna get worse or not."

"Just on his face, or elsewhere?"

"Just on his face."

"So what do you think it is?"

"Poison ivy."

Dr. Baer confirms, "Yeah." Then, to the child, he asks, "How did you get it all over your face like that?"

His mom answers, "He was down at the creek by the school. I've just been baffled as how he just got it on his face. I'm wondering if he was sweating, rubbing his face. Then, when he got home, maybe he got in the tub and washed the rest of it off."

Again, addressing the child, Dr. Baer asks, "How are you doing otherwise?"

"Good."

"How's soccer? Whose team are you on?"

"Blake's [one of Dr. Baer's sons]."

"Oh, are you?" Dr. Baer says excitedly.

Mom: "Saturday's the first game."

"Yeah, I know. Blake is so hyped about this, it's amazing." Then, listening to the boy's back with his stethoscope, Dr. Baer says, "Take a deep breath." He looks at the boy's mother and asks, "He wasn't in smoke or anything?"

"You mean where people were burning outside? No." Checking with her son, she asks, "You weren't, were you? When you were at the ball game?"

"No."

Dr. Baer continues, "We're not usually anxious to give kids steroids, but this is one of the cases where we're pretty much obliged to, so I'm going to give him a short course of prednisone for nine days. As for topical treatment on this, honestly, I wouldn't use anything more than just over-the-counter hydrocortisone. This just blossomed this morning?"

Mom: "No, it started yesterday. But when he got up this morning, his eyes were just little slits, so I didn't know whether to just wait it out or not."

"No, I think it's going to be worse tomorrow. That's part of its future."

Mom: "OK."

"Everything else all right?"

The mother says, "Yeah," but then adds, "although I did want to ask you something else. You may not remember, but I told you once that my father has emphysema and he has that missing gene in his lung."

"Oh, alpha-one-antitrypsin deficiency?"

"Yeah, and I was tested and I was normal. My four brothers were tested and two also have it. Should my son here be tested?"

"You know what, I don't think so. But let me check." Dr. Baer then pulls his handheld pocket computer out of his shirt pocket, turns it on, and looks up the topic in one of the textbooks stored there. Then he reads aloud from the text, " 'There are two autosomal alleles. There is a carrier state with alpha-one-antitrypsin deficiency, and it doesn't manifest itself. If you have both genes, you're at high probability of getting the disease, but if you only have one gene . . .' Basically they're saying you have to have both genes, so that if you were a carrier and your husband was a carrier there is a chance that he could manifest it. He's never had problems with bronchitis or wheezing?"

"No. So, since he's a grandson, he couldn't have it unless I was a carrier? Right? My dad has it and my two brothers have it, but I don't."

"That's what I think. I have to do some more research, but my instincts are for the time being—if he's not manifesting anything, I wouldn't do anything."

"OK."

"Here's the prescription. If in the course of this, he's getting better and then it starts to patch up again, it's because he's getting reexposed. This medicine will accelerate the clearing. But it might still be on shoe laces, the dog, hat bills, belt buckles, balls. It's an invisible oil on the leaf—it stays there for a long time."

"What do we do for the itch? Calamine lotion?"

"Well, that's tough on the face," Dr. Baer answers. "Usually what I recommend is Benadryl, but that causes sedation. But there's nothing better to control the itch than cold compresses and 1% hydrocortisone cream."

Then, Dr. Baer takes out his pocket dictating recorder, and dictates his notes for the chart in front of the patients before they leave. That way, if he forgot to ask any questions, he can still ask. And it also gives the patient another opportunity to hear the recommended treatment plan again.

Mom: "See you Saturday, I guess? Are you coming to the game?"

"Yup. And my wife's going to our older son's game."

Dr. Baer enters the next exam room, and says hello to the patient sitting on the exam table, an older man. He then sits down on the small round stool at the front of the table, and puts his feet on the step at the bottom of the table—his reading glasses perched on the top of his head. He asks the man, "So, what are you doing with your time now?"

"Me? I'm looking for a part-time job, that's what I'm looking for. Hey, Dr. Baer, look at this on the bottom of my heel. It smarts."

"How long have you noticed it?"

"Just the last couple days."

Looking at the man's foot, Dr. Baer asks, "Does it hurt really bad the first step out of bed?"

"Yeah, when I step on it. And I was walking about three miles on it."

Then Dr. Baer looks at the pad that is inside the heel of the man's shoe, and asks, "Did you put this in?"

"I put that in to help it, and it helps some."

"Are you taking anything for it?"

"Just Tylenol."

"Does that help?"

"Not too much, no."

Again trying to see if his description is accurate, Dr. Baer asks, "Well, it's usually that first step of the day that hurts like crazy, it feels like you're stepping on a tack?"

"Yeah, exactly," the patient agrees. Then, when Dr. Baer pushes on the bottom of his heel, the man jumps and says, "Ow! Right there. One place is where it smarts."

"I think you have a heel spur. You were walking three miles in a day?"

"Yesterday and the day before. Yeah, it just started the last couple of days."

"Do you normally walk that much?"

"Yeah, for years."

"Not in these shoes?"

"Oh my God, no. In my joggers, you know."

"What do you say we put a shot in that?"

"Will that help it? I'm going to Washington on Saturday and I need some help. My granddaughter just had her first baby, and I'm going down to visit. I'm a great grandfather. I have two others. I have one that's seven."

"Wow! Yeah, let's put some medicine in that."

"If I can get some help for this, that's what I want."

Looking at his chart, Dr. Baer adds, "Your blood tests were all fine. We did them in March."

"Yeah, you called me."

"OK, let's inject that for you."

"Oh, that would be great. I had it done before."

"Did it hurt the last time?"

"I don't remember—that was 30 years ago."

Looking down at the chart again, Dr. Baer exclaims, "Wow, you're seventy-nine!"

"I'm not telling you how old I am."

"I have it in my chart."

"What are you going to inject it with?"

Joking, Dr. Baer says, "A needle."

"Well I can't have penicillin . . ."

"I know."

"I see these young kids running around, and they think it's great that I walk, as old as I am. But I've done this for twenty-five years—I've walked them three miles."

"Where do you walk?"

"Do you know where the store is on the road north of here near my home?"

"Up that hill?"

"Yes indeed. I go up that hill, then I go clear down through there, and I come up there on the main road, which I don't like too much. Boy, when they told me you were going to be here this morning, that made me feel good."

"Well, thank you."

"I like my doctor. I liked all my doctors. You know, I've been by myself for twelve years now, since my wife died."

"I know." Then pushing on the man's heel to try and find the exact location to inject, Dr. Baer asks, "Is the pain right there?"

"Yeah, punch around there a little bit, I'll tell you exactly where it hurts. Right there, Dr. Baer."

"Don't jump."

"I'm not going to jump. You know I don't jump."

After he begins to inject the heel, Dr. Baer pauses and looks at the patient's face and asks, "Are you doing all right?"

"I'm doing fine."

After he finishes, Dr. Baer rubs the bottom of the man's foot and asks, "How's that feel now?"

"Real good."

"That'll last about a half an hour. It takes the other medicine in the shot a couple of days to kick in."

Then the man remembers another question he had. "I also wanted you to look at this—I have a little spot on my nose there, Dr. Baer."

Looking carefully at the man's nose, Dr. Baer says, "I see that. How long have you had that?"

"Oh, I don't know how long it's been there. I've had too many other things to think about. I can't check up on my nose all the time."

"Does it heal?"

"Oh, it heals. I just pick at it—I know I shouldn't. You know what helps it? Bacitracin seems to help it."

As Dr. Baer examines the sore, his expression turns more serious and he says, "I think you have a little skin cancer there."

"Oh, my God, don't tell me that!"

"Yeah, I do."

"Oh, no wonder. I'm outside all the time. What do I have to do about that?"

"I think it's small enough that I could scrape it out and send a biopsy up, and make sure that that's what it is. But we get a little nervous when skin cancer's on the side of the nose like that, 'cause there isn't a lot there that we can remove, especially in that spot. So I think we should have you see the ear, nose, and throat doctor to take that out."

"Well, right now I'm going home and mow my two acres of ground."

"And you're going down for a visit to Washington, DC?"

"Yeah, just for one day, just for Saturday."

"You're going to have an obvious blemish on your nose when it is taken off."

The man smiles and says, "Oh, no, they'll say, 'He has nose trouble,' and I'll say, 'You're not kidding.' Is that going to hurt to do that?"

"No, he'll numb it up for you. But do you want to do it after you get back?"

"Yeah, I'd rather, if you don't mind. I'll make an appointment, and I'll be right down. He'll put a bandage on there or something?"

"Yeah, you'll have a bandage on your nose, so you may not want to do that till you come back."

"No, I'd rather not. How about the first of next week?"

"How long have you had it?"

"Well, it's been there for a while. My brother that passed away, he had a place on his cheek that he had to have taken care of all the time. We don't have—our family never had no cancer in it—never did. My mother and dad both had heart trouble or something like that. My mom was ninety-something when she died."

Returning to the subject of the man's foot, Dr. Baer recommends, "For the next couple of days on your foot, watch for any sign of infection. It's pretty rare to happen after an injection. But you really ought to take it easy and not walk for a while."

"I won't walk till next week. OK."

Then, while dictating the chart, Dr. Baer stops in the middle and asks, "When you're walking, no chest pain?"

"No, I never get chest pain."

Continuing to dictate, ". . . on the right side of the nose, there's a small pearly edged lesion that appears to be a small basal cell carcinoma. Refer to ENT for biopsy. I injected 2cc of lidocaine into his right heel. . . ."

"OK, Dr. Baer. Thank you."

· · · · ·

Dave agrees with most of the other doctors in this book, that family doctors in rural areas can actually earn a larger income than those in the city. "I've done much better than I ever expected," he relates. "Having said that, I think that's mostly because I think I've tried to live within my harvest. It's a lot easier to spend money in the city. It spends itself. In some ways, I don't have anybody to keep up with. I live a comfortable life—I'm putting away for retirement, I'm saving for the boys to go to college. I'm not going to be rich, but I'm doing everything that I ever wanted to do. What can I say—I'm happy in that regard. I would probably give up income to have more personal time, but I haven't done that yet—that's my fault."

Dave gets home for dinner with his family about two nights a week—"not as much as I would like. Some of that is because the boys now have a crazy schedule. They have karate on Tuesday and Friday, soccer Monday, and they have church Wednesday. So now it's not uncommon that I'm here and they're not. I started the office, and I'm kind of the leader there, so I feel compelled to do that, but I'm trying to back out of the office a little bit. It is a tough thing to do. Medicine is a demanding mistress. But my relationship with my wife is far more important than anything I'm doing in medicine. Having said that, it doesn't mean that I don't get out of bed in the middle of the night and go see patients. I obviously do—fortunately not very often."

Dave also agrees that rural housing costs are much lower. "Where in the world could you do this in Philadelphia? Buy sixty acres with forests and a small pond, and live five minutes from your hospital. Houses are probably half here of what they are in Pittsburgh for similar houses. And a lot of things you take for granted—like no tolls, or parking. And traffic—when I go to Pittsburgh and sit there in traffic five minutes waiting to get through a light, I think, 'This is really crazy!' "

So Dave agrees with Jim Devlin and Thane Turner that you can go home again, "but you cannot recreate the environment in which you grew up. I'm not the same person I was when I started practice here, and I'm certainly not the same person I was when I went away to go to college. Any belief that you're going to crawl into this naïve, warm, bucolic environment is . . . you know, it's medicine. It has to be practiced, and it has to be delivered conscientiously."

· · · · ·

A typical day? Dave says, "I have two nursing homes, but I don't have a lot of patients there, so I go about once a month. Yes, I do home visits, usually in a setting when I know that I'm not going to be calling the ambulance and taking the person to the hospital. I make home visits to a patient of mine just down the road—he's an elderly gentleman. For him, it's really an ambulance trip to the office, so it makes sense in that circumstance. And because the family is saying, regardless of what happens, we don't want to put him in the hospital unless there's something we can do for his comfort. He's ninety-some years old. They're pretty much managing him at home. We also have home nurses who really do a good job. They're kind of our eyes and ears and hands out there in the community. It's a challenge, because a lot of these people are a half hour or forty-five minutes away."

About one-third of Dave's time is spent in the hospital, the rest in the office. One of only three percent of family doctors who do EGDs, he performs about three to four a week, as well as an equal number of colonoscopies. "Pretty much just on my own patients," he explains, "and all the ones in my group. No one else in our group does endoscopy. I enjoy it. Our practice usually has about five to ten patients in the hospital. There are three physicians, a nurse practitioner, and a physician assistant in the office. At one time, I was in line to become the vice president of the Pennsylvania Academy of Family Physicians. But I had a partner who left at the time, and there was no way I could continue with that."

Today, the community is very short of primary care doctors. "I've been recruiting like a maniac for the past six months." Dave says, "We're down four or five family docs right now. But I've been recruiting continuously since 1985. We've also found out we're going to lose our hospitalist [a doctor who works full time in the hospital taking care of inpatients for the entire community]. And, we're short of specialists. Many specialists come here from Johnstown every other week—they really serve us well. I don't know if the community could support many of them full time."

As for managed care, Dave thinks "it's a goner. They managed the money, not the care. It's always been an annoyance for us, although since the university has taken over, it's been less so. I still see my staff struggle with it, though it's not a major problem here. Managed care organizations want large population groups, and there's not a lot of people out here, so we're not a real desirable place for managed care. Still, I sort of resent a lot of the stuff—the paper shuffling, the reporting and all that stuff."

• • • • •

The next patient is an elderly woman from a nearby nursing home, who comes in with her son. She developed pneumonia one month ago, and is getting much better now.

"What can I do for you today?"

Pointing to the center of her chest with one finger, she says, "Well, I have this pain right in here. I'm on the breathing machine, and when I go to breathe in real deep, and blow it out my mouth—well, when I just go so deep, I have a pain, a hard pain, right in here, and I can touch it."

"You can actually put your finger on the pain?"

"Yes."

"What's it feel like?"

"Right here," she points. "It hurts!"

Dr. Baer pushes in the same spot where the patient points, and asks, "Just right here?"

"Yes, right there. Ouch!"

"How long have you had it?"

"Oh, just about a week or so, but it's beginning to bother me. But the other night, she's telling me to take a real deep breath, and that's when it caught me."

"Who told you to take a deep breath?"

"That girl who helps me breathe on the machine."

"Oh, the respiratory therapist."

"And then afterwards, they got a lot of fluid up."

"You haven't fallen or injured yourself?"

"No."

"Do you get short of breath with it?"

"Yes."

Because being short of breath doesn't seem to fit with what he thinks is wrong, Dr. Baer rephrases the question. "Short of breath, or does it hurt to breathe?"

"It hurts to breathe."

"How far *can* you walk before you get short of breath?"

"You know the third floor at the Genesis Home? I walked from 242 down to the elevator. You know, I can't hardly take my breathing lessons, they just catch me so. I have to stop, and I don't know if that's good or not—to stop."

"Have you been coughing a lot?"

"No. But I have a lot of trouble all through my left side."

Dr. Baer corrects her, "That's your right side."

"Well, whatever side it is. And it's under my shoulder, and I can't raise my arm real good. And it hurt me so bad I couldn't lift a cup of coffee."

Looking at her chart, Dr. Baer says, "You're ninety-two. You're full of years."

Laughing, the woman says, "Too many. Oh, I'd like to live a couple years yet, but I don't know. When you have pneumonia, you get pretty sick."

"I hear you. Your EKG today looks the same as it did. You're not having trouble with your memory now are you?"

"I forget a little bit, but I think I have a pretty good memory for my age. They tell me I'm a fighter, and I said 'I'll have to keep on fighting, I guess.' "

"If you didn't have this pain right here, would you have it anywhere else?"

"Yeah, in the back part of my shoulder blade, but I've had that for years. I wish I could get rid of this pain."

Listening to her lungs, Dr. Baer says, "Take a deep breath. Out through your mouth."

"Ow! It hurts in there."

"Have you been eating OK?"

"Pretty good."

Then, listening to her stomach with his stethoscope, Dr. Baer jokes, "It sounds like lunchtime." The patient laughs. Then, Dr. Baer pushes on one spot on her ribs, just to the side of center, where she had complained before.

"Yeah, right there." she says.

"I think what you have is severe costochondritis [an inflammation of the cartilage connecting the ribs]. I'm going to give you some medicine for the pain."

"I don't like taking another pill, but I can't live like this. Some people like to take a lot of medicine, but I'm not one of them."

Her son then asks, "Should she still take her nebulizer treatments?"

"Yes. The trouble here is discerning whether this is lung, heart, or chest wall. This is clearly chest wall—I mean it's right there. I don't think it's also in your lungs, and my instincts are that it's probably not your heart."

"Is there a lot of fluid in my lungs?"

"No, it doesn't sound bad now."

"Then maybe I won't need to breathe quite as deep."

"Well, I think the pain was keeping you from breathing deeply. Also try a heating pad on your chest."

"I guess I'll have to keep on sitting."

"Well, do as much as you can. You're in that 'use it or lose it' phase of life, you know."

"I know. I do as much as I can. Sometimes that isn't very much. I just want to get to the point where I don't feel so lousy all the time."

"I understand, but it's kind of tough right now."

Partly laughing, partly sighing, the patient says, "I guess so."

"Are you taking your medicine for osteoporosis?"

"Oh God, I take how many medicines now?"

"I know."

"I take eight or nine medications now."

Remembering this same conversation from previous office visits, Dr. Baer says, "We've been around this tree before. Are you taking your Fosomax?"

"Yeah, I'm out of it for about two days now, but I've sent for it. But I'm taking all my others. I don't think I have bone problems."

A bit impatient, Dr. Baer says, "Well that's why we have you on the Fosomax."

"Caltrate D—that's for your bones too, isn't it? I take some of that occasionally."

"Occasionally, not every day? Probably every day would be better. Actually, two every day."

"OK. I got a whole bottle of them. I will."

Her son mentions, "She stays alone now. At Genesis."

The woman adds, "Oh, I love it there. OK, thank you very much."

• • • • •

For Dave Baer, living in a rural area is just what he does. "I grew up on a farm. That's pretty much what my expectation is in life. I go to the city to play. Lesley and I get there every couple months. She has folks in Pittsburgh, about two hours away, and when we go, we go to museums and restaurants." While he feels like he doesn't have as much free time as he would like, Dave says that when he does, "I like to bass fish. I can just go down there [pointing to the pond on his property] in five minutes. And, there's some great lakes within an easy driving distance. We take the bass boat out and have some fun with that. We keep the boat down in the barn. I'm easily entertained. In the evenings I can take the bow [and arrow] out back and shoot with the boys. I used to fly—I had my own airplane.

"I enjoy what I do," Dave continues. "I feel God's calling to do it—I really do. I'm doing what I'm supposed to do. Anybody who goes into practice in a rural community, you really feel that sense of belonging to the community. I also see myself as a physician leader in the community now, and continue to have the challenge of morphing medical health care delivery into a model that will attract physicians 'cause we can't continue to keep doing what we've been doing. We're going to need doctors to plug into information systems. Health care is going to be much more complicated as time goes on.

"Some people are talking about a glut of physicians in the country, but now I can't get anyone to come to Bedford County. There are more doctors now then there were ten years ago, but from the perspective of the patient getting to see the doctor, I think it's worse. Most of the primary care doctors in town—three-fourths or more—are from the area. And they're here because this was home to them. I think that speaks to the notion of the PSAP. That's why it works!"

Corry, Pennsylvania

> This confrontation (of patient and doctor) will remain despite
> every convolution which may beset the science and organization
> of patient care. The sick person wants to know what is wrong,
> how he got that way, what will happen to him, whether he can
> be helped and how, and what it will cost him in discomfort,
> money, and personal dignity. In getting the answers, the patient
> wants to be understood as a person in distress and he wants to
> be treated compassionately.
>
> —Edmund Pellegrino, MD

Although Bernie Proy lives and practices family medicine in Corry, Pennsylvania, when he's out of town he tells people that he's from Erie, which is actually 35 miles away. Like most people from small towns, he's learned that "if I tell them I'm from Corry, they're going to say 'Where's Corry?' So I say, 'I'm from Erie.' " Similarly, when you ask him where he grew up, "I tell people Uniontown, because if I say Hopwood, they won't know where it is." Bernie grew up in Hopwood, a very small town about ten miles outside of Uniontown, at the foot of the Chestnut Ridge of the Appalachian Mountains in southwestern Pennsylvania. It was basically farmland, and being at the base of the mountain, timberland and forest. South of Pittsburgh, Hopwood sits near the Mason-Dixon Line, the official separation of the north and south during the Civil War—about 20 miles from the West Virginia border, and 30 miles from the Maryland border.

Bernie's parents were both born and raised in the area, knew each other in high school, went to college, and, "when my father got back from World War II," Bernie says, "he and my mom got married. My father just passed away this past January, they were married fifty-two years. His work was technical— he did refrigeration and air conditioning repair, fixing commercial refrigerators and freezers, like in grocery stores—the produce coolers and those things. I learned the trade and worked with him during summers and weekends. That's how I financed a great deal of my education through college and med school. Also, that's how I got interested in some of the things I do now— woodworking, metalworking. Also, my dad was a hunter, and that was something we always had fun doing. We were rarely successful, but we always kept going back. We just liked being out in the woods together.

"I pretty much knew all along I wanted to be a physician," Bernie recalls. "It was a childhood dream. I even have a picture of me with a stethoscope at Christmas time—I'm about four and my sister's eight. I ended up putting it in my med school yearbook." Then, reflecting on why he decided to be a doctor, Bernie continues, "One of the things that I think must have played a part was my father. He had been a medic in the war, and I remember him saying, 'I wish I could have been a doctor. I wish I had had the opportunity.' But due to circumstances, his home situation, finances, he didn't have an opportunity to do that. He never talked about his experiences during the war. Even when he passed away, I didn't know much of what went on. I think that emotionally it was too trying for him. I'm sure he saw a lot of death and dying on the battlefield, though I'm not really sure. I have his army scrapbook downstairs—he got some medals of honor. But he never showed me the scrapbook, and I just made the decision that until he passed away, I wouldn't look at it. I've recently talked to our congressman, and I'm getting his military transfer orders. He never talked about it, but I think that his medical background had a role in my going into medicine—a caring profession. He was probably a motivation, looking back on it, but at the time it wasn't presented to me like that.

"Also, there was our own family doctor," Bernie continues. "He delivered me. He graduated from Jefferson—he was in the class of 1923. The reason I remember that is that we were talking once and he said, 'When I graduated from medical school, there weren't many things to help people, but that year they discovered insulin.' So that was interesting—I never forgot that. So he was a role model for me. Indirectly, though—not sitting down and talking so much, but by being someone you looked up to. If you needed help, you'd call the doctor. There was always somebody who you could go to, who always had the answer, even though we didn't go to the doctor much. But he was there for us."

After high school, Bernie went to St. Vincent's College in Latrobe. "It was close to home," he explains, "their success rate in getting students into medical school was favorable, and it met my needs. I felt more comfortable in a small college instead of a large university, where maybe I'd get lost in the numbers, and maybe be a little too nervous in that setting." After his first year of college, he had the opportunity to work with a few of the doctors at his local hospital—following them around, "shadowing" them, making rounds in the hospital, and spending time in their offices.

"I think family medicine is always something I wanted to do," he says. "Maybe I was naïve—I thought all doctors were family doctors. And family doctors did everything—that was my vision of what a family doctor was. So really there wasn't much need for a specialist. When I applied to Jefferson, I knew I wanted to be a family physician, so the PSAP was an opportunity to meet my needs in a convenient package. That's why I chose it.

"Similarly," he continues, "I always wanted to practice in a small town.

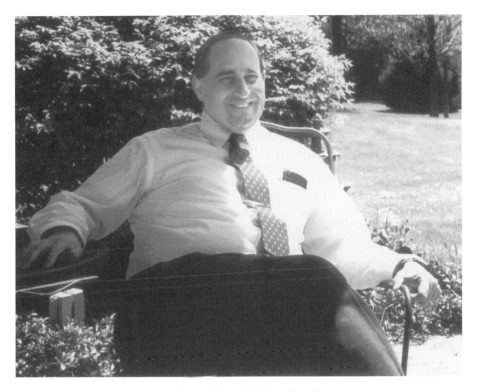

Dr. Bernie Proy in his back yard.

I've never had any interest in urban practice. Actually, I always thought I'd practice in my hometown, but as I went on to residency, opportunities came up, I met some other physicians in a different area, and I was recruited and attracted to Corry. And no one tried to recruit me back in my hometown. That kind of hurt a little bit, because I always thought going into medicine meant going back home. So I said, 'OK, I'll go somewhere where they want me and they need me.' "

• • • • •

When Bernie first came to Philadelphia, it was "Crazy! The traffic—I mean imagine coming from a small town, and coming down the Schuylkill Expressway. It was a memorable experience—I'll never forget it! But once I got settled in my apartment near the medical school, I could walk where I was going, and I adapted real quickly. But I had no interest in staying.

"I enjoyed medical school more than college," Bernie remembers. "In medical school, I felt that I was learning things that I wanted to learn and the pressure of getting into medical school was off my shoulders. So for me it was a good experience. The first two years were a lot of hours, a lot of time, a lot of memorization, academically challenging. Third year was a little difficult, being from a small town and going to the big city—going to the different rotations on mass transit. But after a while I kind of got used to it. Family practice at Latrobe was very good. And having gone to college in the area, I got to renew some friendships there. And family practice was my niche. I felt comfortable with it."

Bernie met his wife Nancy in Philadelphia when he was a second year student. He and a friend were at a local restaurant, and she was there with her sister and friends at a birthday party. "They were having birthday cake," he remembers, smiling "and we asked if we could have some cake, and here we are." At the time, Nancy was attending Temple University and working at a bank. They dated through medical school, and "I graduated June 6, 1980, and we got married June 7, 1980. It was good scheduling—people were already coming in from out of town for the graduation, and it was right before starting my residency in July. It was a lot of adjustment, but we got through it, and we're still here."

For residency, Bernie wanted to go to a community hospital for his family practice training. Studies have shown that the location where doctors take their residency training is oftentimes related to where they end up practicing. Many times, as with a number of the doctors in this book, this is because they choose a residency near where they already know they wanted to practice. In other instances, as with Bernie, the residency leads to a nearby practice opportunity. "Hamot Hospital in Erie [where Joe Nutz also trained] was my first choice," Bernie explains, "and that turned out very well. I liked it there, and it's because of training there that I'm in Corry. There was an opportunity to come down here, so I met the doctors. It was a good match, and they invited me to join them and here I am. In my second year of residency I didn't even know where Corry was. I didn't have a clue. And now I've been in practice here almost twenty years." Bernie and Nancy's first child, Vince, was born during residency, their second, Nick, was born soon after they moved to Corry, and their daughter, Sharon, was born three years later. Today their children are ages 21, 19, and 16.

For Nancy, who was born and raised in Philadelphia, going from Erie to Corry was a huge step. Even going from Philadelphia to Erie was a big change. But she was very adaptable, and that made the transition easier. "That was very important to me," Bernie says. "Even now, for me to be a very good family doctor, I need a very good support system, and she's the keystone for that. She takes care of things when I'm not here, and takes care of things when I am here. For me, having that support helps me be the family physician that I am. Without her, I wouldn't be able to do the things I do. And she likes it here, she honestly likes it here."

• • • • •

Making morning rounds in Corry Hospital, Dr. Proy stops by to see his first patient, a 68-year-old man with asthma. He was started on steroids to treat his wheezing when he came into the hospital, but that has now caused his blood sugar to be elevated. As he sees his patients, Dr. Proy has a very patient-focused approach, going out of his way to explain things in common-sense language, working with the patient to resolve problems, and often asking them if they have any questions. He begins by asking, "How are you doing this morning?"

"I'm doing about the same. I'm coughing, but nothing's coming up. And very wheezy."

"How'd you sleep last night?"

"I slept very well 'cause I took my sleeping pill."

"OK. Well, the one medicine that we're giving you to help your wheezing is making your sugar go up a little bit. So right now I've been giving you some small shots of insulin to bring it down. The best way and easiest way to control it might be to give you some insulin at nighttime—for a short time. Would that be OK with you?"

"Yes."

"That would be easier than a pill, because once you're off these medicines for your lungs, you shouldn't need anything for your sugar."

"OK."

"I'm going to ask the nurses to talk to you more about your sugar, so that you understand it well. Do you have any questions?"

"No."

"Are you having any leg pains?"

"No."

After listening to the patient's lungs, Dr. Proy says, "You're still wheezing—it sounds like an accordion in there. It's a little slow to clear up; it's taking a little longer than we would like."

"Yes, it took a little longer to get in there," the patient responds. Then he coughs about five times—a deep, chesty cough—and brings up some phlegm.

Dr. Proy sits down at his bedside, and writes a note in the chart. Then looking up, he asks, "Any other questions?"

"No. I'm just wondering what triggered my asthma? I haven't had asthma in years."

"Anything from weather changes to . . ."

"Do you think ladybugs have had anything to do with it? I'm loaded with ladybugs."

"Ladybugs cause more of a skin problem."

"They just come in—they're terrible. You have to sweep them up a couple of times a day. It's been a very bad year for ladybugs."

"Once it warms up, they'll stay outside. I'm going to check another chest X-ray."

"OK."

"Because there's still a little more congestion than we want to hear. Have you been walking in the halls, 'cause we don't want you to stay in bed too much."

"Yes, I've been walking three to four times a day."

"Do you have any questions?"

"No."

"OK, so I'm going to make some changes in your steroids to help your breathing, but also do some things to help your sugar. Then we'll see. So you'll have to be here a little longer—till we get those things under control."

"That's OK. I live by myself."

"I'll see you later."

"Thank you, Doctor."

The next patient is a 92-year-old man who came into the hospital in the middle of the night with abdominal pain. He has a history of congestive heart failure and diabetes, and is getting older and frail. He lives alone, and his two children both live about two hours away. So Dr. Proy acts as a sort of mediator and go between. If something goes wrong with "Dad," his kids get a hold of Dr. Proy, who has known the man for a long time, sees him in the office frequently, and has a warm and close relationship with him.

"How are you doing? Not so good?"

Weakly, with a low voice, and grimacing, the man replies, "Oh, I'm so sick. Yesterday morning I got up and felt fine. So I had some toast and tea. Then in a couple of hours, I got so sick."

"I'm sorry to hear that."

"I was in so much pain, I wanted to throw up, but I couldn't. My bowels wanted to move, but I couldn't. I was in so much pain."

"Are you still having a lot of pain this morning?"

"I'm still awfully sore."

"Let me check your tummy. Where does it hurt you? More in the lower part? I'm going to listen." As Dr. Proy pushes his stomach gently with the stethoscope, the patient grimaces. Dr. Proy says, "I'm sorry, it's still a little tender there."

"My tongue's dry. I took my dentures out."

Examining his mouth, Dr. Proy agrees, "Your tongue does look dry. We'll increase your fluids, and get some ice or some swabs for it. I'm going to have another doctor who works with me see you—a surgeon. Because we have to find out what's going on here. And I'll get you something to help your mouth so it's not so uncomfortable. Do you have any questions?"

"No, I just want to get better."

"Well, we both have the same goal, so that's good. You and I go way back too, don't we?"

"Yeah, a long time."

"How far back?"

"About eighteen years," the man answers, starting to smile slightly as he remembers their first meeting. "Maybe longer than that. You were working in the emergency room when they brought me in. And you asked me who my doctor was, and I said I didn't have a doctor 'cause my doctor had moved. And it was too far for us to go down there. So I asked you if you would be my doctor, and you said you would. And so . . ."

"So here we are. I'm glad we could work together."

"I'm glad too. You pulled me through a lot of crises."

"Yeah, we worked hard," Dr. Proy agrees. Then smiling, he says, "I used to have more hair before I met you. Worrying about you, I lost some of it."

"Oh, I wouldn't worry about that," the man responds. "Well, I've lost my teeth, I've lost my sight. I've lost a lot too."

"Well, you haven't lost your sense of humor."

"I hope not."

"Let me straighten the pillow under your head up a little bit. You know, I still have that beautiful set of deer you made for me sitting on the bookshelf in my office—a buck, a doe, and a little fawn. You do nice work, though I know it's kind of hard now."

"I'm going to do some stain work—I can't do any glazing 'cause I can't do the kiln anymore. I couldn't lift things down and lift them out."

"Well, we'll have to get you over this and get you staining."

"Yes, I hope. I planned on cleaning out the shop yesterday, and moving the flowers. My grandson's friend is getting married and he asked if I could help at the reception. So . . ."

"You can't overdo it though. OK, I'm going to have another doctor come see you this morning."

"OK. Thank you, doctor."

The next patient in the hospital is an older man who Dr. Proy has also taken care of for many years. Dr. Proy calls him "Cowboy Bob," saying, "Every time I call him that, he lights up, and he makes some joke of it. You see Bob all over town in his electric wheelchair. He's a really nice fellow with some bad problems. He has valvular heart disease and recurrent congestive heart failure, and is getting sicker. But we're still able to help him. Yesterday, he came into the hospital with a terrible case of pneumonia—he was delirious from the fever, and very short of breath, since the pneumonia aggravated his heart failure." Watching Dr. Proy interact with his patients, one can feel how much he enjoys connecting with them.

As he enters the patient's room, Dr. Proy smiles and says, "Where's your cowboy hat?"

"Back at the apartment."

"How are you getting around?"

"Good. I go all over—to the bank, post office, the grocery store. I even go down to Wal-Mart."

"I remember when—this was a while back—you wheeled down to the local beverage store—the drive through—and got a case of beer and had them put it on the back of the wheelchair. Remember that?"

Laughing, the man says, "That was that nonalcoholic beer."

"Then you came back, some guys were putting a roof on, and here you were outside, drinking beer with the roofing people." Both doctor and patient laugh together at this story. Dr. Proy then asks, "How are you doing today?"

"Better."

"You look better." Then Dr. Proy says, "Cowboy Bob! You used to be a rodeo rider—in Oklahoma. Isn't that right?"

Beaming, the man says, "Yep, that's where my home is."

"When they saw Cowboy Bob coming, they left the rodeo 'cause no one could beat you, could they?"

"No, they didn't. I beat everybody. I have the jacket."

"I know. You showed it to me."

"Yeah. You're a good doctor."

"Well, I'm glad you're feeling better, because you were pretty sick yesterday."

"Yeah, I was kind of sick the night before."

"That was the fever and pneumonia coming on. But now your temperature is down this morning, and you're more alert."

"Uh-huh."

"Where's Paula [his caregiver] today?"

"She might be getting up here."

Then, turning serious, Dr. Proy explains, "You know, your heart valve is leaking more. And it makes your heart pump harder, and in this case when you had the infection, it made the heart pump even harder—and you filled up with some fluid in your lung."

"Yeah."

After listening to the man's lungs with his stethoscope, Dr. Proy reports, "It's still congested on the right side, but it's doing a lot better. So you're going to have to stay with us for a few days."

"OK."

"Until you get better, and we make sure the fever stays down. Do you have any questions?"

"No."

The next patient is a 77-year-old woman who has severe diabetes and related peripheral vascular disease. She had been in a nursing home for three years, but then got better, became independent, and was able to go back to her own apartment. Then, her husband died last year. Recently, she developed cellulitis that was hard to control, and had to have some toes amputated yesterday. Now that she's recovering from that surgery, she has decided that she wants to go back into the nursing home. After discussing this with her, Dr. Proy says that he will help arrange this, and tells her, "We'll work together, we have to. I think it's a good idea." After Dr. Proy leaves her room, he adds, "For her, leaving the nursing home was a big life decision, and going back is also a big decision, because she knows that she'll spend the rest of her life there. Her husband's death has been hard on her."

• • • • •

As Bernie Proy describes the importance that his patient interactions have on his life—and the important role that he has in their lives—you can feel the intense, poignant, and almost palpable powerful emotion that there is nothing in the world that feels as good as helping other people. But, like trying to describe tastes or smells, these are sometimes very hard to put into words or write on paper. "What I like most about being a rural family doctor," he says, "is my chance to make a difference, care for people, and establish long-term relationships with my patients. And the ability to be independent, and make my own decisions about how the practice runs and regarding clinical decisions. I think that's a big plus. So all the way around it meets my needs—professionally, personally, socially, intellectually, spiritually—all the things that are important to me. Also, family doctors in the city don't have the opportunity to be challenged in the same way that I am, because if something a little complex comes up, they're more likely to refer it for one reason or another. So I think I can do more. The patients seem appreciative that they have high-quality care here, and they don't have to leave the area." In small towns, Bernie says his relationship with his patients is also different. "I know them, or I'm getting to know them, or I have known them for a long time. And that allows for trust to be developed. I tell my patients, 'If I don't know the answer I'm going to look it up, or I'm going to ask someone.' And they say thank you a lot.

"I know my patients," he continues, "and I know their past medical history, because I know them. So even though you only spend fifteen minutes with them, I know what to focus on. It's not like I have to ask, 'Do you smoke?' I already know all that. I've spent a lot of time with the patient over the past years developing that relationship, to get to that point. So it's much more efficient to take care of them. That's a luxury for me, as a family doctor, compared to other specialists where all your patients are new and referred in. So even though subspecialists limit themselves to one organ system, they still don't know all the other things about the patient. It adds to the quality of care, because I'm less likely to miss something. There's a story that's being told over time, and I'm following it.

"And I know my patients outside of medicine too," he says. "Like the guy who brought in some drill bits for me today. People drop off fruit. I like that. My patients are very nice folks—that's the reward. Last night, my son had an academic awards banquet at the high school. And a set of twins were there—premature twins that I had taken care of when they were first born. I had done everything from putting in umbilical lines [intravenous lines that are inserted into the blood vessels in the umbilicus in newborns], to intubation, the whole gamut. And it was heartwarming to see these kids walk across the stage and receive academic awards. It was neat!

"So I'm glad that I'm not anonymous," Bernie adds. "I feel that patients have a genuine respect for what I'm doing, how I'm doing it. That's the positive of being in a small town, knowing these people. But, on the other hand, I'd like to be anonymous sometimes—like when I go out to eat with my family, and want to have a nonmedical evening, and just enjoy it with my family. So, yeah, it has some minuses, but you work around it. It's a trade-off. If it were that bad, I wouldn't be in a small town. But on the grand scale, one outweighs the other, so I stay here because for me I value it when patients say thank you, or when you hear people say 'There goes my doctor.' You know, that makes me feel good, that I'm meeting a need, and that I'm able to give back to people."

While Bernie Proy clearly enjoys practicing rural family medicine, as in many small towns, it is very difficult to recruit doctors. And most people don't appreciate how important the presence of even a single doctor is in a small rural town. With only four family doctors in Corry, losing or gaining one doctor has an enormous impact on the care of the people in town. "Right now, we have nine doctors in town. One surgeon is leaving, but another surgeon is coming. An internist is leaving, and we're looking for another. With the issues in medicine in general, and the issues with malpractice in Pennsylvania, many doctors are fleeing the state. Those of us who are remaining are here because we like it, certainly not 'cause it's a hassle-free environment. On the other hand, that's one of the reasons why I'm here—because I wanted to make a difference."

• • • • •

The biggest challenge of rural family practice for Bernie is dealing with the business of medicine. "Even though you can be the best family doctor and offer quality care," he explains, "you still have to be able to maintain a medical practice that's sound in a financial and business sense. Because if it's not sound on either of those, then we would be unable to keep our doors open. And it is becoming harder and harder to do that, with rising costs such as malpractice insurance, nurses' raises—and the reimbursements are not making up the difference. About sixty percent of our patients are in managed care. So it's becoming harder and harder to practice medicine, keeping the business perspective in mind."

On the other hand, his standard of living is quite good, and when he hears that some people have suggested that you can't make a living as a rural family doctor, Bernie counters, "It's totally false. I guarantee you that my cost of living is a lot less than in a city. I can afford a house that meets my needs with less money, the taxes are less, and my commute to and from work is one minute. I'm working while other people are driving back and forth to work. So certainly I'm not spending as much here. And you also readjust your needs—you don't get caught up with the Joneses. But that's a personal thing. For me, our standard of living is certainly plenty—I mean I have a home that I'm comfortable in, my family and my children aren't deprived in any way, I'm sending our children to college. So what it boils down to is, I'm able to do all the things that people in a large city are able to do, but I'm just doing it with less, because I'm spending less on other things. For me, what was important coming out of medical school was how secure I would be. And I am secure. I have a future as long as I work hard. For me, I'm satisfied. In terms of remuneration, I don't think that it's so much that family doctors aren't paid enough, I think it's that specialists are overpaid. That's what I think. You know, we're working hard doing this, and then you say, 'Gee, they're making that much and working from 9 to 5? Wait a minute—I could have done that, but I didn't choose to. Am I less of a physician than that? But I'm happy with what I do.

"One of the other difficult parts of medicine," Bernie adds, "is what I call the paper shuffle. I love patients, I love patient care. I'll do my share of paperwork, but the paperwork is just becoming phenomenally overburdening. I probably spend about three hours a day on paperwork, and that doesn't include all the people I have around me to do paperwork and the people here in the hospital who do paperwork. It may be a necessary thing, but it really detracts from patient care. I don't know how that's going to improve in the future, but something's got to be done. It's just overwhelming. Nowadays, the paperwork is serving the legal profession and the insurance people, but not the patients." Later, when Bernie arrives at his office, he stops by his desk and sees the pile of papers sitting there. "Last night this was empty," he says, "so I'm already on the paper shuffle trail."

• • • • •

The population of Corry is 6,834, about three-fourths of who are patients in the Medical Group of Corry. So Bernie says, "We're providing most of the medical care for the community." The town of Corry, which is a rural HPSA (Health Professional Shortage Area), sits in the far southwestern corner of Erie County, 35 miles from the city of Erie, and only a few miles from the border of very rural Warren County. The economy of the area is mostly blue collar, with a number of small factories—many of which are dependent on the larger auto industry—including one that makes foam for cars and another that makes springs. There is also a plastics plant that makes injected molded plastics, like soap containers, and some small machine shops. Farming is also big—mostly dairy farming—as is the timber industry, with everything from sawmills, to wood grading, and even a furniture factory.

As in many small towns, a Wal-Mart store recently opened, which means that Bernie and his family can now buy socks, underwear, sneakers, and school supplies in town and not drive 45 minutes to get them. The parking lot is packed, and people come from all the small towns in the area to buy food and everything else. The closest movie theater is in Erie, although there is still a drive-in movie in Corry.

• • • • •

"My practice is a private independent practice that was originally established by two physicians back in 1955," Bernie says. "Then another doctor—a local physician who was born and raised here—came back and joined them in 1972, and I joined them in 1983. When I first came, I was concerned about how busy I was going to be. But the other doctors said, 'Hey, just hang your shingle out and you don't have to worry about anything else. The only thing you have to worry about is where to put your shingle.' And that was true—I was fully scheduled in less than a year. When I first came, I worked in the ER part time, partly 'cause they needed help there. I did that for seven years. Full-time office practice *and* the ER at night, which was another twenty to thirty hours a week. I'm not afraid of work.

"We have four physicians now," Bernie continues, "and we're looking for two or three more, but we're having difficulty finding them. We have four midlevels—PAs and NPs—they help with the acute care and with night call. They've been top notch. Very competent and very qualified, good to work with, and a real asset to patient care. There are also two obstetricians, two internists, and a surgeon in town. If someone has a heart attack, we take care of them initially, but usually refer them to the internists to manage in the ICU, or we'll transfer them to Erie because usually they need some type of acute intervention. Other problems that are very complicated, for example premature babies, we send to a tertiary care center. Erie is just about forty-five minutes by ambulance, about ten minutes by air—but during winter they don't fly. Most of our other consultants are in Erie. For surgery, we have a nurse anesthetist here."

A typical day for Bernie starts with making rounds in the hospital at 7:30 AM, where he usually has between three to five patients. Then, he goes over to his office. "There's always paper shuffling in between," he says, "a myriad of forms, and overseeing this, and signing off on that. Then I'll see patients from 9:00 AM to noon. I take off for lunch—I usually bring my lunch, sit down at my desk for peace and quiet, and look over some papers. But I also get up and go for a walk, just to clear my head. Then I'm back in the afternoon—I'm scheduled from 1:00 to 5:00 PM, but usually there are add-ons. From 5:00 to 7:00 PM, I make phone calls to patients, finish some paperwork, and oftentimes go back to see someone in the hospital before I go home. I'm usually home about 7:00 or 7:30 PM. On some Wednesdays, I have the afternoon off. But on the first and second Wednesdays, we go up to our office up in Clymer, New York, which is underserved—we have a PA up there all the time. So my free time is at a premium. We also have a nursing home, there are 120 patients there. One of my associates is the medical director there, and we probably take care of eighty to ninety percent of the patients there. I make rounds there about once a week. I also make house calls about once a month if it's too much of a burden, or too cumbersome for people to get into the office. It's at my discretion, otherwise I'd be running all over the countryside.

"I take care of patients from 'womb to tomb,'" Bernie says. "Birth—I saw a newborn in the hospital today—I attend when babies are born by C-sections. We do adult care, and office surgery. I don't do OB, but have hospital privileges for everything else. We're the team doctor for the school, we do occupational health for the employers, including preemployment exams and take care of work-related injuries, and sometimes tour the plants to better understand and see if we can help cut down on injuries. I usually see thirty to forty patients a day in the office, but because our PAs are more likely to see the acute, short visits, I see the more complex patients who have multiple chronic problems. Of all patients I see, we take care of the bulk of problems, and only refer out five to ten percent of patients—and that's everything including bypass surgery. So we do a little bit of everything. I've been here long enough that my patients are growing older with me. So I still see kids, but not as many as the newest physician in the group.

"We take care of things here that most family doctors in an urban setting wouldn't do—lacerations, fracture care, whatever. And if I have the knowledge and skills, and the patients have the trust . . . and you can't get them in to see the dermatologist. So by necessity I learned how to do things. And I think that's what has kept me active—there's always something challenging. I'd get bored being in a subspecialty. I'd get very bored. We need subspecialists, we need someone to be very narrowly focused, but that's not for me. I have to not know, to be sitting on the edge of my seat, that's what keeps me going.

"My night call is every third night and every third weekend, but the mid-levels take first call all the time and sort out the minor problems. And that's been a big plus. Last night, I only had one call. On a weekend, I have about twenty to twenty-five calls during the entire day on a Saturday or Sunday. On average I get woken up about once a night when I'm on call. It's been a while since I've had to go in to the hospital at night, though—I can't even remember the last time. The PAs have been helpful, and a lot of it we can handle things over the phone. And when you're off, you're off. When I walk out at 7:00 PM and I'm not on call, I'm done. Same on the weekend—if I want to go away, I just go. I don't have to tell anyone."

• • • • •

Bernie Proy has been practicing in Corry for almost 20 years now—about the same time that Chris Dotterer and Dave Baer have been practicing in their communities. In fact, the retention rate of the ten PSAP graduates in this book is 100 percent so far, even higher than the 79 percent for all PSAP graduates. None of the ten has left their practice community, although a few have changed practice arrangements (e.g., left their partner to go off on their own, sold their practice to a hospital system). Together they have practiced an average of more than 11 years in the same rural community, with a range of 3 to 20 years. All entered practice directly following their residency and fellowship training (except for Dave Baer who initially worked in an ER for two years). Depending on when they graduated from medical school—which ranged from 1979 to 1996—six have been in practice for between 10 and 20 years, two from 6 to 7 years, and two of the most recent graduates for only three to four years.

Although the issue of retention is frequently lumped together with that of recruitment, getting doctors to practice in rural areas and getting them to stay are very different phenomena. While it is true that you can't have retention without first getting a physician to come to a small town, the factors that are related to retention are different. While background, plans for family practice, and rural lifestyle factors are most important in recruitment, retention appears to be more related to whether the physician and family are integrated into the community—whether or not they "fit," professionally and personally. While some of this also depends on prior rural background and experiences, practice issues such as income, time commitment, and isolation are often cited by those rural physicians who plan to leave. Whether or not physicians and their spouses are comfortable with rural lifestyle issues, including schools, entertainment, and shopping, it is also a critical reason why small town doctors stay or leave.

• • • • •

Arriving at his office—a one-story brick building located directly behind Corry Hospital—Dr. Proy's first patient is a 62-year-old woman who had open-heart bypass surgery two months ago. She also has high blood pressure and diabetes. Dr. Proy starts off by asking her an open-ended question, allowing her to choose to discuss whatever is on her mind. "How you doing today?"

"Oh, pretty good."

Then, another open-ended question, "How have you been since I've seen you? Any problems?"

"No, nothing really. I like to lie on my stomach at night, and I find I can't lie there all night. It bothers me. And if I pick up something too heavy that I shouldn't have, and turn this way, I can feel it."

Then, probing with more specific closed-ended questions, Dr. Proy asks, "Do you think it feels like it's on the surface? Like bone and muscle? Or deeper, like heart?"

"No, just pressing on it I can feel it."

"So, right where you had the heart surgery?"

"Yeah, its right where the bones were put back together. That's right where I feel it."

"Are you waking up in the middle of the night with any shortness of breath or difficulty breathing?"

"No."

"And is there any discomfort brought on by walking or exertion?"

"No, it's actually when I lay on my stomach—it's from the pressure. Or if I pick up something that's heavy—without thinking. Yeah, its right where they put it back together. And if my grandson—he's very lively—jumps up on me, wham! I can feel that. If I touch it myself, it's right there. Other than that, I feel fine."

"Does your husband still have you out in the yard working?"

"Of course," she says, laughing.

"Does that bring on any chest pain?"

"No."

"So overall, it sounds like you're doing very well."

"Yeah, still shoveling, and doing all the things I did before."

"I see you've also had blood work done. Your cholesterol remains excellent, 155."

"Good."

"No—it's *very* good!"

"OK. Yeah."

"Well, considering it was 278, it's *very* good. You've done excellent. Your lifestyle changes, exercising, your attitude, all the things. Anything else to report?"

"No."

"Any prescriptions you need refilled?"

"I need one for the blood pressure medicine, one for the diabetes."

"Are you having any trouble with your medicines? Any stomach upset?"

"None. Nothing seems to be really bothering me."

"OK, have a seat up here, and let me check you." Then, as Dr. Proy examines her, he explains what he is doing as he goes along. "I'm checking for swollen glands. . . . I'm checking your carotid arteries in your neck. . . . I'm going to listen to your heart. . . . Now, take some big breaths. . . . Show me where you're having the pain."

"It doesn't really hurt. I just feel some pressure—here."

Feeling the area, Dr. Proy says, "Yeah, that's where the step-off is. There's a wire there."

"Well, it was something that I wasn't sure about. And I thought well, I'm going to check it out."

"Good. I want to see you back in three months. Keep doing what you're doing."

"I'm exercising and watching what I eat."

"I can tell that."

"My husband grumbles a little bit, he doesn't always like what . . ."

"Yeah, that's what husbands do."

"Well, he has a choice. Either eat what I prepare, cook it yourself, get peanut butter and jelly, or forget it," she says, laughing.

"Well, he's not going hungry, I know that."

"No."

As Dr. Proy comes out of the room, his PA interrupts him and asks him to help evaluate a 17-year-old who had fractured his index finger six weeks ago playing baseball. Dr. Proy agrees that the finger has healed, and approves a program of increasing activity.

Next, he sees a 69-year-old man who hurt his shoulder. His wife is in the room, sitting next to him.

"Well," Dr. Proy says, greeting the man with a big smile as he walks in the door. "The expert archer [i.e. bow and arrow] and a humble person. How are you?"

"Well I've seen a turkey yesterday, real big like that," the man says, holding his hands apart to show its size. "I bet he had to be about fifteen inches long."

"That's the granddaddy."

"Yeah, he came down off the hill to feed. So if you want to go turkey hunting?"

"Well, thank you, but I don't think I'll be doing that in the near future. So how have you been doing?"

"Pretty good."

"Other than your shoulder, things are going pretty well for you, then?"

"I think I'm doing OK."

Then Dr. Proy turns to his wife and asks, "And how do you think he's doing?"

"He's tired a lot," she says.

"Are you up and about, doing some walking in the woods? Getting around?"

"No."

"Not so much? Well, how about starting on your bow, cut back the pounds, and see if you can start working on it a little bit. Because I think it would be good for your shoulder."

"I think it would."

"Why don't you try it?"

"OK."

"Cut back the pounds. What do you set now? About sixty?"

"About seventy."

"Maybe go down to forty." Then, Dr. Proy turns to his wife, and says, "I think it would be good, kind of get him occupied in some things too. Yeah, because he really enjoys it—that's part of his life." Then, back to the patient, "So we'll get you back into that—that will help. It'll help your shoulder." Checking his heart, Dr. Proy says, "Your heart sounds good. You've come a long way and are continuing to do well. That's why I'd like to see you get back in the bow again."

"I tried that trap over the church; I did pretty good at it. I shot over half a day, and I only missed about six times."

"I'm not surprised. That's great."

Then his wife says, "I think that he started having a problem with his shoulder, though, when he carried the shotgun around in the woods all last fall."

"So we'll have to get it moving. Well, do you think we'll get any summer weather?" Then, examining his shoulder, Dr. Proy remarks, "You're really stiff. If you don't move it, your joint will stiffen up on you. Would you be interested in getting some therapy on it?"

"I don't care."

"I think you should. It's starting to freeze up—and that's not good." Then turning to the wife, Dr. Proy says, "We'll arrange for some therapy, I'll write for it. That's getting tight, and he's going to get a lot of immobility from it." Dr. Proy next explains what's involved in physical therapy. Then he asks, "At night, does it hurt when you sleep on it?"

"Yeah."

"That's one of the main symptoms. Because of your shoulder problem, I want to check you in a month. Any questions?"

"No."

"OK. You have a good day."

"You too."

Dr. Proy then sees a 59-year-old woman who has had ringing in her ears. A few years earlier, Dr. Proy had told her about the difficulty in recruiting new doctors to the area, and the woman said, "You know, my nephew is going to medical school, and I think he would love it here." So Bernie met with her nephew when he was in medical school, and started talking to him about practice in a small town. "And that's how he came here," Bernie recounts, "through his aunt, who is my patient."

Dr. Proy begins, "I have the report from the ear doctor regarding your ringing. And he recommends that you get 'hearing protection.' And he also says that you may need hearing aids down the road."

"Uh-huh. I got that letter. And I took it into my place of employment and gave it to the nurse, and I told them if they were going to put me in a new job with much more noise, then they have to get me hearing protection. They ended up buying me a $300 pair of fancy ear plugs and they cancel out all the noise. They're something else."

"Well, that's what you need. Hearing loss is cumulative. A little bit today, a little bit tomorrow, and it adds up to big hearing loss over time."

"Uh-huh, so that's all documented down at work. They got me those, and I wear those every day. Thank you."

In between patients, Dr. Proy says, "You have to learn who you can spend time with, who needs it. But if you don't keep up the pace, then you can't help as many people. There are a lot of people who need help, especially in underserved areas, so you learn time management skills. You learn efficiency."

The next patient is a 61-year-old man who Dr. Proy has just recently diagnosed with having colon cancer. He also has mild heart disease and high blood pressure.

"Well, I'm glad we picked up that spot in your colon where the cancer is located. The outlook is good once they take care of it. The anemia, the low blood count, will get better. As of now, we don't see any signs of it showing up anywhere else, so those are all good. And they'll take good care of you when you have your surgery at the hospital in Erie."

"I think so too."

"I know they will. That's the best place for you. So they can help you not just with that problem, but also with your blood pressure, your heart problem. We've got to look at the whole picture, not just focus on one thing. That's why I recommended you have your surgery there."

"I'm very satisfied. How's my hemoglobin?"

"9.2."

"Well, that's stayed there for two weeks."

Then Dr. Proy asks, "Looking back, you really didn't have any symptoms, did you?"

"No, not until I took that specimen from my bowels that you had suggested."

"You hadn't noticed any pain or bleeding?"

"No."

"Well, God was watching over you."

"I think so."

"Your blood pressure is good today."

"Should I go back on iron pills?"

"Yes, it will help your iron storage. As long as it doesn't give you an upset stomach or constipation."

"It gave me diarrhea."

"Well that's unusual."

"You said I was a challenge," he says smiling.

"You are a challenge," Dr. Proy agrees, smiling back warmly.

"Well, I'll do what I got to do. My surgery is next week."

"You're tough. And you have everybody hoping and praying and watching over things for you. So you're doing the best you can with things."

"Thank you."

· · · · ·

Despite working very hard, Bernie seems to have a lot of time for his many activities, including metalworking and gardening. Talking about the metalwork, he says, "My dad had the technical skill. But I just got interested in it—I like to make things. I've made some wrought iron things. I made a trailer hitch to pull our tractor. And I made a wood stove for our camp. We cook on it, and it's the main heat source for the camp. I designed it. Its quarter-inch steel, and it weighs about 600 pounds."

Then there's the "camp." As Bernie talks about the camp, he lights up with enthusiasm. "The camp is out in the middle of nowhere, in Warren County— 400 acres. It's basically a place to get away and kind of rough it—and for bonding between the boys and I, and some of the guys we hang around with. My wife and daughter don't want any part of it. We pretend sometimes to hunt and fish, but it's mainly food and beverage, listening to turkeys, and hanging out. We built it from the ground up. It started out to be just a lean-to, but it turned out to be a thirty by sixteen-foot cabin with a cathedral ceiling that sleeps eight. You could live there if you needed to. It's got beds and bunks. I built the stove for that, a lot of the wrought iron hangers for clothes, a ladder to the loft, a lot of the hardware for it. Electricity is there, but we heat it with wood, and have to hand carry water in. And there's no plumbing or bathroom, just an outhouse. We go out there more in the hunting season, in the fall, about once a month. We hunt deer, pheasant, birds. It's not so much the hunting or killing the game, it's just more being out there. I'd probably have just as much fun not carrying a gun, but it's OK. And the game that we shoot, the venison, we eat it. We never let anything go to waste."

Bernie did those things with his father when he was a child. "It's a tradition I passed on to the boys. I made sure the kids know how to check them, and keep them safe. And we do clay pigeons and target shooting just for fun. We try to do a lot of things together. I taught them how to weld—to do metalwork. We also do winter sports. This year we did snowshoeing. The kids have skied since they were two or three years old. I used to. I also used to fly—I learned to fly here in Corry. Then the kids came along, and responsibilities. But now Nick's getting into it, so I'll probably get back into it. So being out here, I don't think we're deprived of anything. We're doing what we want to do. And the way we want to do it."

And when Bernie and Nancy want to get away, they like to go to New York or Philadelphia. But Bernie says, "We go a few times a year. But as soon as you get there, it makes us appreciate coming back."

· · · · ·

Bernie's house is less than a mile from his office and the hospital—and "I can make it out of bed, literally, to the hospital in about two minutes. That's convenient. I have thirteen acres here, all at a fraction of the cost of what this would cost in Philadelphia. The boys and I put in a series of walking trails and sitting areas out back—that took a lot of work. I literally had a farm tractor on it. We cut our own firewood, do our own mulching and fertilizing, put in our own sprinkler system—we dug the holes, put in 2,000 feet of pipe and twenty-six heads, all by hand. I had an Amish man, a carpenter, build the gazebo. They don't come in for medical care, but I do a lot of home visits. That's my barn down there—that's where the forge is, where I do my metalwork. And I have a wood shop in there. I had it put up about five years ago. I like playing outside in the woods, and I have my tractor and some other things in there. We have deer and turkey in the woods back here. So I have all this right here, close to work, and I can be in Erie in thirty-five minutes. It's ideal!"

Sitting out in Bernie's backyard, with their dog Chi-Chi nearby, you can hear water in the background from the fountain that he built. And the yard appears like a huge park with the paths winding through the woods. "It doesn't mean we have to be deprived educationally or socially," Bernie continues. "When we try and recruit doctors or lawyers, some people think they're going to educationally deprive their family, but that's not true. And it doesn't mean I'm a lesser physician just because I don't live in Boston and am not doing heart surgery. This is my niche. This is where I want to be."

• • • • •

The next patient in the office is here to receive the results of his heart tests. Dr. Proy had taken care of the man's father until he had died last year. "How's the beer making?" Dr. Proy asks.

"I was up till 3:00 in the morning. I just started a new batch. I've only been doing it for two years, but I have my own label."

"I know—'Coor-ry Brew.' "

"Yeah, but I'm thinking of a different name."

"So how have you been?"

"Oh, pretty good. I've been thinking about what that stress test, that nuclear stress test, or ECHO, what that showed. Man, what a day that was. My daughter was ready to have a baby, and I'm up half the night, not knowing what to expect from this nuclear stress test, and I had the worst headache."

"Well, it was worth it. It was normal."

"You mean they can tell if I have any blockage?"

"Well, its not 100 percent, but it's the closest I can tell without doing something invasive. The other way would be a catheterization, but why take the risk. So as far I can tell, I don't see any signs of blockage. Which is good. And the ECHO test—since your dad had the valve problem—all that was normal too. So those are two good reports for you."

"That's great! Thank you."

After Dr. Proy walks out of the room, his PA asks him to check a two-month-old boy with an enlarged testicle, which turns out to be a benign fluid-filled hydrocele that will probably resolve on its own.

Dr. Proy then sees the next patient, a 56-year-old woman who comes in with her husband. She has manic depressive disease.

"Is there a problem since I've seen you?"

"No, the only thing is my feet. Right there."

"Are you having trouble walking?"

"Oh, no."

"Let me see you walk," Dr. Proy asks her. Then he asks her husband, "What does she mean when she says that?"

"That they jump."

Dr. Proy turns and asks the woman, "When do they jump the most?"

"Oh, anytime."

"More at nighttime?"

"At nighttime they jump quite a bit. I'm very restless at nighttime."

"Well, that sounds like restless legs syndrome. We've checked your circulation and other things. Your potassium is normal. And all your other tests are normal. And we have to be careful with what medicines to give you, since they may not agree with your other medicines."

"Can you check my weight?"

"It's coming down."

"I'm exercising."

Her husband adds, "She's not eating since they took her off of the other medicine. The psychiatrists are following her."

Then, reviewing her chart, Dr. Proy says, "Your mammogram was normal, but you still need to examine yourself every month."

The patient continues, "Also, I burned my finger."

"Oh, that's not good." Then, looking at the finger, he adds, "But it's healing. When did you burn that?"

"Last week. I didn't know I did it 'cause my fingers are numb."

Examining her finger further, Dr. Proy says, "It doesn't look infected. I think it's best to leave this and watch it." Then, looking at her husband, he adds, "He will help us watch it. He's like old Hawkeye. So we'll just watch it."

After saying goodbye, Dr. Proy heads toward the next room to see another patient, when his office manager catches him in the hall. He informs Dr. Proy that a bomb threat has just been reported! Someone has just called the Corry Fire Department and said that there is a bomb in a public place in town and that it is set to go off by noon. All the businesses in town are being evacuated—even Wal-Mart. The schools are being closed and the kids are all being sent home. And the hospital is locking all its doors and not letting anyone else enter. After a brief discussion, they decide to call and cancel all the appointments for the rest of the day, and Dr. Proy and his PA begin to quickly finish seeing the patients who are already waiting in the office. Although no bomb was ever found, and none went off, it was nevertheless a stark reminder that post–September 11, even small rural towns are vulnerable to terrorism.

Dr. Proy quickly consults with his PA regarding a patient with chest pain, who recently had a negative cardiac catheterization. The man has been diagnosed with GERD (gastroesophageal reflux disease), and they recommend a prescription medicine to stop the acid from developing in his stomach.

Then, after quickly seeing the last two patients in the office, Dr. Proy goes into the hospital and up to the nursery to check a baby boy that was born a few hours ago. He will also perform the baby's circumcision tomorrow, if the parents decide to have it done. As he enters the nursery, crying fills the background.

He asks the nurse how the baby is doing, and she reports that everything is fine. It was the mother's second baby, and a quick delivery—she delivered 22 minutes after she arrived at the hospital. The nurse reports that the baby has already been bathed and had its first stool. Dr. Proy then examines the baby, who is perfectly healthy, and goes to talk to the mother in her room.

"Everything looks very good. His heart, lungs, everything. Do you have any questions?"

"No."

"I heard the feedings have started out really well."

"Yeah. He latched right on to my breast."

"So, I guess you won't be at work tonight?" (The mother works at the restaurant where Dr. Proy and his family have reservations for dinner tonight).

"No, I won't be," she says smiling.

"This is exciting. Your first boy. What's his name?"

"Mark."

"That's really nice. Very good. Congratulations, and you take it easy. If there are any problems, I'll let you know. But I don't anticipate any."

"All right."

"Take care."

"Thank you."

• • • • •

For Bernie, the best things about living in a rural area are the low crime rate, less hustle and bustle on the streets, his house, and the quality of life. "I like the non-crowdedness of it," he says, "the openness, the rural setting. I'm working hard and a lot of hours, so that's probably a drawback. But I set my own schedule, so I look in the mirror and that's the one who sets the schedule. I could say no, but being a caring person, it's hard to say no to patients who want to see me."

And he and Nancy feel that this is a very good area for raising kids, and a very safe community. When she first moved to Corry, Nancy says that she had trouble getting to sleep—it was too quiet. "I had never heard such quiet." But Bernie doesn't feel isolated at all. "I'll give you an example," he says. "Last week I was in Boston, taking a medical course up there. I left Boston on Sunday at 8:45 AM, flew to Pittsburgh, and got the connection up to Erie. I was in the driveway here at 12:45 PM—four hours later. Most people in the city probably drive forty minutes to an airport—or for that matter they drive forty minutes to work each way every day. Yeah, I'm working, while people in the city and suburbs are driving each day. That's an efficiency.

"Sure there are some downsides of living in a rural area," he says. "I don't misbehave, but if I was going to, you can't do it in a small town. We go out to the camp, or go up to Erie to be anonymous, and that's OK. But here I feel very much a part of a community. When my father passed away a few months ago, I was amazed. I got over 300 cards from people from here— cards, people sending fruit baskets, asking what they can do. And that made me feel very good and a part of things. That has value to me. That's the reason I went into family practice—that continuing relationship. The respect of the old family doctor, who's been with people for years, and helps them get through all the trials and tribulations of life—kind of a consultant to help them with their decisions.

"And your kids can't get away with anything," he continues. "People will tell me, 'I saw your son down here.' " Bernie's son, Vince, confirms this, saying, "I don't know who lots of these people are, but they all know who I am." "So, it's a good thing for me," Bernie says laughing. "I know they're not going to act up in town. Maybe somewhere else, but not in town."

Sitting around the table with Bernie and Nancy and their three kids, one hears stories of patients occasionally showing up at the front door sick or injured, sometimes bleeding. And about how patients oftentimes ask Bernie medical questions while the family is at a restaurant. Smiling, Nancy says, "That's just a way of life around here."

• • • • •

As to balancing his professional and personal life, Bernie says, "It's dynamic and ever changing. You have to be true to yourself, you have to just do it. I've never had a patient say, 'Doc, you need a vacation. Why don't you take a week off?' But when I'm off, they say, 'Where were you, I was looking for you?' I need to take care of my own physical and emotional health. I take off a couple of weeks a year. I also made sure that having dinner at home was a priority. It was important for the family to try and eat dinner together, so we do that a lot. Not half the time, but even if the kids have eaten already, they come down and sit down and recap the day's events. I go to the kids' school events whenever I need to be there. That's on the priority list, and it moves up to number one. I make most of their sports events.

"I make the analogy between family practice and farming. It's a lifestyle, and if you ask a farmer why they do it, it's because they want to do it. Certainly, it's not for the money. Money's important, but that's not why they're doing it. In family medicine obviously I'm making a good living and have the financial rewards of working hard. But I'm doing it because I want to do it. That's the main thing. And I'm happy. And it can be done. It depends on what you place value on. For me, it's the relationships. I feel good when people say, 'That's my doctor.' Last night at the awards program, I felt good when I said to myself 'I took care of those kids.' That's the relationship that you're less likely to get in other places, but here you see them every day. That's not to say it doesn't have its minuses—you go down to the grocery store, and people come up to you and say, 'Hey—I've got this rash here.' But that's going to happen anywhere."

As for other community activities, Bernie says, "I serve on the credentials committee, the bylaws committee, the planning committee—all for the hospital. I'm involved in church, but not much more. I had to learn how to say no; otherwise I'd be on every committee in town. And there wouldn't be any time for my family."

· · · · ·

Regarding the future of family practice, Bernie is confident: "There will always be a need. But there has to be a way to get people interested in going into it. It's hard work, and doesn't have the glamour. But it's important because patients need to get care. As to my own future, I plan to keep working as long as God lets me."

When Bernie talks to family doctors interested in practicing in small towns, he asks them, " 'What are you looking for?' If they don't want to work hard, and they just want to make a lot of money, I won't even talk to them. But if you want something that's personally rewarding, if you want to make a difference, if you care, if you like critical thinking, if you like making decisions, if you appreciate patients having respect for you, then I think it's a good choice. And specifically in a rural area, you get to be the kind of physician you want to be—you help shape your own destiny. For me, I would get very bored with a narrow scope of field. I was always like that—it's my personality."

For some time now, Bernie has been mentoring some of the local students from this area, trying to get them to come back one day as family doctors. One young man, who he has been talking to since he was in seventh grade— the grandchild of one of the patients he saw in the office today—is now in medical school, and is planning to return home to practice family medicine. "I took care of him since he was a kid," Bernie relates. "He'd come over and I'd show him how to take a blood pressure. He was here on my back porch with his parents a few years ago, and we talked about medicine, and where he should go to college. That's part of that relationship, and unless you have that relationship, it's really hard to come back. Bernie's own son Vince is also a pre-medical student in college, and expresses hope that he will be able to join his father in practice some day. "Vince asked me yesterday, if I could do it all over again, would I still do the same thing. And I said, 'Yes, exactly.' Sure the scale may have tilted a bit more in the past, but it's still like this [he uses his hands to show an uneven scale, one side higher, one lower]. Sure, he hears me come home and complain sometimes, but he also gets to see me weigh the plusses and minuses, and he's still interested in rural family practice. So that says I really like what I'm doing."

So for Bernie Proy, "Part of my responsibility is finding new doctors here, to make sure there's continuity in medical care here. What better way than to pick the new doctors who will take care of my patients in the future? Then I've done my job!"

CARING FOR THE COUNTRY

Medical service—our usefulness as physicians to society as a whole—is, after all, our reason for existence, and must be the chief object of our policies, as it is the standard by which our worth must be measured.

—William Pusey, MD, 1925

Access to care remains the single most important element for improving quality in rural communities.

—John Coombs, MD, in *Textbook of Rural Medicine*, Geyman, Norris, and Hart

I worked in a bank. You know, it's just paper. It's not real. Nine to five and its shit. You're lookin' at numbers. But I can look back and say, "I helped put out a fire. I helped save somebody." It shows something I did on this earth.

—Fireman Tom Patrick, in *Working*, Studs Terkel

Jim Devlin, Mike Tatarko, Viola Monaghan, Bill Thompson, Christine Dotterer, Catherine O'Neil, Thane Turner, Dave Baer, Joe Nutz, and Bernie Proy. These ten PSAP graduates have all fulfilled their own personal dreams of becoming family doctors in small rural towns, while at the same time serving their patients, and meeting the health care needs of their communities. How many of us have been able to achieve this coalescence of satisfaction and service?

Taken together, these profiles paint a vivid portrait of rural family practice at the beginning of the twenty-first century. They illustrate many of the joys—and the challenges—of rural family practice. And they expose many common myths about rural family medicine, some of which have persisted for decades. That you can't provide high quality medicine practicing in a small town. That you can't be professionally satisfied, and you can't make a good living practicing rural family medicine. And that rural family practice is so overwhelming that you can't have a life outside of medicine. The reality, however, appears to be quite different. Despite what many physicians working in urban academic health centers and medical practices believe, these doctors are providing extraordinarily good care to their patients—competent and personal care that would go far to solving many of the health care problems in the nation if it were available to all Americans. In fact, the care provided by these physicians embody a number of the core competencies described in a recent Institute of Medicine report on health professions education and quality medical care, including delivering patient-centered care, and working as part of interdisciplinary teams. These doctors also appear more professionally and personally satisfied than many of their former teachers and urban colleagues.

What do these profiles tell us about rural family practice, and how it differs from family medicine in urban and suburban areas of the United States? The diagnoses and problems that these doctors care for are similar to those seen in metropolitan areas, except for some farm-related problems. Wherever people live, they have similar diseases and medical problems—high blood pressure, diabetes, heart disease, depression, obesity, respiratory infections, etc. But with fewer subspecialists and medical resources available, most rural family physicians have a much broader scope of practice. Some—like Jim Devlin, Viola Monaghan, and Thane Turner—do obstetrics. Viola Monaghan also does C-sections; Jim Devlin assists at surgery most days; and others like Dave Baer do hospital procedures such as endoscopies and colonoscopies. Most make home visits.

The majority of the 106 patients upon whom the patient-doctor interactions in this book are based were seen as I followed these physicians in their daily practice of family medicine; the others were discussed by them during my visits. The extensive variety of problems and issues that were cared for during that time—collectively representing less than one week of patient encounters in these practices—illustrates the extraordinarily broad scope of rural family practice. The almost 300 problems encountered with these patients also shows how often family doctors deal with multiple problems in the same patient, including those related to their symptoms, their past history, their family history, their diagnoses, and their treatments. As with most family doctors, the patients encountered during these visits were most often seen for physical examinations, well child checkups, routine gynecologic visits, pregnancy, delivery, newborn babies, hypertension, diabetes, arthritis, high cholesterol, depression, and cancer. Additional problems focused on heart disease (chest pain, heart attacks, coronary artery disease, congestive heart failure, arrhythmias, valvular heart disease, cardiac bypass surgery, cardiomyopathies, pericarditis); lung problems (pneumonia, bronchitis, bronchiolitis, chronic obstructive pulmonary disease, asthma, difficulty breathing); gastrointestinal problems (ulcers, irritable bowel syndrome, abdominal pain, rectal bleeding, gastritis, hiatal hernia, difficulty swallowing, gastroesophageal reflux disease, diverticulitis, colostomy, appendicitis); psychological and psychiatric problems (anxiety, depression, schizophrenia, behavioral problems, marital problems, stress, manic depressive illness, obsessive-compulsive disorder); neurologic problems (memory loss, dementia, seizures, multiple sclerosis); skin problems (skin infections, eczema, seborrheic keratoses, skin growths, fungal infections, rosacea, contact dermatitis); vascular problems (stroke, blood clots, arterio-venous malformation, peripheral vascular disease, femoral-popliteal arterial bypass surgery); infections (ear infections, sinusitis, bronchitis, contact with tuberculosis); musculoskeletal problems (osteoporosis, back pain, neck pain, leg pain, foot pain, hip pain, shoulder pain, fractures); urinary problems (pain, blood in the urine, frequent urination, kidney failure); gynecological problems (endometriosis, hysterectomies, irregular periods, tubal ligation, menstrual cramps, abnormal Pap test); procedures (suture removal, joint injections); normal and abnormal lab tests (for cholesterol, blood sugar, prostate cancer, low platelets, anemia, increased urinary bilirubin, cardiac stress test); as well as obesity; smoking; alcoholism; car accidents; fatigue; allergies; congenital hypospadias; fibromyalgia; liver failure; issues around death and dying; school failure; Down's syndrome; alpha-1-anti-trypsin deficiency; B12 deficiency; hypotension; amputation; decreased hearing and hearing aids; burns; hydocele; and restless legs syndrome.

Some of these doctors, like Christine Dotterer, are on call all the time—24/7/365—for their own patients who they know well; others, like Catherine O'Neil, are on call only once a week, but for the much larger group of patients in their entire practice. While rural family doctors work an average six more hours per week than their urban counterparts, they also save an equal amount of time commuting. As Bernie Proy likes to say, "I'm working while other people are driving back and forth to work." Some of the doctors are in solo private practice, while others are in larger groups, or employed by larger hospital systems. But compared to today's physicians practicing in metropolitan areas, each of these doctors appears to have more professional autonomy, and less intrusion from managed care. "One of the nice things about managed care and being in a rural area," Jim Devlin points out, "is that you can kind of control things. . . . And the nice thing here is that they can't sign up with the doctors across the street and the hospital across the street—because there isn't one." Also, because the health care systems in rural areas are smaller and somewhat less complex, these physicians often have more control of their medical practices than those in nonrural areas.

Perhaps the biggest difference between rural and urban/suburban practice, however, is how family doctors are inextricably woven into the fabric of small towns. Rural family doctors provide continuous care to the entire family—sometimes to the entire town—while also living and interacting daily with their patients outside of their office and hospital: at school events, at the supermarket, walking down the street, almost everywhere they go. In fact, the most consistent finding among the doctors in this book is how much they value the relationships that they have with their patients. Christine Dotterer uses the words "mutuality" and "interconnectedness" to describe this. And she often doesn't need to take family histories from her patients, since she frequently knows "more about their family history than they do." As Mike Tatarko explains," There aren't enough adjectives to describe all the interrelationships that are going on." And for Dave Baer, walking through town is "like making rounds." It is exactly this interweaving of one's professional and personal life that makes rural family practice unique. It provides for much of the enormous satisfaction in rural family medicine—as well as some of its difficult challenges.

Another common theme that emerges from these profiles is the feeling among these doctors that they are able to have more of an impact—to make a real difference—in their towns. Not only by providing medical care, but also through their leadership in the medical and overall community. Many serve as president or vice president of their hospital medical staffs, or are on the board of directors of their hospital. Mike Tatarko is the President and CEO of an organization representing over 115 doctors in two and one half rural counties. And Bernie Proy works to identify students from the area who are interested in returning to practice medicine, "to make sure there's continuity in medical care here. What better way than to pick the new doctors who will take better care of my patients in the future." In addition to their medical leadership, many of these doctors are also extremely involved in their community. Mike Tatarko has worked tirelessly to help improve the water supply and clean up the environment in Nanty Glo and the surrounding area. Jim Devlin led the community-wide effort to build the main park and playground in Brockway. Joe Nutz is chair of the board of directors of the local bank. And Chris Dotterer helped get fluoride into the local water supply after she was elected to borough council. As Jefferson President Paul Brucker explains, "These are good doctors who are there because they think they belong there, and they enjoy being there. They want to do a good job and make a difference in their community. In fact, to be a good physician, you have to know what's going on in the community."

Each of these doctors also treasures his or her unique rural lifestyle, including varied outdoor activities. They see their towns as wonderful places to raise their children. They also enjoy a high standard of living—in some ways higher than their urban counterparts, especially considering the much lower housing costs. All appear to be doing very well financially, although—as with Chris Dotterer and Bill Thompson, who made conscious decisions to work fewer hours and spend more time with their families—their income clearly depends on how hard and long they work. All of the doctors indicated that their standard of living is among the highest in their community, and most expressed surprise when they heard that some have questioned whether rural family doctors could make a good living. These PSAP graduates also have a rich and fulfilling life outside of medicine with their families, and for themselves. From Jim Devlin's giant pumpkins, to Chris Dotterer's baby pheasants and bonsai, and Mike Tatarko's 100 mile marathons. From Bill Thompson serving on the local ski patrol, to Bernie Proy's metalwork and "camp," and Joe Nutz's boat. These doctors are homeschooling their children, hunting, fishing, flying airplanes, and farming. Bernie Proy captures this spirit of independence when he says, "We're doing what we want to do. And the way we want to do it."

Although these ten family physicians are generally very happy and satisfied with their personal and professional lives—and clearly emphasize the positive aspects of their life and practice—they also point out the negatives. Listening to them, you can hear these doctors express what they feel are some of the biggest challenges in practicing family medicine in small rural towns: the medical isolation, the business side of medicine (which though it also exists in urban areas, can be more problematic due to the lower reimbursements in rural areas), the struggle to maintain their personal life and family, and their concerns about keeping up with the changes in medicine. Dave Baer remarks, "It gets pretty lonesome out here at times, when the only other person . . . who can see the patient is another family doctor." For Bernie Proy, the biggest challenge is maintaining a "practice that's sound in a financial and business sense." And Mike Tatarko worries about "trying to make sure that you keep up to date on everything," and expresses what he feels is the biggest challenge of rural family practice, "I watch all my friends' family and parents die, and that is really tough!" These rural physicians are also increasingly dealing with many of the same pressures and hassles that all doctors now face—decreasing autonomy, rising malpractice insurance costs, decreasing reimbursement from government and insurance companies, managed care, and mounting paperwork and regulation. However, compared to their peers practicing in nonrural areas, the degree of these problems is somewhat less. Bernie Proy says it best, when talking about his son, "Sure the scale may have tilted a bit more in the past. . . . Sure, he hears me come home and complain sometimes, but he also gets to see me weigh the plusses and minuses, and he's still interested in rural family practice. So that says I really like what I'm doing."

Many of these doctors also struggle with the boundary between their professional and personal life as do many other Americans nowadays. Bill Thompson talks about trying to "maintain relationships with my family," and Thane Turner about "the time thing . . . how overwhelming rural medicine really is. It's everywhere." Jim Devlin expresses one of his major challenges is "trying to give 110% all the time," and Joe Nutz feels that the biggest challenge is "when you're tired, and you want private time [with family]." But like the others, Joe then adds, "That's just part of being a small town family practitioner." And people in town "come by and help me out when I need it." Of course, not all aspects of living in small towns are idyllic. Crime does exist, as do problems like drugs and violence in the schools—just in smaller doses than in the city and suburbs. These doctors also acknowledge some of the negative aspects of rural living, as when Chris Dotterer says, "There's not all the entertainment possibilities." And of course, the lack of shopping.

So rural family practice is like family practice everywhere, but also very different. What these ten doctors clearly demonstrate is that practicing family medicine in small rural towns is neither inherently good nor bad, but rather is dependent on the match between the person and this unique profession. The same issues that make rural family practice attractive for some, are viewed as disadvantages by others. As Joe Nutz says, "The best thing about living in a small town is the same thing I don't like about it. It's a double-edged sword." Many rural physicians report that the rural lifestyle is a major reason for their career choice. They describe rural areas as a great environment in which to live, to raise a family, to participate in outdoor activities, and to become an active member of a close-knit community. But while rural areas have the advantage of lower crime rates, less traffic, and less time spent commuting, they also lack the cultural amenities of urban living. So while rural and urban physicians seem to agree on the specifics of what their locales provide, they differ in how they personally value and weigh the importance of these factors. Urban doctors shy away from rural areas because they have small populations and lack anonymity, while rural doctors love knowing everyone in town. And urban physicians don't want to raise their children in small towns, while rural doctors think it's a great place to raise kids.

In many ways, the picture of rural family medicine that emerges from these profiles represents a professional and personal life that many doctors today would find extremely attractive—more professional autonomy, a more satisfying relationship with their patients, less managed care, lower malpractice insurance premiums, a higher standard of living, less crime, less traffic, and less expensive housing with more land. From Mike Tatarko's perspective, "you wonder why people aren't running out here, rather than living in Philly or Pittsburgh." However, one also needs to be comfortable with the negative aspects of rural practice—including having fewer medical resources, being more isolated, having less anonymity, and having access to fewer cultural activities. Rural family practice is not ideal. And the future of rural family practice remains undefined in many ways, as does much of medicine. But for the right person, the right fit, it can be a great profession, a wonderful life, and at the same time serve an important societal need.

• • • • •

For most of the past century, rural Americans—as with those living in rural areas in almost every country in the world—have not had their fair share of physicians, with resultant problems in access to health care. Currently, rural areas of this country have about half as many physicians per given population as do nonrural areas, and the distribution of physicians in rural areas is worsening. Overall, there are more than 20 million people who live in rural areas of the United States without an adequate supply of primary care doctors— almost half the number of Americans that have no health insurance, the other national health care shame in this country. But while providing health insurance to everyone in this country is a critically important goal, it will not solve the access problem for those living in rural America.

Nevertheless, little attention is paid to the rural physician shortage, or to rural areas in general. Today, the common image of rural America alternates between the negative impression of an impoverished, socially marginal setting and the positive vision of a romantic and idyllic place. Although there is some truth in both of these pictures, neither is very accurate. While small rural towns have been forgotten or ignored by much of the nation, the reality is that one out of every five Americans lives in a rural area, and the rural population is actually increasing. Although this growth is not as fast as in metropolitan areas, it is estimated that the rural population will still be 19 percent of the total US population in 2020, down only slightly from its current 20 percent.

While not all rural areas suffer from a lack of physicians, almost 40 percent of the rural population lives in a physician shortage area. And even the majority of those rural areas that currently have an adequate physician supply will soon need more, as their current family doctors leave or retire—as two-thirds of non-shortage rural counties have an adequate supply *only* because of the family doctors who are currently there. That is the nature of providing health care to areas with a small population with only a few doctors in town—the loss, or gain, of only one or two physicians has a major impact on access to health care. Of the ten towns where the doctors in this book practice, five are in federally designated primary care HPSAs, and four others also report a need for more family doctors. The tenth town has an adequate supply only because of the PSAP graduate who is practicing there. These physicians also play a key role in stabilizing the physician supply in their towns, serving a role that sociologists call "anchorpersons." As a result of their long term and strong commitment to the area, they have been very influential in recruiting and retaining other physicians and health care providers. New doctors are unlikely to move to a small town if they are concerned that the current physicians may leave. Likewise, some doctors, especially those who have recently arrived in town or those nearing retirement, are more likely to leave if other physicians in town also decide to move. So having a long-term committed physician—like these PSAP graduates—is oftentimes the glue that holds a town's health care system together.

• • • • •

While there has long been widespread agreement that many rural areas have a serious shortage of physicians, especially primary care physicians, there is no such agreement on how to resolve this problem. For most of the past century, the role of medical schools in addressing the rural primary care shortage has remained controversial. Some have felt this role to be limited. Clearly, many forces outside of the academic environment have had an important impact on physicians' choice of specialty and practice location. In addition, there has been concern for decades that preferential medical school admission of applicants from rural areas will not work, contending that since metropolitan areas have obvious professional, financial, and living advantages, rural-raised students will end up choosing to practice in metropolitan areas, similar to their urban colleagues. There is also longstanding concern that these types of medical school programs to increase the supply of rural physicians are too small to have a significant impact, and that they will decrease the quality of physicians.

What has been learned from the PSAP—and from these ten rural family doctors—regarding the role of medical schools in addressing the rural physician shortage? The wide variation among medical schools in the proportion of their graduates practicing in rural areas, ranging from 2 percent to 41 percent, suggests that schools can have an important impact on the geographic location of their graduates. However, the clearest evidence comes simply from the success of the PSAP and other similar programs. Between one-fourth and three-fourths of the graduates from these programs are practicing in rural areas (depending on the definition of rural used), and two-thirds have chosen a primary care specialty (mostly family practice). And of critical importance, the PSAP retention rate is the highest ever reported—79 percent for rural family doctors during the eleven to sixteen years they have been followed so far—almost double the rural retention rate of the NHSC.

There are also concerns that these programs do not totally resolve the shortage of rural physicians, and that not all of the PSAP graduates fulfill their commitment. While no program is perfect, the PSAP does address the problem more than any other policy or program has yet demonstrated. Not only were PSAP graduates eight times as likely to become rural family doctors as their peers, but even of those PSAP graduates who did not practice rural family medicine, almost all practiced either in rural or the smallest metropolitan counties or in one of the primary care specialties. Only 16 percent of PSAP graduates were thus considered "failures," that is, practicing a nonprimary care specialty in a large metropolitan area. What about the concern that these medical school programs produce so few doctors that their overall impact is negligible? This fails to take into account the disproportionate impact of even a very small number of physicians on a small town. Here again, the PSAP outcomes have shown the importance of this small program on the state's rural physician workforce, accounting for one of every eight family doctors in rural Pennsylvania. In fact, if each of the 146 US medical schools graduated just five to ten additional family doctors each year who practiced in underserved rural areas, that would be enough to eliminate the rural primary care physician shortage—which has persisted for most of the past century—in less than ten years.

As to the question of whether preferentially admitting rural-raised individuals will produce inferior doctors, studies have shown that PSAP students have had academic admission credentials similar to their classmates. Even so, medical school admission decisions have never been based purely on academic criteria, but are always made in combination with nonacademic factors. In addition to college grades and Medical College Admission Test (MCAT) scores, medical schools almost always require that applicants are motivated, have prior experience with the medical profession, and have appropriate interpersonal and communication skills. Among applicants meeting these qualifications, selection is then frequently made by also taking into consideration letters of recommendation and personal interviews, and such other criteria as leadership experiences, extracurricular activities, helping activities, research activities, life experiences, race and ethnicity, and alumni status. Geographic background, most often state residence, has also been an important factor for most public, as well as many private medical schools. The PSAP admission process differs from the traditional admission process in that, among those academically and otherwise qualified applicants, selection is primarily based on an applicant's likelihood for rural family practice, as determined by his or her rural background and commitment to rural family medicine. By broadening the admission criteria in this way, the PSAP results in a different group of medical students than would otherwise be admitted. As University President Paul Brucker explains, "We were committed to making sure that the people in this program were academically equivalent to other people in the class. But there was also an appreciation of the cultural differences between rural and urban areas. That you just can't say to someone 'go to a rural area,' unless you fit with that rural area, and your family fits with that rural area." More important than admission criteria, however, is the quality of the physicians graduating from the program. Again, the medical school attrition rate of PSAP students, and their academic performance during medical school and residency training has been similar to their peers. Any program of preferential admission in an educational environment is extremely controversial. In undergraduate education, it is essential to make sure that the admission process is fair, and it is also important to enrich the educational environment of all students with a diverse student body. For medical and other professional schools, however, there is another critical factor that must be considered and balanced—the potential contribution to society. Here, the PSAP and other similar programs have clearly produced a physician workforce that better meets the health care needs of the population.

While medical school programs such as the PSAP are the most effective way to increase the rural physician supply, the solution to this long-standing and serious problem clearly requires multiple approaches. The NHSC and other loan repayment and service programs also represent critically important ways to improve the health care needs of many rural communities. It is also crucial to provide increasing practice support—addressing key issues such as malpractice insurance, reimbursement, and regulations—in order to facilitate recruitment of rural physicians and to help them stay.

· · · · ·

In order for our experience with the PSAP to be most helpful for others, however, it is not sufficient to merely prove *that* the program works, it must also be shown *why* the PSAP works, and *how* it works. The common themes that emerge from the ten PSAP graduates profiled in this book strongly reinforce our prior research studies in this area. Their stories add important personal perspectives to those statistical outcomes, and give a clearer sense of the characteristics of those people who are best suited to practice rural family medicine and to remain. They also provide a deeper insight into why the PSAP has been so successful, namely, that rural background and entering medical school with plans to become a family physician are clearly the most important factors related to becoming a rural family doctor. In fact, despite the myriad of factors that obviously go into a person's career decision, these two characteristics—rural background and plans for family practice—are so powerful that seven out of every eight Jefferson graduates practicing rural primary care have at least one of them. Conversely, fewer than two percent of all graduates entered rural primary care if they lacked these two factors.

Nine of the ten doctors interviewed in this book, like almost all of the PSAP graduates practicing rural family medicine, grew up in rural areas and love being back there. For decades, rural background has consistently been found to be the most important predictor of rural practice. And while it is true that many rural-raised people do want to leave small towns, and some even seek a career in medicine as a way to help facilitate this, it is relatively easy to distinguish those rural-raised individuals who want to return, from those who want to leave. Asking students about their background, culture, and interests provides valuable information. Listening to why these ten doctors decided to practice rural family medicine, one gets a better sense of the importance of rural background, and why it is key. For only by spending a significant portion of your life in a small rural town can one really understand how you will feel living there, and how you will be able to balance the positive and negative aspects of the rural lifestyle.

What about the common perception that most medical students enter medical school wanting to be family doctors, but everyone changes their mind regarding specialty choice? The commitment to family practice of the ten PSAP graduates in this book has been remarkably consistent. When you read what these physicians wrote on their medical school applications—some more than 25 years ago—you have to be impressed with how similar their life has turned out to those original dreams and goals. Overall, while research has shown that many medical students do change their precise specialty plans, this does not mean that there is no relationship between these initial career plans and their eventual specialty, or that all students enter medical school equally likely to enter every discipline. In fact, most students eventually enter one of their top initially planned specialties; and, the overall stability rate for family practice is higher than for most other specialties. For those wanting to live in rural America, family practice is the most natural medical discipline. In fact, the specialty of family practice is tightly linked to rural health care. For not only do family doctors provide the majority of primary care in rural areas, but also rural practice is the only area where family medicine is irreplaceable by other specialists. In fact, entering medical school with plans to be a family doctor is the second most predictive factor for rural practice, and the combination of this with rural background has a cumulative effect, where having both factors is twice as powerful as having either one.

The greatest proof that rural background and initial interest in rural family medicine are predictive of eventual rural family practice, however, is simply that the PSAP and other similar programs have been able to accurately select medical students who eventually became—and remained—rural family physicians. Considering that the PSAP has been so successful at Jefferson—a large, urban, private medical school in the northeastern United States, characteristics generally related to a low output of rural family physicians—it is likely that this type of program would have an even greater impact in other medical schools and in other areas of the country.

What have we learned from the PSAP about the role of other primary care physicians and of nonphysician providers in caring for rural populations?

Most importantly, that people living in rural areas need all the primary care providers they can get—irrespective of their discipline. Having said that, the fact remains that family doctors are much more likely to practice in small rural towns than are general internists or general pediatricians. And family practice is the only planned specialty choice at entrance to medical school that is predictive of practicing any type of rural primary care. In fact, entering medical school with plans for general internal medicine is inversely related to practicing rural primary care, and initial plans for general pediatrics is unrelated. It is also important to acknowledge that while the PSAP addresses the shortage of primary care physicians, many rural areas also need additional nonprimary care specialists, including general surgeons.

As for nurse practitioners (NPs) and physician assistants (PAs), they also have a critical role in caring for rural America. Six of the ten doctors in this book work with NPs or PAs, as do 28 percent of all rural primary care doctors. Some have gone so far as to advocate that NPs and PAs should become the major providers of primary care in rural America, since not enough physicians practice there. In reality, however, fewer than one-fourth of PAs and NPs practice in rural areas, and the majority of PAs work in nonprimary care areas of medicine. Nationally, NPs and PAs together are involved in only 3 percent of all visits to primary care doctors. So, even with the increase in NPs and PAs being trained today, there are not even close to the overall numbers that are needed to provide all the rural primary care. In some states, including Pennsylvania, NPs and PAs can not legally practice medicine independent of physicians. Nevertheless, as seen in the profiles in this book, nonphysician providers do make a major contribution to the rural primary care workforce, and substantially increase access to care for people living in rural areas.

While men in general are more likely to practice rural primary care, women in the PSAP—like Viola Monaghan, Christine Dotterer, and Catherine O'Neil—are equally likely to do so, an outcome also reported by another similar program. The important role of one's spouse on practice location has also been well documented—in medicine and in other areas—and can also be seen with many of these doctors. Having an NHSC scholarship, and taking a senior family medicine rural preceptorship are also predictive of rural primary care. However, as seen with Viola Monaghan for the NHSC, and with Bill Thompson and four of the other physicians who took a rural preceptorship, these personal narratives appear to reinforce our prior preliminary data that the most important role of these programs is in confirming the already existing career plans of these doctors.

The role of economic factors in selecting a career in rural primary care, though very concerning, remains unproven. Previous research has shown that neither a medical student's expectation of future income, nor their medical school level of debt were predictive of practicing rural primary care. Among the ten doctors I interviewed, a number followed through on their career plans to practice rural family medicine despite their high debts. On the other hand, the rapidly increasing debt of more recent graduates—now averaging more than $100,000, with many physicians owing over $150,000—raises serious questions as to whether this will become a more important factor in the future. Certainly many of the physicians in this book expressed deep concerns that this increasing level of debt will further limit the number of family doctors in small rural towns.

Regarding the critically important issue of retention, our outcome studies have shown that the only two predictive factors are being in the PSAP and attending a rural college—both of which all ten of these doctors did. This fits with the increasingly accepted theory that rural retention is very different than rural recruitment, and is most related to the integration and preparedness of physicians and their families to the rural environment.

Over the years, most of the PSAP students have generally expressed positive feelings about the program. Their major concerns have focused on the limited financial support. Some who decided not to become rural family physicians have been reluctant to complete the PSAP curriculum during medical school. Nevertheless, most of the graduates have been appreciative of the program and its role in helping them fulfill their personal career goals.

· · · · ·

A major policy issue that needs to be raised regarding the rural physician shortage is: If programs like the PSAP work—and they clearly do—then why haven't more medical schools developed similar programs? With the research that has been published, and after reading these narrative stories, the reason for the PSAP's success is available for all to see. The likely explanation as to why most other schools do not develop similar programs is that increasing the supply and retention of rural family doctors is not as important as the three major missions of medical schools—education, research, and patient care. This is in contrast to what is happening in other countries, including Canada and Australia, where new rural medical schools have recently been developed. It is not surprising, however, considering the enormous financial pressures that US medical schools and academic health centers are facing as a result of the increasingly competitive health care environment. This has forced most medical schools to try and explicitly link their supporting dollars to their budgeted activities. For the rural physician shortage, and for programs like the PSAP, this represents a major problem, since although medical schools are responsible for developing and implementing these programs, the major beneficiaries of the PSAP are the people living in rural communities—not the medical schools. As such, medical schools are unlikely to develop them without explicit financial support. As former Jefferson Dean Joseph Gonnella says, "There are no incentives for a medical school to have this type of program. If you put the burden on the medical school, they will not be developed." In fact, Jefferson is the only private medical school in the country to have such a program entirely supported by the university, and there are only a handful of public medical schools with similar programs. This disconnect between the mission of the medical schools, which hold the key to these programs but lack explicit funding for them, and the needs of the rural communities that these programs serve, means not only that other schools are unlikely to develop these types of programs, but that some schools that already have them in place may be forced to discontinue them unless specific financial support is provided. Who should pay for these programs? Unless supported by state and federal governments, these programs will not be replicated. It would be a shame if these important programs—that have been proven to work, have the highest retention ever reported, with graduates who are professionally and personally satisfied, and that provide high-quality care for their patients and their communities—are not developed or continued.

What is the proper role of government in supporting programs that improve the supply and retention of rural doctors? Is this goal a public good, deserving of public support? Or should it be left to the marketplace to address the rural physician shortage, as it has been, unsuccessfully, for decades? Today, almost all of the current forces that impact a physician's decision regarding his or her medical specialty and practice location—from admission and educational decisions within medical schools, to financial and practice support issues—are working against choosing rural family medicine. In fact, these forces are actually leading to an increase in the number of subspecialty physicians practicing in affluent urban and suburban areas, at the expense of rural family doctors. And with market forces having an increasingly important effect on health care policy, there remains serious concern for those living in rural areas who have less force in the market. It is hard to imagine a scenario where rural areas will ever have an adequate supply of doctors, without strong government support for programs that have been proven to improve this problem.

Another important policy issue that needs to be faced in order to address the rural physician shortage is medical school debt. Combined with the increasing financial restrictions also impinging upon rural providers, including lower reimbursement rates and rapidly increasing malpractice insurance premiums, the tenuous financial balance of rural primary care could rapidly reverse in many small towns. The issue of the uninsured in this country also hits rural Americans particularly hard, a group of people that has been described as being in "triple jeopardy—rural, poor, and uninsured."

Finally, the future of the rural physician workforce also depends heavily on the future of the specialty of family practice. For as family practice goes, so goes rural primary care. When the number of US medical school graduates entering family practice increased during the 1990s, rural areas were a prime beneficiary. But with the numbers entering family practice having decreased over the past six years—though family practice still represents one of the most popular medical specialties, chosen by eight to ten percent of US graduates—rural areas will be adversely affected.

These critical issues require that policy makers focus specifically on what works in rural areas. Because rural areas are not just small urban areas anymore than children are just small adults. They are also qualitatively different, with very different needs and requiring different solutions. Often, health care programs are designed to solve urban problems but ignore rural areas. This invariably results in more problems for people living in rural areas. It is therefore imperative to explicitly consider the impact of all health care policies on rural Americans.

• • • • •

During the past few decades, the majority of programs to increase the number of physicians practicing in rural areas have focused on urban and suburban-raised medical students, exposing them to clinical experiences in rural areas, or providing financial support for their education and practice. Taking a different perspective, the PSAP was developed based on the key observation that despite the seemingly significant barriers that exist, some physicians nevertheless still choose to practice rural family medicine. And they do so primarily because of their background, lifestyle preferences, interest in family practice, and their commitment. The importance of this is highlighted by a recent survey of physicians completing their residency training showing that the top consideration for selecting a practice for three-fourths of them was "geographic location/lifestyle," greater than other choices of finances, call schedule, loan forgiveness, or specialty support. So, rather than primarily focusing on decreasing the major barriers to rural family practice, the PSAP instead attempted to increase the number of those physicians highly likely to practice rural family medicine.

Today, the results are clear. For those policy makers and educators who want to increase the supply and retention of rural primary care physicians, the greatest impact, by far, will be achieved by increasing the selection of medical students who grew up in rural areas and are committed to practice rural family medicine. In fact, any program that does not do this may have limited success. This is also the most economical strategy to address the problem. While this admissions component—responsible for 75 percent of the success of the PSAP—is necessary, however, it is not sufficient. Educational experiences, mentoring, and practice support should also be provided to maximize success even further. While medical schools hold the key to making these programs happen, they won't develop them unless there is financial support and incentives available from state and federal governments. And by becoming more accountable for public problems such as the need for rural physicians, medical schools could justify new and increased public funding to support their social mission.

• • • • •

Even in today's complex and changing world, the work that we do and the place where we live are vitally important. For physicians, selecting a medical specialty and choosing where to practice are among the most important decisions they make. These ten PSAP graduates became family doctors in small rural towns, and in doing so have been able to fulfill their professional aspirations and achieve their personal goals while at the same time making a difference in their communities. Their stories provide important lessons for all of us about what is significant in work, and in life. They also teach us about the rewards and difficulties—and the fit—of rural family practice and about meeting the need for medical care that exists in thousands of small rural towns. For in the end, we all want to feel like Thane Turner: "It's very satisfying . . . It's all here!" And like Catherine O'Neil: "I love it. . . . It worked out perfect!" And like Bernie Proy: "All the way around it meets my needs— professionally, personally, socially, intellectually, spiritually." And like Chris Dotterer: "I don't think there's any other job like it!" And like Mike Tatarko: "I couldn't have asked for it to work out any better."

From a personal perspective, it has been a wonderful opportunity to be part of this unique program during the past 27 years. It has also been personally rewarding to have gotten to know the individual PSAP students and graduates of the program, as they are a wonderful group of individuals. In visiting the ten PSAP graduates for this book, I not only had the pleasure to reacquaint myself with them and visit them in their current lives, but I had the extraordinary opportunity to observe them take care of their patients. Watching my former students practice family medicine in their small rural towns was a unique experience, and I came away from it with a great sense of fulfillment. For me, the excellent and personal care they are providing to the people in their rural communities is the greatest measure of the success of the PSAP.

And what of the future of rural family practice and of the PSAP? Like all of medicine, rural family practice faces serious challenges. Despite this, it is hard *not* to be optimistic about the future when I look at the recent PSAP graduates and the current PSAP students from the classes of 2004 to 2006. These students and graduates are every bit as dedicated, motivated, and committed as those in the past. And I have little doubt that should my successor visit these doctors in another 27 years—in 2030—he or she will find a program that has continued to have an important impact on the rural physician workforce and a group of rural family doctors who are as satisfied, fulfilled, and committed as those who are profiled here.

• • • • •

This book, then, has told the story of the PSAP of Jefferson Medical College, through the professional and personal lives of its graduates. The PSAP has been successful because it identifies, recruits, admits, supports, mentors, and trains students who grew up in rural areas and are intent on becoming rural family doctors. After graduation from medical school, a large proportion of these physicians then gravitate to rural areas to follow their professional and personal goals and do what they have always wanted to do. Not surprisingly, almost all stay.

A few years ago, I came upon a cartoon that accurately captures the dilemma of the rural physician workforce. There are two frames. On the left side, a patient is sitting on the exam table in a doctor's office, partially undressed. There are two doctors standing in front of him, and the caption underneath says "Over Supply." On the right frame, above a caption that reads "No Supply," an identical-looking patient is sitting on the same table, but this time he is entirely alone. There is no one else in the picture—no doctor. This cartoon shows the stark but simple reality facing people living in rural areas—that there aren't enough doctors. And while there are certainly negative impacts of having too many physicians—it is likely to result in unnecessary health care services and increased costs—not having any doctor at all is simply unacceptable.

If the United States is truly serious in its commitment to provide medical care to each of its citizens, it must address the shortage of physicians in rural areas. This nation long ago committed itself to provide equally difficult yet important services to people living in rural areas—services such as highways, schools, telephones, electricity, and mail service—and it is imperative that the nation do the same with medical care. Only then can we assure that every American will have access to health care.

EPILOGUE

Changes continue to occur in all of our lives. In the year or so since I visited the ten PSAP graduates profiled in this book, half have experienced significant changes—in their personal lives, in their practices, and in medicine. Thane Turner and his wife have a happy and healthy new son, Benjamin. With Catherine O'Neil's practice now staffing the University Health Service, she has taken on the added role of medical director of Bloomsburg University. Catherine and her husband also moved into their new house, further up the hill, and are expecting their second child. And Joe Nutz moved into his new computerized office and was joined by his new partner.

Viola Monaghan decided to make a major career change. After completing her four-year commitment with the NHSC, she decided to join a new practice in the town of Ithaca, New York that focuses on the medical and surgical treatment of venous diseases, including deep vein thrombosis and thrombophlebitis (blood clots and inflammation of the veins), varicose veins, chronic venous insufficiency, and venous leg ulcers. She and her family also moved to a new house in the nearby small rural town of Trumansburg.

And as for Bernie Proy, whose motivation to become a doctor was, in part, related to his own father's lack of opportunity to do so, and who has been mentoring other young people in his community to return home as family doctors, Bernie just heard that his oldest son, Vince, has been accepted into the class of 2007 of Jefferson's PSAP! Vince will be the first child of a PSAP graduate to also be in the PSAP—planning to follow in his father's footsteps and become part of the next generation of rural family doctors, caring for the country.

REFERENCES

Ackermann RJ, Comeau RW. Mercer University School of Medicine: a successful approach to primary care medical education. *Fam Med.* 1996;28:395–402.

Adams DP. *American Board of Family Practice: A History.* Lexington, Ky: American Board of Family Practice; 1999.

Adkins RJ, Anderson GR, Cullen TJ, et al. Geographic and specialty distribution of WAMI Program participants and nonparticipants. *J Med Educ.* 1987;62:810–817.

Agency for Health Care Policy and Research. *Improving Health Care for Rural Populations: Research in Action Fact Sheet.* AHCPR Publication No. 96-P040. 1996. Available at: http://www.ahrq.gov/research/rural.htm. Accessed August 6, 2003.

Agency for Healthcare Research and Quality. *AHRQ Focus on Research: Rural Health Care.* AHRQ Publication No. 02-M015. 2002. Available at: http://www.ahrq.gov/news/focus/focrural.htm. Accessed August 6, 2003.

American Academy of Family Physicians. Table 59: Performance of diagnostic procedures in family physicians offices, May 2002. In: *2003 Facts about Family Practice.* Kansas City, Mo: AAFP; 2003. Available at: http://www.aafp.org/x821.xml. Accessed February 16, 2004.

American Academy of Family Physicians. Table 61: Hospital admission privileges of family physicians, by census division, May 2003. In: *2003 Facts about Family Practice.* Kansas City, Mo: AAFP; 2003. Available at: http://www.aafp.org/x823.xml. Accessed February 16, 2004.

American Academy of Family Physicians. 2003 MATCH information sheet. 2003. Available at: http://www.aafp.org/match/nrmpinfo.html. Accessed August 10, 2003.

American Board of Family Practice. Diplomate Statistics. 2003. Available at: http://www.abfp.org/about/stats.aspx. Accessed August 11, 2003.

Babbott D, Baldwin DC, Jolly P, et al. The stability of early specialty preferences among US medical school graduates in 1983. *JAMA*. 1998;259:1970–1975.

Barnett, BL. From cradle to rocker: Providing care across the human life cycle. In: Sloane, PD, Slatt LM, Curtis P, eds. *Essentials of Family Medicine*. Philadelphia: Lippincott Williams & Wilkins; 1998.

Bedford County Chamber of Commerce. Community Information: History. 2003. Available at: http://www.bedfordcountychamber.org/?orgid=4&storyTypeID=& sid=&. Accessed August 9, 2003.

Berwick DM. *Escape Fire*. New York: The Commonwealth Fund; 2002.

Blumenthal D, Campbell EG, Weissman JS. The social missions of academic health centers. *N Engl J Med*. 1997;337:1550–1553.

Boulger JG. Family medicine education and rural health: a response to present and future needs. *J Rural Health*. 1991;7:105–115.

Boulger JG. Successful Duluth program narrows the gender gap. Letter to editor. *Fam Med*. 2001;33:6–7.

Brazeau NK, Potts MJ, Hickner JM. The Upper Peninsula Program: a successful model for increasing primary care physicians in rural areas. *Fam Med*. 1990;22:350–355.

Brennan TA. Luxury primary care—market innovation or threat to access? *N Engl J Med*. 2002;346:1165–1168.

Bryan JE. The Role of the Family Physician in America's Developing Medical Care Program. Private communication with EB White. St. Louis: Warren H. Green, Inc.; 1968.

Buchbinder SB, Wilson M, Melick CF, et al. Estimates of costs of primary care turnover. *Am J Managed Care*. 1999;5:1431–1438.

Carline JD, Greer T. Comparing physicians' specialty interests upon entering medical school with their eventual practice specialties. *Acad Med*. 1991;66:44–46.

The Center for Rural Pennsylvania. Newsletter. July/August 2002. Available at: http://www.ruralpa.org/news0702.html. Accessed August 11, 2003.

Cohen JJ. Why doctors don't always go where they're needed. *Acad Med*. 1999;73:1277.

Columbia Montour Chamber of Commerce. Welcome to Bloomsburg, Pennsylvania, 2003. Available at: http://townhall.bafn.org/Government/bloomsburg/history.htm. Accessed February 16, 2004.

Colwill JM, Cultice JM. The future supply of family physicians: implications for rural America. *Health Aff*. 2003;22:190–198.

Cordes SM. Come on in, the water's just fine. *Acad Med*. 1990;65:S1–S9.

The core content of family medicine: report of the committee on requirements for certification. *GP*. 1966;34:225.

Council on Graduate Medical Education. *Physician Distribution and Health Care Challenges in Rural and Inner City Areas: Tenth Report to Congress and the Department of Health and Human Services Secretary*. Rockville, Md: Health Resources and Services Administration, US Department of Health and Human Services; 1998.

Cullen JC, Hart LG, Whitcomb ME, et al. The National Health Service Corps: rural physician service and retention. *J Am Board Fam Pract*. 1997;10:272–279.

Cullison S, Reid C, Colwill JS. Medical school admissions, specialty selection, and distribution of physicians. *JAMA*. 1976;235:502–505.

Cutchin MP. Community and self: concepts for rural physician integration and retention. *Soc Sci Med*. 1997;44:1661–1674.

Donaldson MS, Yordy KD, Lohr KN, et al., editors, for the Institute of Medicine.

Primary Care: America's Health in a New Era. Washington, DC: National Academy Press; 1996.

Eberhardt MS, Ingram DD, Makuc DM, et al. *Urban and Rural Health Chartbook. Health, United States, 2001* Urban and Rural Health Chartbook. Hyattsville, Md: National Center for Health Statistics; 2001.

Ernst RL, Yett DE. *Physician location and specialty choice.* Ann Arbor, Mich: Health Administration Press; 1985.

Federal Office of Rural Health Policy. Facts about . . . rural physicians. 1997. Available at: http://www.shepscenter.unc.edu/research_programs/rural_program/phy.html. Accessed August 6, 2003.

Flexner, A. Medical Education in the United States and Canada: A Report to the Carnegie Foundation for the Advancement of Teaching. Washington, DC: Science and Health Publications; 1960. (Original printing, 1910).

Fryer GE, Dovey SM, Green LA. The United States relies on family physicians, unlike any other specialty. *Am Fam Physician.* 2001;63:1669.

Gamm L, Hutchison L, Bellamy G, et al. Rural healthy people 2010: identifying rural health priorities and models for practice. *J Rural Health.* 2002:18;9–14.

Geyman JP. *Family Practice: Foundation of Changing Health Care.* 2nd ed. Norwalk, Conn: Appleton-Century Crofts; 1985.

Geyman JP, Norris TE, Hart LG. *Textbook of Rural Medicine.* New York: McGraw-Hill; 2001.

Gonnella JS, Hojat M, Erdmann JB, et al. Assessment measures in medical school, residency, and practice: the connections. *Acad Med.* 1993;68:S3–S106.

The Graduate Education of Physicians: The Report of the Citizens Commission of Graduate Medical Education. Chicago: American Medical Association; 1966.

Graham R, Roberts R, Östergaard DJ, et al. Family practice in the United States: a status report. *JAMA.* 2002;288:1097–1101.

Greiner AC, Knebel E, eds. Institute of Medicine. Health Professions Education: A Bridge to Quality. Washington, DC: The National Academies Press; 2003.

Hart GL, Salsberg E, Phillips DM, et al. Rural health care providers in the United States. *J Rural Health.* 2002;18:211–232.

Hart JT. The inverse care law. *Lancet.* 1971;i:405–412.

Health Is a Community Affair. The Report of the National Commission on Community Health Services. Cambridge, Mass: Harvard University Press; 1966.

HHS Rural Task Force: Report to the Secretary. One Department Serving Rural America. Washington, DC: HHS; 2002.

Hojat M, Gonnella JS, Veloski JJ, et al. Jefferson Medical College longitudinal study: a prototype for evaluation of changes. *Educ Health.* 1996;9:99–113.

Hooker RS, McCaig LF. Use of physician assistants and nurse practitioners in primary care, 1995–1999. *Health Aff.* 2001;20:231–238.

JAMA study proves that PSAP brings family physicians to underserved areas. *Jefferson Medical College Alumni Bulletin.* 1999;49:27–28.

Jolly P, Hudley DM, eds. *Association of American Medical Colleges Data Book: Statistical Information Related to Medical Education.* Washington, DC: AAMC; 1998.

Kassebaum DC, Szenas PL. Medical students' career indecision and specialty rejection: roads not taken. *Acad. Med.* 1995;70:937–43.

Kassebaum DC, Szenas PL. Rural sources of medical students, and graduates' choice of medical practice. *Acad Med.* 1993;68:232–236.

Kidder, Tracy. *Hometown.* New York: Random House; 1999.

Kronick R, Goodman DC, Wennberg J, et al. The marketplace in health care reform: the demographic limitations of managed competition. *N Engl J Med.* 1993;328: 148–152.

Linzer M, Slavin T, Mouth S, et al. Admission, recruitment, and retention: finding and keeping the generalist-oriented student. *J Gen Intern Med.* 1994;9:S14–S23.

Ludmerer KM. *Time to Heal: American Medical Education from the Turn of the Century to the Era of Managed Care.* New York: Oxford Press; 1999.

Madison DL. Managing a chronic problem: the rural physician shortage. *Ann Intern Med.* 1980;92:852–854.

Mattson DE, Stehr DE, Will RE. Evaluation of a program designed to produce rural physicians. *J Med Educ.* 1973;48:323–331.

Mayers L, Harrison LV. *The Distribution of Physicians in the United States.* New York: General Education Board; 1924.

McPhee J. *Heirs of General Practice.* New York: The Noonday Press; 1984.

Medical Student Education: Cost, Debt, and Resident Stipend Facts. Association of American Medical Colleges. Washington, DC: AAMC; 2003. Available at: http://www.aamc.org/students/financing/debthelp/factcard03.pdf. Accessed February 16, 2004.

Meeting the Challenge of Family Practice. The Report of the Ad Hoc Committee on Education for Family Practice of the Council on Medical Education. Chicago: American Medical Association; 1966.

Merritt, Hawkins & Associates. Summary Report: 2003 Survey of Final-Year Medical Residents. 2003. Available at: http://www.merritthawkins.com/merritthawkins/pdf/MHA2003residentsurv.pdf. Accessed August 12, 2003.

Mills OF, Tatarko M, Bates JF, et al. Telemedicine precepting in a family practice center. *Fam Med.* 1993;31:239–243.

Oklahoma State University Center for Health Policy Research. 25+ Years: Oklahoma Physician Manpower Training Commission. 2001. Available at: http://www.osu-med.com/telemedicine/Pub/chpr/chpr.0201pmtc.pdf. Accessed August 12, 2003.

Pathman DE. Medical education and physicians' career choices: are we taking credit beyond our due? *Acad Med.* 1996;71:963–968.

Pathman DE, Konrad TR, Ricketts TC. The comparative retention of National Health Service Corps and other rural physicians. *JAMA.* 1992;268:1552–1558.

Pathman DE, Steiner BD, Jones BD, et al. Preparing and retaining rural physicians through medical education. *Acad Med.* 1999;74:810–820.

Peabody FW. The care of the patient. *JAMA.* 1927;88:877–882.

Pellegrino E. The generalist function in medicine. *JAMA.* 1966;198:541.

Pennsylvania Department of Health. *Health Profile, 1996: Pennsylvania Counties.* Harrisburg, Pa: Pennsylvania Dept of Health; 1996.

Phillips DM, Dunlap PG, eds. *Physician Recruitment and Retention.* Washington, DC: National Rural Health Association; 1998.

Phillips RL, Green LA. Making choices about the scope of family practice. *J Am Board Fam Pract.* 2002;15:250–254.

Pisacano NJ. General practice: a eulogy. *Am J Gen Pract.* 1964;19:173–179.

Pusey WA. Medical education and medical service. *JAMA.* 1925;84:281–285.

Rabinowitz HK. A program to recruit and educate medical students to practice family medicine in underserved areas. *JAMA.* 1983;249:1038–1041.

Rabinowitz HK. The precision phase: seven years experience with a required family medicine clerkship for third-year medical students. *Fam Med.* 1983;15:168–172.

Rabinowitz HK. The effect of a required residency based student clerkship on resident selection. *Fam Med.* 1986;18:287–289.

Rabinowitz HK. Estimating the percentage of primary care rural physicians produced by regular and special admissions policies. *J Med Educ.* 1986;61:588–600.

Rabinowitz HK. The relationship between medical student career choice and a required third-year family practice clerkship. *Fam Med.* 1988;20:118–121.

Rabinowitz HK. The relationship between US medical school admission policy and graduates entering family practice. *Fam Pract.* 1988;5:142–144.

Rabinowitz HK. Rural applicants. Letter to editor. *J Med Educ.* 1988;63:732–733.

Rabinowitz HK. Evaluation of a selective medical school admission policy to increase the number of family physicians in rural and underserved areas. *N Engl J Med.* 1988;319:480–486.

Rabinowitz HK. The change in specialty preference by medical students over time: an analysis of students who prefer family medicine. *Fam Med.* 1990;22:62–63.

Rabinowitz HK. Recruitment, retention and follow-up of a program to increase the number of family physicians in rural and underserved areas. *N Engl J Med.* 1993; 328:934–939.

Rabinowitz HK. The role of the medical school admissions process in the outcome of generalists. *Acad Med.* 1999;74:S39–S44.

Rabinowitz HK, Diamond JJ, Hojat M, et al. Demographic, educational, and economic factors related to recruitment and retention of physicians in rural Pennsylvania. *J Rural Health.* 1999;15:216–220.

Rabinowitz HK, Diamond JJ, Markham FW, et al. A program to increase the number of family physicians in rural and underserved areas: impact after 22 years. *JAMA.* 1999;281:255–260.

Rabinowitz HK, Diamond JJ, Markham FW, et al. Critical factors for designing programs to increase the supply and retention of rural primary care physicians. *JAMA.* 2001;286:1041–1048.

Rabinowitz HK, Diamond JJ, Veloski JJ, et al. The impact of multiple predictors on generalist physicians' care of underserved populations. *Am J Pub Health.* 2000;90: 1225–1228.

Rabinowitz HK, Paynter NP. The role of the medical school in rural graduate medical education: pipeline or control valve? *J Rural Health.* 2000;16:249–253.

Rabinowitz HK, Rosenthal MP, Diamond JJ, et al. Alternate career choices of medical students: their relationship to choice of specialty. *Fam Med.* 1993;25:665–667.

Rogers DE. The challenge of primary care. In: *Doing Better and Feeling Worse.* Knowles JH, ed. New York: WW Norton & Company; 1977.

Rosenblatt RA, Whitcomb ME, Cullen TJ, et al. Which medical schools produce rural physicians? *JAMA.* 1992;268:1559–1565.

Rosenthal MP, Turner TN, Diamond J, et al. Future income expectation of first-year medical students as a predictor of family practice specialty choice. *Acad Med.* 1992; 67:328–331.

Rosenthal TC, McGuigan H, Osborne J, et al. One-two residency tracks in family practice: are they getting the job done? *Fam Med.* 1997;30:90–93.

Rowland D, Lyons B. Triple jeopardy: rural, poor, and uninsured. *Health Serv Res.* 1989;23:976–1004.

Selinsgrove Chamber of Commerce. Welcome to Selinsgrove. 2002. Available at: http://www.selinsgrove.org/. Accessed August 11, 2003.

Shi L. The relation between primary care and life chances. *J Health Care Poor Underserved.* 1992;3:321–335.

Shi L. Primary care, specialty care, and life chances. *Int J Health Serv.* 1994;24:431–458.

Shi L, Starfield B, Kennedy B, Kawachi I. Income inequality, primary care and health indicators. *J Fam Pract.* 1999;48:275–284.

Starfield B. *Primary care: Concept, Evaluation, and Policy.* New York: Oxford Press; 1992.

Starfield B. Primary care: is it essential? *Lancet.* 1994;344:1129–1133.

Starfield B. Is US health really the best in the world? *JAMA.* 2000;284:483–485.

Stearns JA, Stearns MA, Glasser M, Londo RA. Illinois RMED: a comprehensive program to improve the supply of rural family physicians. *Fam Med.* 2000;32:17–21.

Stegner W. *Angle of Repose.* New York: Ballantine Books; 1971.

Strasser R, Rourke J, Anwar I, et al. *Policy on Training for Rural Practice.* Victoria, Australia: World Organization of Family Doctors; 1996.

Terkel S. *Working: People Talk About What They Do and How They Feel About What They Do.* New York: The New York Press; 1997.

Tornquist C, corresp. Program to bring doctors to small towns successful, study says. CNN Web site. 1999. Available at: http://www.cnn.com/HEALTH/9902/14/small .town.doctor/. Accessed August 10, 2003.

Town of the week: Boswell, Pennsylvania. Michael Feldman's Whad'ya know? Web site. 1998. Available at: http://www.notmuch.com/Features/Town/town-080898 .html. Accessed August 11, 2003.

US Bureau of the Census. *1990 Census of Population and Housing: CPH-L-79, States and Counties by Urban/Rural Population.* Washington, DC: US Bureau of the Census; 1991.

US Department of HHS. About NHSC: Our Achievements. NHSC Web site. Available at: http://nhsc.bhpr.hrsa.gov/about/our/where.cfm. Accessed August 6, 2003.

Verby JE, Newell JP, Andresen SA, et al. Changing the medical school curriculum to improve patient access to primary care. *JAMA.* 1991;266:110–113.

Welcome to Lock Haven: The history of Old Town. Available at: http://www.kcnet .org/history/oldtown/history1.htm. Accessed August 11, 2003.

White K, Williams TF, Greenberg BG. The ecology of medical care. *N Engl J Med.* 1961;265:885–892.

Wielawski IM. Practice sights: state primary care development strategies. In: *To Improve Health and Health Care, Volume VI: The Robert Wood Johnson Foundation Anthology.* Issacs SL, Knickman JR, eds. San Francisco: Jossey-Bass; 2003.

Williams WC. The practice. In: *The Autobiography of William Carlos Williams.* New York: Random House; 1951.

Willoughby TL, Arnold L, Calkins V. Personal characteristics and achievements of medical students from urban and nonurban areas. *J Med Educ.* 1981;56:717–726.

Wirth L. *Urbanism as a Way of Life.* Chicago: Chicago University Press; 1964.

WWAMI Rural Health Research Center. Rural-Urban Commuting Area Codes (RUCAS). 2002. Available at: http://www.fammed.washington.edu/wwamirhrc/. Accessed August 6, 2003.

Xu G, Veloski JJ, Hojat M, et al. Factors influencing physicians' choices to practice in inner-city or rural areas. *Acad Med.* 1997;72:1026.

Xu G, Veloski JJ, Hojat M, et al. Factors influencing primary care physicians' choice of practice in medically underserved areas. *Acad Med.* 1997;72:S109–S111.